Social Indicators Research Series

Volume 60

This series aims to provide a public forum for single treatises and collections of papers on social indicators research that are too long to be published in our journal *Social Indicators Research*. Like the journal, the book series deals with statistical assessments of the quality of life from a broad perspective. It welcomes the research on a wide variety of substantive areas, including health, crime, housing, education, family life, leisure activities, transportation, mobility, economics, work, religion and environmental issues. These areas of research will focus on the impact of key issues such as health on the overall quality of life and vice versa. An international review board, consisting of Ruut Veenhoven, Joachim Vogel, Ed Diener, Torbjorn Moum, Mirjam A.G. Sprangers and Wolfgang Glatzer, will ensure the high quality of the series as a whole.

More information about this series at http://www.springer.com/series/6548

Filomena Maggino
Editor

A Life Devoted to Quality of Life

Festschrift in Honor of Alex C. Michalos

Springer

Editor
Filomena Maggino
Dipartimento di Statistica, Informatica, Applicazioni "G. Parenti" (DiSIA)
Università degli Studi di Firenze
Firenze, Italy

ISSN 1387-6570 ISSN 2215-0099 (electronic)
Social Indicators Research Series
ISBN 978-3-319-20567-0 ISBN 978-3-319-20568-7 (eBook)
DOI 10.1007/978-3-319-20568-7

Library of Congress Control Number: 2015953836

Springer Cham Heidelberg New York Dordrecht London

Printed on acid-free paper

Springer International Publishing AG Switzerland is part of Springer Science+Business Media (www.springer.com)

Preface

I believe that anyone has one or more guides ("maestro," in Italian). I feel to be lucky since I had very few maestri and Alex is one of them.

I met alex for the first time in 1999 in Rome, at the presentation of a collective book which I also contribute to. I immediately felt a strong scientific affinity and perceived a great humanity. The presentation was done in Italian but it seemed that he understood everything. The message that he transmitted was clear to me: apart from the individual scientific position, the language in the field of quality of life has no limits and boundaries.

From that moment, I kept in touch with him and followed in parallel the development of the International Society for Quality of Life Studies.

I have no need to remark Alex's high scientific level. In this respect, Alex represented always an important guide for me. But he was an example for me also from the personal point of view.

I noticed that in any conference I attended and where Alex was present, he attended sessions by paying to any presentation always a great attention independently of who was the speaker, famous or young, academic or practitioner, by giving precious suggestions and advices, and by giving encouragements, supports, and opportunities. And there I realized the difference between being a great scholar and being a great maestro.

With time, the initial feelings of affinity and humanity increased more and more. This happened also in particular occasions and difficult moments, when I asked for his suggestions and advices. I felt always being understood and supported.

Chance decided that I had to fill two positions that were previously (and successfully) filled also by him, presidency of ISQOLS and direction of Social Indicators Research journal. In these positions I tried and try to be inspired by his example. I am not sure if I was and am successful in interpreting that inspiration, but I will be keeping on being inspired by him.

Firenze, Italy | Filomena Maggino

Contents

Part I
Quality of Life in Different Segments of Population

Chapter 1
Children, Adolescents and Quality of Life: The Social Sciences Perspective Over Two Decades

Ferran Casas

Introduction

I met alex Michalos personally for the first time in July 1990, at the ISA conference in Madrid. Before that moment he was only a name I had quoted many times, particularly in my doctoral dissertation on indicators of social risk situations for children.

My second personal contact was in 1996 in Prince George, Canada, when he kindly invited me to participate in the first international conference of the ISQOLS (International Society for Quality of Life Studies) he was chairing. That was a great occasion to meet some of the best-known researchers on quality of life at the time. There, I presented a paper on children's rights and children's quality of life, and he encouraged me to write an article and send it to the journal *Social Indicators Research*, of which he was the editor. The article was accepted and published in 1997 (Casas 1997). In a personal communication Alex wrote me "we need more papers like this".

Although by that time I had already published a certain number of articles in English, particularly on children's problems and children's rights, the words Alex addressed to me were deeply encouraging. I felt more committed to my work on identifying indicators for children's rights, of children's quality of life and, particularly, of children's subjective well-being (SWB).

In 1997, I accepted the post of Director at the newly-created Quality of Life Research Institute at the University of Girona (Casas and Planes 2014) and left my position as professor at the University of Barcelona. Due to my previous experience organising international conferences when I was Director of the Childhood Studies Centre in Madrid (1990–1993), Alex proposed I organise the second international

F. Casas (✉)
Research Institute on Quality of Life, University of Girona,
Plaça Sant Domènec 9, 17071 Girona, Spain
e-mail: ferran.casas@udg.edu

F. Maggino (ed.), *A Life Devoted to Quality of Life*, Social Indicators Research Series 60, DOI 10.1007/978-3-319-20568-7_1

ISQOLS conference at the University of Girona in July 2000. I accepted, and we managed it with the support of Joe Sirgy, Don Ratz and many other ISQOLS colleagues. There I met the few "missing" big names that had been unable to attend the Prince George conference. I published the proceedings with Carme Saurina (Casas and Saurina 2001).

After devoting a session to children's and adolescents' quality of life at the ISQOLS conference in Frankfurt in July 2003, Alex offered me, together with other colleagues, the opportunity to be co-editor of a book on research into children's and adolescents' quality of life, and it became a reality 1 year later (Dannerbeck et al. 2004).

In 2006, Alex invited Asher Ben-Arieh to write a monographic issue of the SIR on child well-being, which finally became two volumes, and for which I was invited to present two articles (Casas et al. 2007a, b).

That year, together with a research team colleague I also submitted an article to *Applied Research in Quality of Life* on kinship foster care and the satisfaction of the different stakeholders involved. Shortly after being informed that the article had been accepted (Montserrat and Casas 2007), I received another personal communication from Alex, telling me that he had been trying to obtain similar data for Canada, but had been unsuccessful – and he therefore very much appreciated our efforts in obtaining the data and publishing the results.

As far as I know, Alex has never published much on children's and adolescents' well-being or quality of life. However, after this telegraphic sequence of dates in my personal history it is very easy to realise that Alex has always "been there" and has constantly and proactively been particularly supportive on this topic.

A good deal of the advances I have been able to contribute to in this field have had Alex as a reference. With this I would like to say thanks, Alex, for continuously guiding and supporting us in this minority field of children's and adolescents' quality of life!

Indicators, Children's Well-Being and Children's Quality of Life

The definition of "well-being" and "quality of life" is particularly important in the field of children's and adolescents' studies. We know that for many authors in health sciences these two constructs are more or less synonymous. However, that is not the case for most authors in the social sciences. That fact makes the literature review confusing. There is a long history of social debates and changes in the meaning of child well-being (see Sandin 2014, for a description); however, the history of children's quality-of-life studies is very short.

Although they have followed different paths in different countries and political regimes, just to highlight a few of the changes that aid understanding of children and their well-being in the Western world, one important turning point seems to appear after the Second World War, when criticism of the authoritarian political regimes supported a developmental ideology based on the individual child within a democratic family and democratic society. Children's happiness replaced more socially-oriented topics from before the war, such as child labour, failing educational provisions and immigration, for example (Sandin 2014). Another turning point is symbolised by the adoption of the UN Convention on the Rights of the Child and subsequent new topics of discussion: Do children have the same human rights as other human beings, or do they have different rights? The forming of concepts such as "the best interest of the child" and "a child's perspective" mobilised children as citizens and legal subjects and emphasised children's autonomy from the family (Sandin 2014).

As Sandin (2014) says, *a long-term shift involves a movement away from the idea of children that emphasizes their vulnerability and fragility toward a view of children that emphasizes the similarity of children's needs as individuals to those of adults. (...). The notion of children as having separate rights is consequently eroded.*

According to Sandin (2014), *the understanding of well-being is expressed both through the institutions of education and care created for children and through discussions about what is good for children that are voiced by professional groups that claim precedence in the defining of well-being.* Therefore, the concept of well-being is not homogeneous across countries, cultures or political regimes and is linked to the understanding of what "good life" means in each society.

The concept of "quality of life" was born with the "social indicators movement" in the 1960s, and was intended as a much broader concept than well-being, involving the use of both objective and subjective indicators to assess any reality. "Subjective indicators" include people's *perceptions, evaluations and aspirations* (Campbell et al. 1976). Although the inclusion of subjective indicators using data provided by adults was accepted and promoted from the very birth of the social indicators movement, a generalised acceptance of the inclusion of data provided by children in any indicators system was delayed until the twenty-first century. Debates and reluctances appearing during the 1960s against including subjective data in the measurement of social change using "adults' data" at a macro social level have repeatedly appeared in relation to children's and adolescents' subjective indicators over the past two decades.

Andelman et al. (1999), in their review of the literature on children's quality of life, pointed out that although a large amount of research uses the key words "quality of life" and "children", most of it has been developed from a health perspective, in clinical contexts and with small samples of children with some specific health problem. According to these authors, the availability of data from larger samples and non-clinical populations was very scarce and happened in very few countries up to that period. Additionally, a good deal of the research with these key words was evaluating children's QOL without collecting data on children's own assessment of their lives.

The landscape did not change noticeably when other reviewers added other key words to their search, such as "well-being" (Pollard and Lee 2003) or "life satisfaction", or even "adolescents" (Huebner 2004).

The use of statistical data and indicators to analyse the well-being of the overall population of children began before the "social indicators movement", particularly with the publication of the "State of the Child" reports in the US in the 1940s (Ben-Arieh 2000, 2006, 2008; Ben-Arieh et al. 2001). The "social indicators movement" arose within a climate of rapid social change and with the belief among social scientists and public officials that well measured and consistently collected social indicators could provide a way of monitoring the condition of groups in society at a particular moment and over time, including the conditions of children and families (Land 2000).

A glance at the number of this kind of reports published recently reveals that children's well-being and its indicators are fields of growing scientific interest. Much of this new and enhanced activity can be accounted for by UNICEF's *State of the World's Children* annual report, as well as the Annie E. Casey Foundation's *Kids Count* initiative in the United States. The UN's CRC, through its global ratification and reporting and monitoring mechanism, has also played an important role in increasing interest in reporting on children's situations (Ben-Arieh 2012).

Ben-Arieh has contributed to two seminal compilation studies that presented data from a wide spectrum of studies and experiences on the monitoring and measurement of the "state of children" in large populations (Ben-Arieh and Wintersberger 1997; Ben-Arieh et al. 2001) and have united a previously completely disjointed field of study at the international level.

The same author (2008) suggested that the birth of what he called "the child indicators movement" is related to the convergence of five global trends (Casas 2011):

- Recognising children's rights, with the approval of the United Nations Convention.
- The "new" sociology of childhood.
- The ecology of child development (Bronfenbrenner and Morris 1998).
- New methodological perspectives in child studies: valuing the subjective viewpoints of child participants, accepting children as a unit of observation, and systematically collecting child statistics in certain countries.
- The desire to improve policy decisions by collecting and disseminating improved data on all areas of child and adolescent life.

At present, there are many data series and indicators from which to form opinions and draw conclusions on children's well-being in the industrialised countries (Bradshaw et al. 2007). The rapidly growing interest in children's well-being indicators stems, in part, from a movement toward accountability-based public policy, which demands more accurate measures of the conditions children face and the outcomes of various programmes designed to address those conditions. At the same time, rapid changes in family life have prompted an increased demand from child development professionals, social scientists, and the public for a better picture of children's well-being and their quality of life (Ben-Arieh et al. 2014).

The recent scientific literature on macro-social child and adolescent well-being and quality of life may be identified more easily in the literature databases using the descriptor "child indicators". A recent review by Ben-Arieh (2008) allows us to appreciate the breadth and diversity of this literature, which has even led to the creation of a new international journal, *Child Indicators Research.*

In summarising the history of child indicators, Ben-Arieh has suggested that, initially, most systems only included "survival indicators": rates of mortality, disease, and social problems affecting children (for instance, deschooling, illiteracy, school failure, etc.). During the 1990s, more child well-being researchers emphasised the need for "positive" indicators and, particularly, "subjective" indicators, due to the increased focus on quality of life (Casas 1997, 2011).

Many of these attempts to improve child well-being focused on children's futures: "that they may experience well-being when they reach adulthood". This adult-centred orientation has too often caused people to disregard the value of childhood itself, postponing children's well-being to a later generation. The result is that a large number of policies have not addressed well-being but rather *well-becoming*.

By way of a summary, from a global perspective, the availability of indicators on different aspects of children's lives is still greatly limited to (a) negative indicators; (b) objective indicators, and with the exception of UNICEF's reports and those of a few other international agencies, to (c) a few countries.

One of the recent major contributions to the international debate on children's "positive" conceptualisation of well-being has been the Handbook of Child Well-Being, edited by Ben-Arieh et al. (2014). This handbook includes 114 chapters (more than 238 authors from 32 different countries) on the state-of-the-art in international and transdisciplinary perspectives. This handbook presents a wide range of different theoretical, disciplinary and methodological approaches to child well-being.

Conceptualising Children's Subjective Well-Being

What did constitute a truly new initial contribution by the social indicators movement was the inclusion of subjective indicators as a key component in appropriately assessing the quality-of-life construct. This inclusion when referring to children's and adolescents' quality of life was generally also postponed until the twenty-first century.

Conceptual debates on what constitutes subjective well-being have been intense in recent decades due to the existence of two competing constructs: subjective well-being and psychological well-being. However, there is also a third construct in the scientific international arena: HR-QOL (health-related quality of life).

Definitions of children's well-being found in the HR-QOL literature are very heterogeneous. As mentioned previously, the health sciences focus on clinical populations with very diverse backgrounds. The assessment of children's well-being frequently has one crucial aim: to evaluate changes after any health programme or intervention. Therefore, in this context, child well-being is an expected output.

The definition of children's well-being in the tradition of psychological well-being (the *eudemonic* tradition) is very problematic. Research in this tradition has mainly focused on adults. Their measurement instruments are usually very abstract in nature and therefore include a language not appropriate for use with children. Attempts to include *eudemonic* items in children's questionnaires have only started in recent years, and not always successfully; to date, there does not seem to be any consensus regarding an available reliable instrument to be used with children cross-nationally.

With children and adolescents, only one tradition has in fact contributed much in empirical terms to the study of children's well-being using large samples: the *hedonic* tradition, using the subjective well-being (SWB) construct. This is a clear limitation, which will probably be overcome in the next few decades, but which represents the current situation in the field of research.

Therefore, the key word "subjective", when discussing children's SWB, has a dual meaning: (a) it refers to subjective data, collected using subjective measuring techniques; (b) it usually refers to the *hedonic* tradition in research on well-being.

In the *hedonic* tradition, SWB is usually defined as having three components: positive affect, negative affect and life satisfaction. There is general consensus that life satisfaction should be measured using two procedures: (a) by assessing overall life satisfaction – using either one single item scale or context-free psychometric scales; and (b) by assessing satisfaction with the most relevant life-domains – there are different theoretical positions about which are the most relevant domains in children's or adolescents lives. In fact, the few existing domain-based instruments have very different characteristics, and include notably different domains.

Although *happiness* is considered by many authors to be synonymous with *life satisfaction* (see Veenhoven 2000), some authors consider it not to be exactly the same and say it is important to explore the consistency of answers to happiness items in relation to answers to items on overall life. Happiness is often considered a major component of positive affect. Some recent research results even suggest that positive affect is by far the most important component of SWB (Cummins 2014).

Data Provided by Children and the Increasing Interest in Children's and Adolescents' SWB Indicators

Throughout the history of the human sciences many scientific researchers have devoted great effort to questioning *individual* children in order to "discover" how they function. For example, developmental psychologists have been very interested in finding out about children's personality, intelligence, motivation, capacities, and so on. However, very seldom have data provided by *large samples* of children been considered of any interest, meaning they have rarely been collected. While adults' surveys received great interest in the last century as it became obvious that adults' opinions are of major political relevance, children's and adolescents opinions have never raised much interest, with the sole exception of that of advertisers interested in selling products to them, who have taken this kind of data collection very seriously indeed.

When social scientists began to collect data from large samples of children, it was for diverse reasons; nevertheless, the results were often unexpected (a few examples are explained in Casas 2011). This evidence forced social researchers to face the fact that we were only now "discovering" that our child population has some different characteristics than these we thought. In other words, the majority of children sometimes do not perceive, think or have the opinions or evaluations on their life and on their world that adults believe they have. Many adults' attributions on children's worlds may be wrong. Even our social representations of children and adolescents, shared by the majority of people, may be wrong (Casas et al. 2013a). This happens simply because we never went to ask representative samples of children what do they really think. In the history of the human sciences there are far more studies asking mothers or teachers about children's satisfaction with school than studies asking children about their own satisfaction with school.

In the academic world, children are slowly being recognized as key informants and competent informers on their own lives. Consequently, their voices, their evaluations and their points of view are increasingly more accepted as key sources of information in scientific research.

The availability of children's subjective indicators is growing – albeit only slowly. At present, most existing cross-national comparisons including subjective indicators of children's well-being or quality of life are still using data from only two international databases containing children's self-reported information on different aspects of their own lives: the HBSC (www.hbsc.org) and the PISA (www.oecd.org/pisa).

To adopt a perspective that focuses on the positive aspects of childhood "at present", we need additional databases including data on more areas of child well-being and quality of life. Researchers have up to now focused exclusively on health, education, demographics, and social services, but should now expand their interests to totally "new" topics in the child population: satisfaction with services and life aspects, values, social skills, leisure time, interests and activities involving new technologies, social participation, etc.

Although, as several authors have indicated, research in the area of child and adolescent well-being is lagging far behind the wide availability of adult qualitative and quantitative findings, this does not justify a continued lack of interest or credibility, at the population level, in data obtained from young people using instruments that, like instruments for adults, need to be improved over time and compared across cultures (Casas 2011).

What is surprising is that while "subjective adult satisfaction" with services and life conditions has become a very important policy issue, the satisfaction of children and adolescents continues to be treated as irrelevant. Too often, in the social and human sciences, the low reliability and validity of data obtained from children and adolescents are used as an excuse to avoid collecting such data, when curiously, only advertisers and marketing experts appear to be interested in this population and to have "overcome' difficulties concerning validity and reliability (Casas 2011).

In addressing child well-being and quality of life, we must not forget that by definition, quality of life includes the **perceptions, evaluations, and aspirations** of everyone involved, and those of children and adolescents are therefore essential. In other words, we must not confuse child well-being with **adult opinions of child well-being**. Both are important, but they are not the same, and both are a part of the complex social reality we call child well-being. Therefore, we face the challenge of filling the large information gap concerning the younger population's point of view of the social reality that affects humanity.

Only in the last few decades have scientists become interested in studying children's and adolescents' well-being **from their own perspective**. Until very recently, it was assumed that solely adult evaluations on children's well-being data would be valid enough.

Assessing Children's and Adolescents' SWB

Different kinds of information have been collected and published on the assumption they are related to children's well-being. However, one of the most solid ways of systematically assessing children's and adolescents' well-being is reflected in the use of standardised instruments with large samples of children, which are psychometrically demonstrated to be **valid, reliable and sensitive**. After finding evidence that such instruments are valid, reliable and sensitive in a concrete language and/or cultural context, they can also be tested for their use across languages and cultures.

At present, researchers have a number – although not many – of such psychometric instruments available. A few **specific scales** for assessing child well-being have already been developed (Casas 2011). Some examples are:

- *Perceived Life Satisfaction Scale* (PLSS) (Andelman et al. 1999).
- *Students' Life Satisfaction Scale* (SLSS) (Huebner 1991).
- *Multidimensional Students' Life Satisfaction Scales* (MSLSS) (Huebner 1994).
- *Quality of Life Profile – Adolescent version* (QOLP-Q) (Raphael et al. 1996).
- *Comprehensive Quality of Life Scale – Students version* (Com-QOL Students) (Cummins 1997; Gullone and Cummins 1999).
- *Brief Multidimensional Students' Life Satisfaction Scale* (BMSLSS) (Seligson et al. 2003).
- *Personal Well-Being Index – School Children* (PWI-SC) (Cummins and Lau 2005).

However, in some research **general scales to assess well-being** for the whole (adult) population have also been successfully used on adolescent samples, including:

- *Satisfaction with Life Scale* (SWLS) (Diener et al. 1985) (although several adaptations for children have also been proposed).

- *Personal Well-Being Index* (PWI) (Cummins et al. 2003; International Wellbeing Group 2006).
- *Fordyce's Happiness Scale* (FHS) (Fordyce 1988).
- *Cantril's Ladder* (Cantril 1965).
- *Overall Life Satisfaction* (Campbell et al. 1976).

The last three scales are single-item. The psychometric characteristics of some of the other scales may be found in Bender (1997) and Gilman and Huebner (2000). The correlations between these scales are moderate to high.

The most frequently used scale with adolescents in the psychological scientific literature to date is probably the OLS, although its use can be found with a range of different wordings. That said, Cantril's Ladder is probably the most quoted scale, it being the one included in the HBSC international database, the only one that provides data for international comparison across many countries and results are therefore those usually included in studies by UNICEF and other international agencies. However, different authors have pointed out that using a single-item measure for international comparison of such a complex construct as SWB reflects too weak a methodological position.

In principle, the scores obtained using any of these scales can be consistently adopted as subjective indicators at the population level in countries that have versions adapted to their language and culture. Nevertheless, multi-item scales are a much more robust alternative.

Most of the original scales used within these instruments are 5- or 7-point Likert-like scales, which are commonly used to assess psychological constructs. However, it is well-known that data related to SWB – at least in industrialised countries – are negatively skewed, which means that most people will respond only to a restricted portion of the conventional scale. Therefore, crucially these scales need to be not only valid and reliable, but also particularly **sensitive**. Moreover, when subjective quality-of-life measures are used as outcomes, scale sensitivity becomes a critical concern since this construct has a high trait component, and small deviations are highly meaningful. As suggested by Guyatt and Jaeschker (1990), it is really quite curious that this crucial fact regarding the sensitivity of SWB scales has been virtually ignored so often. The only solution to such a challenge is to expand the number of possible responses (Cummins and Gullone 2000).

Such expansion would not appear to systematically influence scale reliability, and is therefore psychometrically feasible, but is made difficult by the convention of naming all response categories. It has been argued that this naming is quite unnecessary and actually detracts from the interval nature of the scale (Cummins and Gullone 2000). The solution adopted by different researchers has been that of using 11-point, end-defined scales. These offer a form of rating (0–10) which lies within the common experience of children and adolescents (and adults) in most countries and produces increased sensitivity of the measurement instrument. This solution has also been discussed with groups of adolescents (Casas et al. 2013b) and adopted by different researchers when administering these scales to children and adolescents, resulting in good understanding (Casas et al. 2012).

As already mentioned, another ongoing debate is that regarding which domains are relevant to assess children's and adolescents' life satisfaction. The two most frequently used scales with adolescents structured by life domains are probably the BMSLSS (Seligson et al. 2003) and the PWI (Cummins 1998; Cummins et al. 2003) or, alternatively, for younger ages, the PWI-SC (Cummins and Lau 2005). These scales usually display rather high correlations with one another (.610 between BMSLSS and PWI in Casas et al. 2012c; ranging from .662 to .756 depending on the country between BMSLSS and PWI-SC, in Casas et al. 2015); however, if we read the items included on them they look very different and such a high correlation even looks strange. While the PWI includes 7 rather abstract items (on health, standard of living, achievements in life, personal safety, community, security for future, and relationships with other people), the BMSLSS includes 5 rather concrete items (on family, friends, school, oneself, and the place you live in). This leads to the idea that they are complementary rather than alternative scales, and that the two together can be merged into a single scale. This idea has been explored in Casas et al. (2014). However, there is another persistent observation in the field of positive psychology, which also contributes to explaining these results: all positive constructs tend to be positively correlated, raising a doubt about the existence of a positive "supra-construct" (Stones and Kozma 1985; Diener et al. 1999). When analysing children's answers to SWB scales, their tendency for extreme positive options is even more evident than among adults, suggesting their **life optimism** tends to be "extreme".

When the tendency to give positive answers becomes "constant" for many participants, as is the case with many items in children's samples, we face a serious methodological problem: extreme answers distort the mean and decrease the variance, raising problems for statistical calculations and interpretations. For this reason, some authors recommend checking and deleting the extreme constant answers (International Wellbeing Group 2006). In some samples of children, this has meant deleting more than 14 % of the subjects (Casas et al. 2012b). However, children's extreme positive feelings are "real" and we need to find solutions in order to listen to and believe children rather than deleting them from our databases. Some researchers of children's SWB have explored an alternative approach to decide which cases in their database should be deleted. It has been observed that even the most optimistic children tend NOT to give extreme positive answers about satisfaction with services in their neighbourhood, for example with the library, public transport or local policy. Therefore, the adopted solution has been to check for extreme positive answers in all satisfaction-related items and not only in the items on the psychometric scales. Children giving extreme positive answers to all satisfaction items have been deleted and those only giving extreme positive answers on psychometric scales have not, because they are considered reliable enough (Casas et al. 2012a).

The fact that all of these scales display lower explained variances among children or young adolescents than among older adolescents or adults raises still another debate: we may be missing life domains which are relevant for children but not for older adolescents or adults. For example, satisfaction with "achievements" in life may be very much related to work among adults, but not at all among children and adolescents.

In recent years, different research articles have made the proposal of including new items on existing scales, demonstrating that the new items contribute to the construct with unique explained variance, and significantly improve the overall explained variance. For example, Tomyn and Cummins (2011) have proposed including a new item on satisfaction with school for adolescents using the PWI-SC; Casas et al. (2011) proposed a new item on satisfaction with time use in the PWI; and Vaqué et al. (2015) have tested a new item on satisfaction with food with younger children using the PWI-SC.

The Need for More Available International Data: The *Children's Worlds* Research Project

One of the outstanding on-going projects to obtain more data from children is the *Children's Worlds* project, the International Survey of Children's Well-Being (ISCWeB) (http://www.isciweb.org/). This study aims to collect data on children's lives and daily activities, their time use and in particular on their own perceptions and evaluations of their well-being, from as many countries and in as representative a way as possible. The purpose is to improve children's well-being by raising awareness of it among children, their parents and their communities, but also among opinion leaders, decision makers, professionals and the general public.

The project began in 2009 when a group of researchers, mainly from the International Society for Child Indicators (ISCI), held a meeting hosted by UNICEF-Geneva to discuss the potential need for the survey. The group agreed that such a survey would fill an important gap in knowledge about children's lives internationally. One of the products of the meeting was an early version of a survey questionnaire. This first draft questionnaire was tested and piloted in the summer and autumn of 2010 in six countries – Brazil, England, Germany, Honduras, Israel and Spain – and a second draft version was piloted in the first half of 2011 in five countries – Germany, Romania, South Africa, Spain and Turkey.

In October 2011, members of the research group reviewed the learning from the second pilot and drew up a third set of the survey questionnaires with separate versions for children aged 8, 10 and 12. These questionnaires were then in the first large-scale wave of data collection.

The first wave of data collection took place between the winter of 2011 and the winter of 2012 in 14 countries from around the globe. The countries involved in this stage were: Algeria, Brazil, Canada, Chile, England, Israel, Nepal, Romania, Rwanda, South Africa, South Korea, Spain, Uganda and United States. Around 34,500 children in mid-childhood participated in this wave of the survey and the questionnaires were translated into a wide range of languages including – Arabic, Basque, Catalan, Galician, Hebrew, Hungarian, Korean, Nepali, Portuguese, Romanian, several versions of English and several versions of Spanish.

The sample is based on school, and therefore the classes (grades) of the majority of children in the targeted age groups were sampled in each country. In half of the countries (Algeria, Brazil, Chile, Israel, Romania, South Korea and the US) all three age groups were sampled, in two countries (Canada and Uganda) only two of the age groups were sampled and in five countries (England, Nepal, Rwanda, South Africa and Spain) children from only one age group were sampled. Most of the samples were convenience-samples except for Chile, South Korea and Spain, in which a representative sample was obtained.

Some preliminary findings from this wave of data collection were presented in November 2012 at a meeting hosted by UNICEF Innocenti Research Centre in Florence, and at the ISCI conference in Seoul in May 2013.

The second wave of the survey was conducted during the winter of 2013 and spring of 2014, with representative samples of children aged 8–12 in 15 countries around the globe – Algeria, Colombia, England, Estonia, Ethiopia, Germany, Israel, Nepal, Norway, Poland, Romania, South Africa, South Korea, Spain and Turkey, with the support of the Jacobs Foundation. Each participating country surveyed a representative sample of at least 1000 children in each of three school year groups – around the ages of 8, 10 and 12 (Rees and Main).

A representative sample of children in mainstream schools in the whole country or a specific region was obtained for each country. The sampling strategy varied from country to country, subject to the characteristics of each. More detailed information on this can be found in each of the country's reports. Results are planned to be presented in May 2015 and the database will be made public available 1 year later.

The final format of the ISCWeB questionnaire includes three versions for the different age groups – one questionnaire for children around eight, another for those around ten and a third for those around 12 years of age. The three questionnaires all cover the following key aspects of children's lives:

- Basic characteristics (age, gender, country of birth)
- Living situation, home and family relationships
- Money and economic circumstances
- Friends and other relationships
- Local area
- School
- Time use
- Self
- Overall subjective well-being
- Children's rights

The questionnaires for the older two age groups also cover two further topics – recent changes in children's lives and qualities aspired to for the future.

The question items fall into four basic types:

1. Fact-based items – e.g. age, gender, household possessions.
2. Agreement items. These consist of statements (e.g. *'I feel safe at home'*). In most cases children are asked to respond on a five-point scale labelled 'I do not agree',

'Agree a little', 'Agree somewhat', 'Agree a lot', 'Totally agree'. There is also a 'Don't know' option. Some of the agreement items in the questionnaires for 10-year-olds and 12-year-olds use an 11-point numbered (0–10) scale with the end points labelled 'Don't agree at all' and 'Totally agree'.

3. Frequency items. These mostly consist of questions about various aspects of time use, but also experiences of bullying and worries about family money. These items are all on a four-point scale with descriptions of frequencies relevant to the topic – e.g. 'Rarely or never', 'Less than once a week', 'Once or twice a week', 'Every day or almost every day'.
4. Satisfaction items. These consist of questions about satisfaction with various aspects of life and with life as a whole. In the versions of the questionnaire for 10-year-olds and 12-year-olds these items all use an 11-point (0–10) response scale with the end points labelled as 'Not at all satisfied' and 'Totally satisfied'. In the questionnaire for 8-year-olds, taking into account children's typical levels of cognitive and linguistic development at this age, these questions are phrased as being about 'happiness' rather than 'satisfaction' and a shorter five-point scale is used with each point on the scale being represented by a symbolic facial expression (emoticons).

The length of the questionnaire (total number of items to answer) was determined through the piloting process and as a result the questionnaire contains fewer items for younger age groups. In total, there are 112 items in the questionnaire for 12-year-olds, 104 items for 10-year-olds and 71 items for 8-year-olds.

Among the items described above, the questionnaires contain versions of three previously tested psychometric SWB scales. First, there is a context-free scale intended to measure cognitive SWB comprising five items which form a short modified version of the Student Life Satisfaction Scale (SLSS, Huebner 1991). Then there are two scales made up of domain satisfaction items – the seven-item Personal Well-being Index – School Children (Cummins and Lau 2005) and a modified version of the five-item Brief Multidimensional Student Life Satisfaction Scale (Seligson et al. 2003). As well as the previously tested scales, two new sets of items are included. The first is a set of six items on positive affect which are influenced by Russell's Core Affect Scale (Russell 2003). The second is a set of six items designed to represent various aspects of psychological well-being based on a framework proposed by Ryff (1989).

A key issue for the project has been to try to ensure that the various versions of the questionnaire in the different languages spoken by children in the participating countries are as compatible as possible. With this aim, the translation process has been as follows. Each country started with the standard English-language version of the questionnaires. The questionnaires were then translated into the relevant languages and then, independently of the original translation, translated back into English. Each back-translated English version was compared with the original English version and this comparison was used to highlight any discrepancies or issues. Any identified issues were then resolved by revising the translations as required (Rees and Main 2015).

Research Results: Many New Findings in Just a Few Years

The increasing interest in exploring how different SWB psychometric scales work with children and adolescents in different countries and using different languages has led to a series of new debates throughout the present century. However, we must highlight a particularly crucial new question that has appeared: why is SWB constantly decreasing between approximately 10 and 16 years of age in almost all countries?

This is a new question because researchers have never before asked large samples of children or adolescents whether they are satisfied with their own lives using a sensitive scale. It was previously an irrelevant question for leading researchers: only a few started asking this question to a few children in very few countries before the beginning of the new century. As a consequence, we have remained ignorant and now the evidence looks very surprising. A few data collections by Huebner in a southern state of the US are among the few exceptions to this situation. Park & Huebner appear to have been the first researchers to compare children's SWB between two countries using multi-item psychometric scales (Park et al. 2004; Park and Huebner 2005).

Throughout this century different research results in different countries have begun to highlight this constant decrease (Goldbeck et al. 2007). We did not previously know when it starts or finishes; now we have some evidence that it may start at 10 and perhaps finish around 16, or perhaps 18, depending on the country. We are not yet sure if this decrease happens in different countries in the same way. In Brazil, the few data we have from a local sample seem to suggest a decrease only up to 15, while in Romania it seems to continue after 18. At present, we have evidence of such a decrease in most European countries (Currie et al. 2012), and also in Algeria, Australia, Brazil, and Chile, using several psychometric instruments (Holte et al. 2014).

Some of these research results are suggesting that the decrease is gender sensitive. Boys' decrease in life satisfaction seems to be more influenced by a decrease in all school-related aspects, while girls' is more related to their own body, doing sports and physical exercise.

Several explanations have been suggested by different colleagues. These are alternative hypotheses to be tested in the next future:

- Stress increases with age among adolescents, particularly because of school requirements.
- Depression increases throughout adolescence, particularly in urban contexts and in industrialised countries.
- As adolescence progresses, the starting point of "extreme optimism" slowly changes into a "more realistic evaluation of the world".
- This phenomenon is one of the "natural" characteristics of adolescence that has always existed. We simply did not know about it, and it is nothing to worry about.

Besides the impressive amount of new knowledge accumulated using quantitative methods over a couple of decades, it is worth pointing out that the relevant aspects of current knowledge on children's well-being is also coming from the emerging qualitative approaches. On the one hand, it is difficult to believe that all aspects related to a "good life" can be quantified; on the other, many aspects of what children consider well-being may happen that have never been included in any of the existing instruments that assess children's well-being. Some authors argue that we should not only ask children about their well-being in a more open way, but also let them lead the kind of research needed to accumulate knowledge from children's points of view. According to Mason and Watson (2014) children have been *traditionally marginalized in the formal processes of knowledge production, which have positioned them as "objects" of change processes. Advocates for children's involvement as participants in research argue that positioning children as subjects in the research process increases their control in the production of knowledge about their lives.*

Even some traditional quantitative research may be improved accepting children as advisers of adult researchers. For example, before deciding the format in which well-being psychometric scales would be administered to children in the pilot survey of the Children's Worlds project in Catalonia, researchers explored the already existing formats. They identified 14 different formats in just a few European countries. Researchers found that they did not have a solid criterion to decide which format was best for children and decided to ask children themselves, showing them these existing formats. The children in question immediately said some of the most frequently used formats were not appropriate for use with children of their age – and they reorganised and improved a few of the existing formats, finally suggesting a new format for each age group.

Some Reflections on the Future of Indicators of Children's and Adolescents' SWB

At present, normative data on children's or adolescents' SWB do not seem to be available from any country, although this is an aim of the Children's Worlds project. Scores from psychometric scales on SWB on representative samples of children and adolescents would be robust normative data if available from all ages and from as many countries as possible.

However, if children are so extremely optimistic and therefore tend to score so high in overall life satisfaction, does it make sense to have macro-social data? Is there any political decision or intervention programme that makes sense in order to improve their situation? The million-dollar question is probably this: can the constant decreasing tendency of SWB between 10 and 16 years of age be changed? Our answer is surprisingly YES, it does make a lot of sense. We have many subgroups of children and adolescents whose overall life satisfaction is far below the mean. Some of them have already been pointed out in different studies, but much more research is needed in more countries in order to identify such groups and suggest appropriate actions to overcome these situations.

Having normative data is a pre-requisite to be able to compare against any population subgroup. For example, research teams in different countries (Brazil, Israel and Spain) have recently started to collect data on life satisfaction and satisfaction with different life domains among children placed out-of-home (i.e., foster care, residential care or kinship care). In order to know how far the SWB of these subgroups lies from the SWB of the overall population we need to compare the results with the normative data.

A second crucial need is the availability of more data from longitudinal studies in order to better understand the evolution of SWB throughout childhood and adolescence. The few ongoing longitudinal studies on children's subjective well-being are suggesting that not all children's SWB decreases dramatically from the age of 10–16. Transition periods (i.e. from primary to secondary school) seem to impact the subjective well-being of many children but not all – and much more boys than girls. This impact can probably be buffered. On the other hand, the social and cultural context seems to have an important role in increasing or buffering the path of the decrease: for example, the decrease from 12 to 16 years of age is much more noticeable among adolescents in the region of Oran, in Algeria, than among adolescents in Catalonia, Spain (Casas et al. 2013c).

In summary, the field of study of indicators of children's and adolescents' SWB is very young in terms of history, but is showing an increasing energy and productivity. This activity is quickly contributing to new knowledge from the point of view of children and adolescents, and some of its results are challenging traditional beliefs regarding the youngest generation. However, there is still much more work to be done than the work already published in scientific journals in order to answer some of the basic new questions generating important debates in the international arena, and particularly to demonstrate which kind of social environments and supportive actions may increase children's and adolescents' SWB, or, in some cases, slow down its dramatic decrease. We hope this short paper may stimulate more researchers to join us and also stimulate the assuming of new challenges for those already on board.

Acknowledgements Thanks are due to Barney Griffins for editing of the English text.

References

Andelman, R.B., Attkisson, C.C., Zima, B.T., & Rosenblatt, A.B. (1999). Quality of life of children: Toward conceptual clarity. In M.E. Maruisch, *The use of psychological testing for treatment planning and outcomes assessment*. London: LEA.

Ben-Arieh, A. (2000). Beyond welfare: Measuring and monitoring the state of children – New trends and domains. *Social Indicators Research, 52*(3), 235–257.

Ben-Arieh, A. (2006). Is the study of the "State of Our Children" changing? Revisiting after five years. *Children and Youth Services Review, 28*(7), 799–811.

Ben-Arieh, A. (2008). The child indicators movement: Past, present and future. *Child Indicators Research, 1*, 3–16.

Ben-Arieh, A. (2012). How do we measure and monitor the "State of Our Children"? Revisiting the topic in honor of Sheila B. Kamerman. *Children and Youth Services Review, 34*, 569–575.
Ben-Arieh, A., Casas, F., Frønes, I., & Korbin, J.E. (2014). *Handbook of Child Well-Being*. Dordrecht: Springer.
Ben-Arieh, A., & Wintersberger, H. (Eds.) (1997). *Monitoring and measuring the state of the children: Beyond survival. Eurosocial Report, 62*. Vienna: European Centre for Social Welfare Policy and Research.
Ben-Arieh, A., Kaufman, N.H., Andrews, B.A., Goerge, R., Lee, B.J., & Aber, J.L. (2001). *Measuring and monitoring children's well-being*. Dordrecht: Kluwer.
Bender, T.A. (1997). Assessment of subjective well-being during childhood and adolescence. In G. Phye, *Handbook of classroom assessment: learning, achievement and adjustment* (pp. 199–225). S. Diego (Ca): Academic Press.
Bradshaw, J., Hoelscher, P., & Richardson, D. (2007). An index of child well-being in the European Union. *Social Indicators Research, 80*, 133–177.
Bronfenbrenner, U., & Morris, P. (1998). The ecology of developmental processes. In W. Damon & R. Lerner: *Handbook of child psychology: Theoretical models of human development, 1*. New York: Wiley.
Campbell, A., Converse, P.E., & Rogers, W.L. (1976). *The quality of American life: Perceptions, evaluations, and satisfactions*. New York: Russell Sage.
Cantril, H. (1965). *The pattern of human concerns*. New Brunswick (N.J.): Rutgers Univ. Press.
Casas, F. (1997). Children's rights and children's quality of life: conceptual and practical issues. *Social Indicators Research, 42*, 283–298.
Casas, F. (2011). Subjective social indicators and child and adolescent well-being. *Child Indicators Research, 4(4)*, 555–575.
Casas, F., Alfaro, J., Sarriera, J.C., Bedin, L., Grigoras, B., Bălţătescu, S., Malo, S., & Sirlopú, D. (2015). El bienestar subjetivo en la infancia: Estudio de la comparabilidad de 3 escalas psicométricas en 4 países de habla latina. *Psicoperspectivas Individuo y Sociedad, 14*(1), 6–18.
Casas, F., Bello, A., González, M., Aligué, M., Bertrán, I., Montserrat, C., Navarro, D., González-Bueno, G., & von Bredow, M. (2012a). *Calidad de vida y bienestar infantil subjetivo en España. ¿Qué afecta al bienestar de niños y niñas españoles de 1 de ESO?* Madrid: UNICEF España. Retrieved from https://www.unicef.es/actualidad-documentacion/publicaciones/calidad-de-vida-y-bienestar-infantil-subjetivo-en-espana.
Casas, F., Bello, A., González, M., & Aligué, M. (2012b). Personal Well-Being among Spanish Adolescents. *Journal of Social Research & Policy*, 3(2), 19–45. Retrieved from http://www.jsrp.ro/content/JSRP-Vol3_Iss2_CASAS
Casas, F., Figuer, C., González, M., & Malo, S. (2007a). The values adolescents aspire to, their well-being and the values parents aspire to for their children. *Social Indicators Research, 84*, 271–290.
Casas, F., Figuer, C., González, M., Malo, S., Alsinet, C., & Subarroca, S. (2007b). The well-being of 12- to 16-year-old adolescents and their parents: Results from 1999 to 2003 Spanish samples. *Social Indicators Research, 83*(1), 87–115. doi: 10.1007/s11205-006-9059-1.
Casas, F., González, M., & Navarro, D. (2013a). Social psychology and child well-being. In A. Ben-Arieh, F. Casas, I. Frønes, & J.E. Korbin, *Handbook of Child* Well-Being (pp. 513–554). Dordrecht: Springer.
Casas, F., González, M., Navarro, D., & Aligué, M. (2013b). Children as Advisers of Their Researchers: Assuming a Different Status for Children. *Child Indicators Research, 6*, 193–212. doi 10.1007/s12187-012-9168-0.
Casas, F., & Planes, M. (2014). The IRQV (Research Institute on Quality of Life, University of Girona, Spain). In A.C. Michalos (Ed.), *Encyclopedia of Quality of Life Research* (pp. 3389–3392). Dordrecht: Springer.
Casas, F., Sarriera, J.C., Abs, D., Coenders, G., Alfaro, J., Saforcada, E., & Tonon, G. (2012c). Subjective indicators of personal well-being among adolescents. Performance and results for

different scales in Latin-language speaking countries: A contribution to the international debate. *Child Indicators Research, 5*, 1–28.

Casas, F., Sarriera, J.C., Alfaro, J., González, M., Malo, S., Bertran, I., Figuer, C., Abs da Cruz, D., Bedin, L., Paradiso, A., Weinreich, K., & Valdenegro, B. (2011). Testing the Personal Wellbeing Index on 12–16 year-old adolescents in 3 different countries with 2 new items. *Social Indicators Research, 105*, 461–482.

Casas, F., Sarriera, J.C., Alfaro, J., González, M., Bedin, L., Abs, D., Figuer, C., & Valdenegro, B. (2014). *Reconsidering life domains that contribute to subjective well-being among adolescents with data from three countries. Journal of Happiness Studies*. doi 10.1007/s10902-014-950-20.

Casas, F., & Saurina, C. (Eds.) (2001). *Proceedings of the Third Conference of the International Society for Quality of Life Studies (ISQOLS)*. Universitat de Girona: Diversitas, 14.

Casas, F., Tiliouine, H., & Figuer, C. (2013c). The Subjective Well-being of Adolescents from Two Different Cultures: Applying Three Versions of the PWI in Algeria and Spain. *Social Indicators Research, 115*, 637–651. doi 10.1007/s11205-012-0229-z.

Cummins, R.A. (1997). *Comprehensive Quality of Life Scale – Student (Grades 7–12): ComQol-S5 (Fifth Edition)*. Melbourne: School of Psychology, Deakin University.

Cummins, R.A. (1998). The second approximation to an international standard of life satisfaction. *Social Indicators Research, 43*, 307–334.

Cummins, R.A. (2014). Understanding the well-being of children and adolescents through homeostàtic theory. In A. Ben-Arieh, F. Casas, I. Frønes, & J.E. Korbin, *Handbook of Child Well-Being* (635–662). Dordrecht: Springer.

Cummins, R.A., Eckersley, R. Pallant, J., Van Vugt, J., & Misajon, R. (2003). Developing a national index of subjective wellbeing: The Australian Unity Wellbeing Index. *Social Indicators Research, 64*, 159–190.

Cummins, R.A., & Gullone, E. (2000). Why we should not use 5-point Likert scales: The case for subjective quality of life measurement. *Proceedings Second International Conference on Quality of Life in Cities*, 74–93. Singapore: National University of Singapore.

Cummins, R.A., & Lau, A.L. (2005). *Personal Wellbeing Index – School Children. Manual (Third Edition)*. Melbourne: School of Psychology, Deakin University.

Currie, C., Zanotti, C., Morgan, A., Currie, D., de Looze, M., Roberts, C., & Rasmussen, V.B. (2012). Social determinants of Health and well-being among young people. In W.A.R. of Europe (Ed.): *Health Policy for Children and Adolescents, 6*. Copenhagen: WHO Regional Office for Europe.

Dannerbeck, A., Casas, F., Sadurní, M., & Coenders, G. (Eds.) (2004). Quality-of-life research on children and adolescents. *Social Indicators Research Series, 23*, 1–195. Dordrecht: Kluwer.

Diener, E., Emmons, R., Larsen, R., & Smith, H.L. (1985). The satisfaction with life scale. *Journal of Personality Assessment, 49*(1), 71–75.

Diener, E., Suh, E.M., Lucas, R.E., & Smith, H.L. (1999). Subjective well-being: Three decades of progress. *Psychological Bulletin, 125*(2), 276–302.

Fordyce, M.W. (1988). A review of research on the happiness measures: a sixty second index of happiness and mental health. *Social Indicators Research, 20*(4), 355–381.

Gilman, R., & Huebner, E.S. (2000). Review of life satisfaction measures for adolescents. *Behavior Change, 17*, 178–196.

Goldbeck, L., Schmitz, T.G., Besier, T., Herschbach, P., & Henrich, G. (2007). Life satisfaction decreases with age. *Quality of life research, 16*, 969–979.

Guyatt, G.H., & Jaeschker, R. (1990). Measurement in clinical trials: Choosing the appropriate approach. In B. Spilker (Ed.), *Quality of life assessment in clinical trials* (pp. 37–46). New York: Raven.

Gullone, E., & Cummins R.A. (1999). The Comprehensive Quality of Life Scale: A psychometric evaluation with an adolescent sample. *Behaviour Change, 16*, 127–139.

Holte, A., Barry, M.M., Bekkhus, M., Borge, A.I.H., Bowes, L., Casas, F., … Zachrisson, H.D. (2014). Psychology of child well-being. In A. Ben-Arieh, F. Casas, I. Frønes, & J.E. Korbin, *Handbook of Child Well-Being* (pp. 555–631). Dordrecht: Springer.
Huebner, E.S (1991). Initial development of the Students' Life Satisfaction Scale. *School Psychology International, 12*, 231–240.
Huebner, E.S. (1994). Preliminary development and validation of a multidimensional life satisfaction scale of children. *Psychological Assessment, 6*(2), 149–158.
Huebner, E.S. (2004). Research on assessment of life satisfaction of children and adolescents. *Social Indicators Research, 66*(1–2), 3–33.
International Wellbeing Group (2006). *Personal Wellbeing Index Manual (4th ed.).* Retrieved from http://www.deakin.edu.au/research/acqol/instruments/wellbeing-index/pwi-a-english.pdf
Land, K. (2000). Social indicators. In E.F. Borgatta, & R.V. Montgomery (Eds.), *Encyclopedia of Sociology* (pp. 2682–2690). New York: Macmillan.
Mason, J., & Watson, E. (2014). Researching children: Research on, with, and by children. In A. Ben-Arieh, F. Casas, I. Frønes, & J.E. Korbin, Handbook of Child Well-Being (pp. 2757–2796). Dordrecht: Springer.
Montserrat, C., & Casas, F. (2007). Kinship foster care from the perspective of quality of life: Research on the satisfaction of the stakeholders. *Applied Research in Quality of Life*, 1(3–4), 227–237.
Park, N., Huebner, E.S., Laughlin, J.E., Valois, R.F., & Gilman, R. (2004). A cross-cultural comparison of child and adolescent life satisfaction reports. *Social Indicators Research, 66*, 61–79.
Park, N., & Huebner, E.S. (2005). A cross-cultural study of the levels and correlates of life satisfaction among adolescents. *Journal of Cross-Cultural Psychology, 36*, 444–456.
Pollard, E., & Lee, P.D. (2003). Child well-being: A systematic review of the literature. *Social Indicators Research, 61*(1), 59–78.
Raphael, D., Rukholm, E., Brown, I., Hill-Bailey, P., & Donato, E. (1996). The Quality of Life Profile-Adolescent Version: Background, description, and initial validation. *Journal of Adolescent Health, 19*, 366–375.
Rees, G., & Main, G. (2015). Children's views on their lives and well-being in 15 countries: An initial report on the Children's Worlds survey, 2013–14. Children's Worlds. Retrieved from http://www.isciweb.org/?CategoryID=176&ArticleID=108
Ryff, C.D. (1989). Happiness is everything, or is it – Explorations on the meaning of psychological well-being. *Journal of Personality and Social Psychology, 57*(6), 1069–1081.
Russell, J.A. (2003). Core Affect and the Psychological Construction of Emotion. *Psychological Review, 110*(1), 145–172.
Sandin, B. (2014). History of Children's Well-Being. In A. Ben-Arieh, F. Casas, I. Frønes, & J.E. Korbin, *Handbook of Child Well-Being* (pp. 31–86). Dordrecht: Springer.
Seligson, J.L., Huebner, E.S., & Valois, R.F. (2003). Preliminary validation of the Brief Multidimensional Students' Life Satisfaction Scale (BMSLSS). *Social Indicators Research, 61*(2), 121–145. doi: 10.1023/A:1021326822957.
Stones, M.J., & Kozma, A. (1985). Structural relationships among happiness scales: A second order factorial study. *Social Indicators Research, 17*, 19–28.
Tomyn, A.J., & Cummins, R.A. (2011). The Subjective Wellbeing of High-School students: Validating the Personal Wellbeing Index—School Children. *Social Indicators Research, 101*, 405–418.
Vaqué, C., González, M., & Casas, F. (2015). Does Satisfaction with Food Matter? Testing the Personal Well-Being Index-School Children (PWI-SC) with an Additional Item on Satisfaction with Food on a Sample of 10 to 12-Year-Olds. *Child Indicators Research, online first.* doi 10.1007/s12187-015-9301-y.
Veenhoven, R. (2000). The four qualities of life, *Journal of Happiness Studies, 1*, 1–39.

Chapter 2
Measuring Trends in Child Well-Being and Child Suffering in the United States, 1975–2013

Kenneth C. Land, Vicki L. Lamb, and Qiang Fu

Introduction

Every generation of adults, and American adults in particular, is concerned about the well-being of their children and youth (Moore 1999; Land 2012). From the stagflation and socially turbulent days of the 1970s in the US through the decline of the rust belt industries and transition to the information age in the 1980s to the relatively prosperous *e*-economy and multicultural years of the late-1990s followed by the digitized-roboticized, economically uncertain, and politically anxious early years of the twenty-first century, Americans have fretted over the material circumstances of the nation's children, their health and safety, their educational progress, and their moral development. Are their fears and concerns warranted? How do we know whether circumstances of life for children in the United States are bad and worsening, or good and improving? On what basis can the public and its leaders form opinions and draw conclusions?

To systematically address these and related questions, for the past 15 years the Child and Youth Well-Being Index (CWI) Project at Duke University has developed and studied the CWI as an instrument for measuring trends over time in

K.C. Land (✉)
Department of Sociology and Center for Child and Family Policy, Duke University, Duke box 90088, Durham, NC 27708, USA
e-mail: kland@soc.duke.edu

V.L. Lamb
Department of Human Sciences, North Carolina Central University, 1801 Fayetteville Street, Durham, NC 27707, USA
e-mail: vlamb@nccu.edu

Q. Fu
Department of Sociology, The University of British Columbia, Vancouver, BC V6T 1Z1, Canada
e-mail: fu.qiangsoc@gmail.com

F. Maggino (ed.), *A Life Devoted to Quality of Life*, Social Indicators Research Series 60, DOI 10.1007/978-3-319-20568-7_2

the well-being of America's children and youth. Since 2004, the Project also has published an annual update and report on the Index, most recently in December 2014 (Land 2014). This chapter commences with a review of the conceptual foundations of the CWI, its composition and methods of construction, and empirical findings on trends in the Index and its components at the national level.

The CWI has been motivated by the well-being question: "How are the kids doing?" Reversing the spectrum of this question, it becomes "Are the kids suffering?" As with the well-being question, adults might be able to answer these questions for their own children or those in their immediate surroundings, and many children could provide information about their own well-being/suffering or those of other children. However, applied to large populations of children, suffering questions are more challenging and merit systematic research attention. The second part of this chapter describes our recent work on the conceptualization, construction, and calculation of a Child and Youth Suffering Index (CSI) to measure trends in levels of suffering of America's children and youth. Comparisons of findings from the CSI and CWI round out the chapter.

Conceptualizing and Measuring Child Well-Being

How can the notion of child and youth well-being be conceptualized?[1] What is meant by well-being? Assuming this term can be defined, how can it be measured? These are generic, foundational questions to which no simple, definitive, and immutable answers can be given. Rather, they will continue to motivate research and researchers for decades to come. As Ben-Arieh and Frones (2007) note, however, recent studies in the sociology and psychology of childhood conceptualized children's well-being during childhood as a separate and distinct phase in life rather than simply a period of preparation for adulthood. This conceptualization has led to two innovative approaches to the measurement of child well-being.

A Phenomenological/Ethnographic Positive Well-Being Approach

One of these, illustrated by the work of Fattore et al. (2007) on children's conceptualization of their well-being, places children centrally as research participants in the articulation of their understandings of what contributes to their *positive well-being*. Following the approach advocated by Ben-Arieh (2005), the explicit aim of this approach is to facilitate input from children about what for them constitutes well-being and about the factors they identify as contributing to this well-being.

[1] This section and parts of the next section are adapted from Land (2012).

The approach employs a qualitative methodology from the phenomenological/ ethnographic research tradition, which, according to Denzin and Lincoln (1998, p. 3), attempts "to make sense of, or interpret, phenomena in terms of the meanings people bring to them."

According to Fattore et al. (2007, p. 18), the child-participatory approach leads to the conclusion that *children's well-being is defined through feelings*, in particular *happiness*, but that integrating sadness is also relevant. For example, well-being is about *feeling secure*, particularly in social relations, when relations are harmonious. Well-being also has a *moral quality* – being a moral actor in relation to oneself (when making decision's in one's best interests) and in behaving towards others. Adults are considered as behaving morally when they make decisions in children's best interests.

A Quantitative Positive Psychology Approach

The qualitative research approach and empirical findings of Fattore et al. (2007) complement the *positive psychology* approach of Huebner (1991, 2004), which uses more traditional quantitative, psychometric research designs. Huebner noted that various psychologists recently have called for greater attention to a science of positive psychology, which focuses on studying conditions that promote optimal human and societal development (e.g., McCullough and Snyder 2000; Seligman and Csikszentmihalyi 2000). To contrast with the previous emphasis on pathological conditions, the development of positive psychology requires constructs and measures that reflect the full range of human functioning, incorporating indicators of high levels of wellness as well as psychopathological functioning.

Huebner (2004) observed that one such construct, *life satisfaction*, has been studied extensively in adulthood (see Diener et al. 1999), but had gained attention in psychological studies with children and adolescents only in the 1990s (see Bender 1997; Huebner 1997). Since the early work of Andrews and Withey (1976) and Campbell et al. (1976), *global life satisfaction* has been defined as a cognitive evaluation of one's life as a whole (Shin and Johnson 1978). Although affect can influence life satisfaction reports, life satisfaction is distinguished from transitory affective states. Emotions refer to specific momentary reactions to specific events that occur in people's lives, such as anger, joy, anxiety, and so forth. Life satisfaction reports typically refer to more general, enduring background appraisals encompassing one's overall life or major facets of one's life (Diener et al. 1999; Lazarus 1991). Although experiences of frequent positive emotions, infrequent negative emotions, and life satisfaction tend to intercorrelate, suggesting a higher-order subjective well-being factor, affective and life satisfaction reports can diverge over time and demonstrate different determinants (see Diener 1994).

Based on an extensive review of research studies of children and youth (ages 8–18), Huebner (2004, pp. 22–24) concluded that life satisfaction appears to be a useful psychological construct that is related to, but separable from, a variety of other well-being constructs. Global life satisfaction does not represent an isolated characteristic or appraisal tendency of children and/or youth, but has broad implications for their intrapersonal and interpersonal adaptation in a variety of life contexts, encompasses the full range of subjective appraisals from very negative to very positive, and complements well-being measures that are limited to negative well-being indicators, such as reports of psychopathological symptoms.

The Child and Youth Well-Being Index (CWI)

In brief, different research approaches have led to the conclusion that *the well-being of children and youth can be defined in terms of the two traditions that have come to dominate subjective well-being studies of adults – those based on feelings, especially happiness, and those based on life satisfaction assessments.* The challenge, however, of using this foundation of research on well-being to address questions pertaining to changes in the well-being of America's children and youths, such as those stated at the beginning of this chapter, is that there are virtually no continuous, consistently collected, nationally-representative databases on subjective well-being that extend beyond a single cross-section sample of a segment of this population.

An alternative approach, pursued by Land and colleagues (Land et al. 2001, 2007, 2012), *is to use the results of subjective well-being studies to inform the selection of time series of demographic, social, and economic statistics for use in the construction of a social indicator – the Child and Youth Well-Being Index (CWI) –* that can be calculated annually and used to monitor overall well-being as well as its major components. The general nature and rationale of the CWI will be described in the following paragraphs. In order to position the CWI as a social indicator, however, we begin with a review of the two major traditions of social indicators research.

The Objective Social Indicators Tradition

The term *social indicators* was born and given its initial meaning in an attempt, undertaken in the early 1960s by the American Academy of Arts and Sciences for the National Aeronautics and Space Administration, to detect and anticipate the nature and magnitude of the second-order consequences of the space program for American society (Land 1983, p. 2; Noll and Zapf 1994, p. 1). Frustrated by the lack of sufficient data to detect such effects and the absence of a systematic conceptual framework and methodology for analysis, some of those involved in the Academy project attempted to develop a system of social indicators with which to detect and anticipate social change as well as to evaluate specific programs and determine their impact. The results of this part of the Academy project were published in a volume (Bauer 1966) bearing the name *Social Indicators* and the following definition:

> ... *social indicators* – statistics, statistical series, and all other forms of evidence – that enable us to assess where we stand and are going with respect to our values and goals... (Bauer 1966, p. 1)

Thus, efforts to develop "objective" social indicators began with the initial wave of identity and interest in the topic in the 1960s and extend to the present. The emphasis in this tradition is on the development of statistics that reflect important "social conditions" and the monitoring of trends in a range of "areas of social concern" over time. The key undefined terms here require the identification of:

- the "social conditions" to be measured, and
- the "areas of social concern" for which trends are to be monitored. Since the 1970s, the primary approach to the identification and definition processes has been through the creation of "expert" panels of social scientists, statisticians, and citizens.

These panels have applied a variety of approaches to their work, such as:

- the "indicators of social change" approach (Sheldon and Moore 1968);
- the Swedish "level of living" approach (Erickson 1974); and
- the "goals commissions" approach (e.g., the *U.S. Healthy People 2010* Goals; see U.S. Department of Health and Human Services 2000).

A key element of this approach (Noll 2002, p. 175) is that the experts must achieve consensus on:

- the conditions and areas of concern to be measured;
- good and bad conditions; and
- the directions in which society should move.

These, of course, are strong requirements. And, in its reliance on "expert" panels, the objective social indicators tradition is always open to the criticism that the conditions identified have not been corroborated as relevant to how people actually experience happiness, life satisfaction, and subjective well-being. This criticism motivates the other major tradition of work on the measurement of the quality of life.

The Subjective Well-Being Indicators Tradition

The subjective well-being indicators tradition commenced with the Campbell et al. (1976) and Andrews and Withey (1976) volumes cited above. As noted there, this approach uses various social science research techniques, including in-depth interviews, focus-group discussions, clinical studies, and sample surveys to study how people define their happiness and satisfaction with life and the social conditions of life that they experience on a day-to-day basis.

In the four decades since the publication of the path-breaking studies by Campbell et al. (1976) and Andrews and Withey (1976) volumes, many studies of subjective well-being have been conducted. As noted above in the review of recent research on the subjective well-being of children and adolescents, these studies show that subjective well-being is an individual's summary of the positive experiences in life, consisting of three components (Diener 1994):

- global life satisfaction,
- positive affect, and
- negative affect.

In brief, we today are the beneficiaries of these many subjective well-being studies, including studies of children and adolescents such as those reviewed above. As a result, we know a lot more about what makes people, including children and adolescents, happy and satisfied with life today than in the early-1970s. In particular, Cummins (1996, 1997) reached the following conclusions about the quality of life based on comparisons of findings across numerous subjective well-being studies:

- there is a potential for tremendous variety of assessments of satisfaction with life experiences, with individuals often differing in their ratings of importance of the key elements associated with their life satisfactions and happiness;
- but, at the same time, the accumulation of findings across many studies shows that certain domains of well-being occur over and over again;
- there also is a fairly high degree of similarity among individuals on the relative weightings given to these domains in determining overall life satisfaction;
- and, perhaps most interestingly, there is a lot of similarity between the domains of well-being identified in subjective well-being studies and the areas of concern identified by expert panels in objective social indicators studies.

Intersecting the Two Traditions and the Child and Youth Well-Being Index

This naturally leads to the question: Can the empirical findings from subjective well-being studies about domains of well-being be used to inform the construction of summary quality-of-life indices? That is, rather than relying solely on the opinions of expert panels, can we use the accumulated body of empirical findings from subjective well-being studies in a manner similar to the use of research findings or best evidence to inform decisions in clinical and public health in modern evidence-based medicine (see, e.g., Jenicek 2003)? In other words: Can subjective well-being studies be used to make composite or summary quality-of-life/well-being indices more evidence-based not only in the use of empirical data, but also in the selection of the domains of well-being and indicators used in their construction? Put more figuratively, can we bring these two social indicators/quality-of-life research traditions into intersection so that we may construct composite social indicators based on objective social indicators (demographic, social, and economic statistics) of specific aspects of social life that are more firmly grounded in what we have learned about subjective well-being over the past three decades?

The answer to these rhetorical questions offered by Land et al. (2001, 2007, 2012) is "yes" with respect to the development of a composite index of child and youth well-being. The *Child and Youth Well-Being Index (CWI)* is:

- a composite measure of trends over time in the well-being of America's children and young people,
- that consists of several interrelated summary indices of annual time series of numerous social indicators of the well-being of children and youth in the United States.

The general objective of the CWI summary indices is to:

- give a sense of the overall direction of change in the well-being of children and youth in the U.S. as compared to values observed in certain base years.

The CWI is designed to address questions such as the following:

- Overall, on average, how did child and youth well-being in the U.S. change in the last quarter of the twentieth century and beyond?
- Did it improve or deteriorate?
- By approximately how much?
- In which domains of social life?
- For specific age groups?
- For particular race/ethnic groups?
- For each of the sexes?
- And did race/ethnic group and sex disparities increase or decrease?

The approach to the assessment of child and youth well-being taken in the construction of the CWI, thus, is that of the development of an evidence-based social indicator that can be used to address these and related questions.

In brief, the *Child and Youth Well-Being Index (CWI)* is an *evidence-based composite or summary measure of trends over time in the quality of life/well-being of America's children from birth up to the 18th birthday.*[2] The CWI is evidence-based in two senses (Land et al. 2012). First, the Index is based on demographic, social, and economic statistical time series of empirical data on the Key Indicators. Second, the Domains of Well-Being and the choices of the Key Indicators within each Domain are based on decades of studies of well-being, including both quantitative and qualitative research on the well-being of children, adolescents, teenagers, and young adults.

The Index is calculated and updated annually from the time series data in order to track changes in the well-being of children annually compared to 1975 base-year

[2] Or, as stated using Census/demographic notation, ages 0–17 at last birthday. Some of the Key Indicators in the CWI use slightly higher or slightly lower upper bounds, because of the age intervals in which the Indicators are reported. Our analyses, however, have found that the main focus of the CWI – the measurement of trends over time – is not greatly affected by these small differences in upper-age boundaries.

values.[3] As a composite[4] index of changes over time, the most important information to be found in the CWI is in the direction of change in Indicators and Well-Being Domains: Are the indices up and thus indicative of overall improvements? Down and thus indicative of deterioration? Flat and thus indicative of little or no change?

Children and youth live unique lives; each experiences a range of social conditions at different points. The Index comprises Key Indicators associated with different stages of the first two decades of life. Different Indicators capture children and youth at different stages of life. During the early childhood years, for example, PreKindergarten enrollment is an Indicator of early schooling participation, while the violent crime victimization rate is indicative for ages 12–17.

The overall CWI organizes the following 28 Key Indicators[5] into *seven Quality-of-Life/Well-Being Domains*.[6] These seven Domains have been well-established, having recurred time after time in more than three decades of empirical research in numerous subjective well-being studies. They also have been found, in one form or another, in studies of the well-being of children and youth. Each Domain represents an important area that affects quality of life:

Family Economic Well-Being Domain[7]

1. Poverty Rate (All Families with Children Ages 0–17)
2. Secure Parental Employment Rate (All Families with Children Ages 0–17)
3. Median Annual Income (All Families with Children Ages 0–17)
4. Rate of Children with Health Insurance (All Families with Children Ages 0–17)

Safe/Risky Behavior Domain[8]

1. Teenage Birth Rate (Ages 10–17)
2. Rate of Violent Crime Victimization (Ages 12–19)[9]
3. Rate of Violent Crime Offenders (Ages 12–17)
4. Rate of Cigarette Smoking (Grade 12)[10]

---

[3] The geographical focus of the CWI in this Report is the U.S., that is, the nation as a whole; hence, it is termed the National CWI. The conceptual framework and methodology of the CWI also has been applied at the level of the 50 U.S. states (O'Hare et al. 2013) and to regions within the states (Lee et al. 2009).

[4] The averaging method used in construction of the CWI is described below in the Methods of Construction section.

[5] Unless otherwise noted, indicators refer to children ages 0–17.

[6] Some Key Indicators can be assigned to more than one Well-Being Domain, but, for purposes of Domain-Specific and Overall Index construction, each is included in only one Domain.

[7] The label "Material Well-Being" has also been used for this Domain.

[8] The label "Safety/Behavioral Concerns" has also been used for this Domain.

[9] The upper age limit of 19 is used for this indicator, as the data series for this Key Indicator are not available for ages 12–18 separately.

[10] The Monitoring the Future (MTF) Project is the source of time series data for five of the Key Indicators (Rates of Cigarette Smoking, Binge Alcohol Drinking, and Illicit Drug Use in this Domain, as well as Rate of Weekly Religious Attendance and Percent Who Report Religion as

5. Rate of Binge Alcohol Drinking (Grade 12)
6. Rate of Illicit Drug Use (Grade 12)

Social Relationships Domain

1. Rate of Children in Families Headed by a Single Parent (All Families with Children Ages 0–17)
2. Rate of Children Who Have Moved Within the Last Year (Ages 1–17)

Emotional/Spiritual Well-Being Domain:

1. Suicide Rate (Ages 10–19)[11]
2. Rate of Weekly Religious Attendance (Grade 12)
3. Percent Who Report Religion as Being Very Important (Grade 12)

Community Engagement Domain[12]

1. Rate of Persons Who Have Received a High School Diploma (Ages 18–24)[13]
2. Institutionally Disconnected Youth Rate (Ages 16–19)[14]
3. Rate of PreKindergarten Enrollment (Ages 3–4)
4. Rate of Persons Who Have Received a Bachelor's Degree (Ages 25–29)[15]
5. Rate of Voting in Presidential Elections (Ages 18–24)[16]

Educational Attainment Domain

1. Reading Test Scores (Averages of Ages 9, 13, and 17)
2. Mathematics Test Scores (Average of Ages 9, 13, and 17)

Health Domain

1. Infant Mortality Rate
2. Low Birth Weight Rate

Being Very Important in the Emotional/Spiritual Well-Being Domain). The MTF Project originally began as the High School Senior Survey in 1975, with surveys of national samples of seniors (modal age 18) in U.S. high schools taken in the spring of the academic school year. Samples of 8th graders (modal age 14) and 10th graders (modal age 16) were added in 1991. In studies of time series of MTF data on these five Key Indicators, we have found substantial covariation over time among the 8th, 10th, and 12th grade responses. For this reason, and because the 12th grade data extend back to the principal base year of the CWI Project, 1975, we use the 12th grade time series as data for these five Key Indicators.

[11]The upper age limit of 19 is used for Suicide Rate (Emotional/Spiritual Domain) as well as Mortality Rate and Rate of Obese Children and Adolescents (Health Domain), as these data series are not available for an upper age limit of 18.

[12]This Domain includes participation in educational, economic, and political institutions. The labels "place in community" and "community connectedness" also have been used for this Domain.

[13]Since some youth are delayed in completing the requirements for high school diplomas or General Education Equivalent (GED) degrees, a higher upper age limit is used for this Key Indicator series.

[14]The rate of those ages 16–19 who are not working and not in school. The upper age limit of 19 is used for this Indicator, as the data series is not available for an upper age limit of 18.

[15]Similarly to the use of a higher age limit for the high school diploma Key Indicator, a higher age limit is used for this series, in order to index trends in commitment to, and participation in, higher education institutions.

[16]Since the legal voting age for presidential elections is 18, ages 18–24 are used to represent trends in youth voting behavior.

3. Mortality Rate (Ages 1–19)
4. Rate of Children with Very Good or Excellent Health (Ages 0–17, as reported by parents)
5. Rate of Children with Activity Limitations due to Health Problems (Ages 0–17, as reported by parents)
6. Rate of Obese Children and Adolescents (Ages 6–19)

In sum, the CWI builds on a base of subjective well-being empirical research in both identifying which Domains of Well-Being to measure and assigning Indicators to those Domains. It can therefore be viewed as an evidence-based measure of trends in averages of the social conditions encountered by children and youth in the United States across recent decades.[17]

Methods of Index Construction

After assembling annual time series data (from vital statistics and sample surveys) were assembled on the 28 national-level Key Indicators in the seven Quality-of-Life/Well-Being Domains[18] identified above, the first step in the calculation of the CWI is to index each of the time series by a base year (1975). The base-year value of the Indicator is assigned a value of 100 and subsequent values of the Indicator are taken as percentage changes in the CWI. The directions of the Indicators are oriented so that a value greater than 100 in subsequent years means the social condition measured has improved relative to its observed value in the base year, while a value less than 100 in subsequent years means the social condition has deteriorated.

Numerical values of the 28 indexed Key Indicator time series then are grouped into the seven Domains of Well-Being by equal weighting to calculate the Domain-

[17]The basic CWI that is the subject of this report is focused on the population of all American children and youth. As part of our research on child well-being, however, we also have studied time trends in the CWI for children classified by gender, race/ethnicity, family income levels, and immigrant status (Land et al. 2012; Hernandez et al. 2012). These studies generally show that, when the overall CWI changes (increases, decreases) by 1 unit, the CWI for children from African-American and Hispanic families and from families in the lowest quintile of the income distribution correspondingly changes (increases, decreases) by 1.5 to 2 units. That is, children from African-American and Hispanic families and from families in the lowest quintile of the income distribution, on average, benefit more than the total child and youth population when the CWI increases and are negatively affected more than the total child and youth population when the CWI decreases. Part of the reason for these multipliers being larger than 1 is that children from white and Asian families and from families in the upper parts of the income distribution generally fare better on the well-being outcomes measured by the CWI and have less to gain during periods of overall increasing child well-being than those from other race/ethnic groups and at lower levels of the family income distribution.

[18]Those Key Indicators that do not directly measure outcomes for children and youth are *proxy indicators* of those outcomes. For instance, data are not available on direct measure of the poverty status of children, only on the poverty status of families that have children up to age 18. However, it is not strained to infer that a child living in a family whose income falls below the poverty line has a poverty-level economic well-being. Thus, the poverty status of the family is used as a proxy Indicator for the poverty status of the child.

Specific Index values for each year. The seven Domain-Specific Indices then are grouped into an equally-weighted CWI value for each year. The CWI Project uses an equal-weighting strategy for constructing its composite indices for two reasons. First, it is the simplest and most transparent strategy and can easily be replicated by others. Second, statistical research done in conjunction with the CWI Project (Hagerty and Land 2007) has demonstrated that, in the absence of a clear ordering of the Indicators of a composite index by their relative importance to the composite index, and with a high degree of consensus in the population, an equal weighting strategy is privileged in the sense that it will achieve the greatest level of agreement among the members of the population – in statistical terminology, the equal-weighting method is a *minimax estimator.*

Long-, Medium-, and Short-Term Changes in the CWI and Its Seven Domain Indices, 1975–2013

Figure 2.1 charts annual percentage changes from 1975 to 2013 in the overall composite CWI, with the value of the CWI in the base year 1975 set equal to 100. Observed data on all 28 of the 28 Key Indicators currently (December 2014) are available for the year 2011; observations are available on 22 of the 28 Key Indicators for 2012, and on 13 of the 28 Key Indicators for 2013. In order to calculate values of the CWI through 2013, the remaining Indicators were projected for 2012

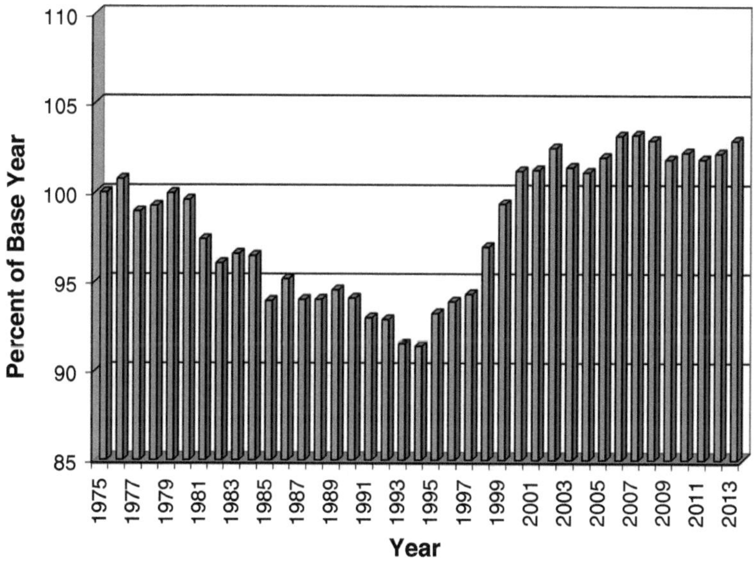

Fig. 2.1 Child and Youth Well-Being Index, 1975–2013

and/2013 by use of statistical time series models.[19] Trends in the overall, composite CWI give a sense of changes in child and youth well-being both in the short-term (the last few years) and the long-term (since the base year 1975). The latter time frame yields a historical perspective, as values of the Index for the late 1970s and early 1980s now pertain to individuals who were children at that time but are part of today's parental cohorts.

Over the *long-term* of 38 years (1975–2013), the CWI shows periods of both deterioration and improvement. Through the late 1970s, the CWI oscillated at levels near the base year value of 100; then shows a decline beginning in 1980 and ending in 1994 with a value of 91.37. The roots of this decline (Land et al. 2012) were in the economic recession of the early 1980s (which negatively affected the Family Economic Well-Being Domain); in changing family structures (toward more single-parenting); in an upturn in risky behavior (especially increases in teenage childbearing, illicit drug use, and violent crime victimization and offending); and in the beginnings of the trend towards an increasing prevalence of obese children (which negatively impacted the Health Domain).

In the *medium-term* of the past 20 years from 1994 to 2013, the CWI increased through the late 1990s, reaching a peak of 102.49 in 2002. This period of increase was associated with the rapidly expanding economy of the late-1990s, the stabilization of family structures, and downturns in risky behavior (Land et al. 2012). Since 2002, the Index has oscillated at or near this peak, with values of 101.85 in 2011, 102.19 in 2012, and an initial estimate of 102.90 for 2013. The CWI since 2002 exhibits the imprint of the economic expansions and contractions of the first decade of the twenty-first century, especially the Great Recession of 2008–2009.

As evident from Fig. 2.1, the long-term trend in the CWI, taking into account the improvements in some Well-Being Domains and Key Indicators and deteriorations in others, yields values of the Index in the most recent years 2011, 2012, and 2013 slightly above the 100 base year value. In other words, the predominant long-term trend in the CWI is indicative of a small overall improvement in 38 years. By comparison, medium-term changes in the CWI over the past 20 years show substantial improvements, from 91.37 in 1994 to 102.90 in 2013.

Focusing on *short-term changes* in the CWI, the past 6 years 2008–2013 were a turbulent time for our nation, with the impacts of the Great Recession in 2008–2009 and the slow recovery in 2010–2013. For these most recent years, Fig. 2.1 shows that:

- The CWI decreased by 1.34 %, from 103.22 in 2007 to 101.84 in 2009, the years of impact of the Great Recession.
- The CWI then is 102.23 for 2010, the last year for which data are available on all 28 Key Indicators.
- In the following years, the CWI shows partially projected values of 101.85 in 2011, 102.19 in 2012 and 102.90 in 2013.

In sum, these recent annual numerical changes in the CWI indicate that the declines of 2008–2009 did not continue in the four most recent years. However, the annual

[19] For a description of the autoregressive integrated moving average (ARIMA) models used to project each individual Key Indicator time series, see Land et al. (2012).

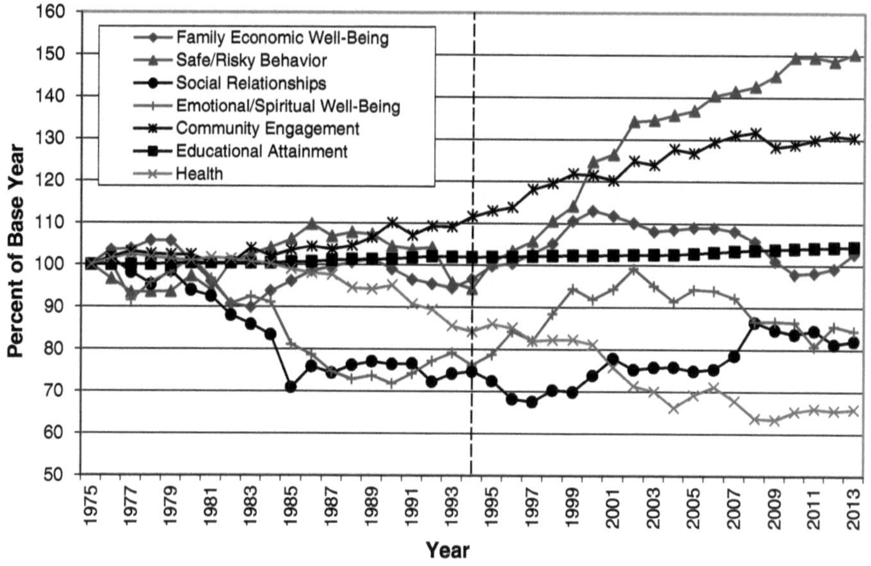

Fig. 2.2 Domain-specific summary indices, 1975–2013

changes for 2010 through 2013 are not statistically significant and are indicative of small short-term improvements in overall child and youth well-being.

The CWI can alert us to recent changes and emerging trends in overall child and youth well-being. We also can study both long-term and medium-term trends and cycles in the seven Well-Being Domains and their component Key Indicators. This section of the chapter focuses on these trends, especially in the medium-term since the year 1994. Regarding long-term changes, Fig. 2.2 displays annual percentage changes since 1975 in the seven CWI Well-Being Domains, with the value of each series in the base year 1975 set equal to 100.

Focusing on medium-term trends (for assistance in visually identifying this time period, a vertical dashed line is inserted in Fig. 2.2 at the year 1994) over the past 20 years, 1994–2013, the seven Well-Being Domain Indices in Fig. 2.2 show diverse patterns:

- the Family Economic Well-Being Domain Index cycles up and down with expansions and contractions in the national economy;
- the Safe/Risky Behavior and Community Engagement Indices show substantial improvements;
- the Educational Attainment Index shows slight increases;
- two Domain Indices with long-term declines, Social Relationships and Emotional/Spiritual Well-Being, have slight medium-term improvements and subsequent declines; and
- one Domain Index with long-term declines, Health, further declined in the medium-term.

Comparisons with a Child Suffering Index (CSI), 1975–2013

As noted in the Introduction to this chapter, the Child Well-Being Research Project team recently has focused on the extent to which its Key Indicators can be used to assess trends U.S. in child and youth suffering.[20] This section reports our initial explorations as a first step towards that objective.

Most generally, *suffering* refers to barriers to the realization of child well-being and happiness. Anderson (2014) identifies three types of suffering, namely, distress resulting from threat or damage to one's physical being (*physical suffering*), distress originating in one's cognitive or affective self-identity (*mental suffering*), and distress cumulating from threat or damage to one's social identity (*social suffering*). Applying this conceptual scheme to the 28 Key Indicators of the CWI, we tentatively have assigned the following 15 Key Indicators to the Physical Suffering, Social Suffering, and Mental Suffering categories[21]:

Physical Suffering

1. Rate of low birth weight
2. Infant Mortality rate
3. Mortality rate, ages 1–19
4. Percentage of children ages 0–17 with Very Good or Excellent health (as reported by parents)
5. Percent of children ages 0–17 with Activity Limitations (as reported by their parents)
6. Obesity rate, 6–19

Social Suffering

1. Percent of Children Ages 0–17 living in families below the poverty line
2. Percent of Children Ages 0–17 living in families with secure parental employment
3. Percent of Children Ages 0–17 living in families with health insurance
4. Percent of Children Ages 0–17 Living in Single-Parent families
5. Rate of Residential Mobility of Children Ages 0–17
6. Percent who have received high school diploma, Ages 18–24
7. Percent not working or in school, Ages 16–19

---

[20] At the level of international comparisons of child suffering indicators, our work is reported in Land et al. (2015).

[21] As with the CWI (see footnote 6), some Key Indicators can be assigned to more than one category of suffering. For purposes of Index calculation, however, each is included only in one category. An example is the Violent Crime Victimization Rate Key Indicator. Being victimized by a violent crime can result in both physical and mental suffering and thus this indicator could be included in both categories. Since, in most cases of violent crime victimization of children and youths ages 12–17, mental suffering (anxiety, anguish, depression, etc.) is a longer term consequence than physical suffering, we have included this Key Indicator in the mental suffering category.

Mental Suffering

1. Violent Crime Victimization rate, Ages 12–17
2. Suicide rate, Ages 10–19

To construct a U.S. Child and Youth Suffering Index (CSI) on a basis comparable to the CWI, we indexed these 15 Key Indicator time series to the 1975 base year and recoded them in such a way that *an increase indicates an increase in suffering*. As with the CWI, the 15 indexed time series then were composed into equally-weighted category-specific indices which then were composed into an equally-weighted overall CSI the metric of which is annual percentage changes from the base year 1975 value of 100. These 15 Key Indicators are a core part of the CWI. Therefore, when coded such that an increase in the indicators is indicative of an increase in suffering, it is expected that the resulting Child and Youth Suffering Index will have a negative correlation with the Child and Youth Well-Being Index. However, the CWI includes a number of other indicators that are reflective of child well-being/flourishing. Therefore, the CSI will not be perfectly negatively correlated with the CWI.

Two variations on the resulting CSI are shown in Fig. 2.3, one that includes the obesity Key Indicator and one that does not. Because the long-term obesity trend from 1975 has been so large – quadrupling from the mid-1970s to the 2010s, it has a very large impact on the CSI if it is included. The result is a CSI series in Fig. 2.3 that rises above the base year value of 100 in 1975 very quickly in the 1980s, reaches a peak of 124.6 in 1994 followed by a decline to a low point of 104.4 in the year 2000, and then oscillates in the 2000s with values in the 102–104 range in the years 2001–2009, and then climbs to 107.6 in 2012 and 108.4 in 2013. If the obesity series is not included, then Fig. 2.3 shows that the impacts of the decline in violent crime victimization bring the series down to less than the base year 100 value in the late 1990s. It then stays in 91–94 range from 2001 to 2013.

As expected, there is an inverse relationship between trends in the CWI and the CSI. And, as expected, the correlation is not perfect, which is to say that there are

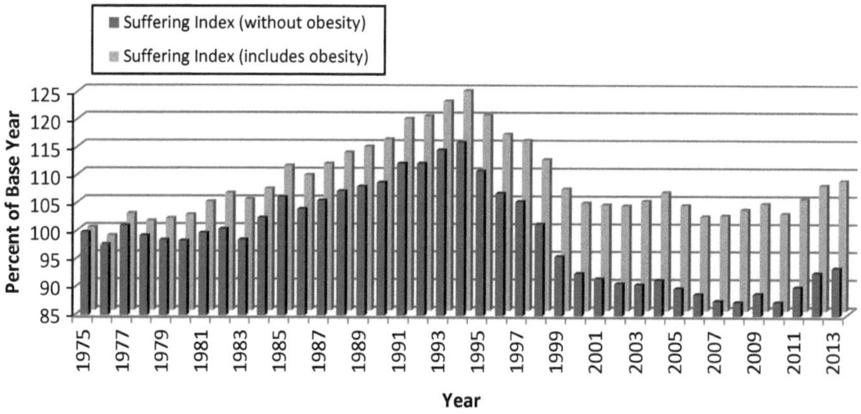

Fig. 2.3 Child Suffering Index, without and including obesity indicator, 1975–2013

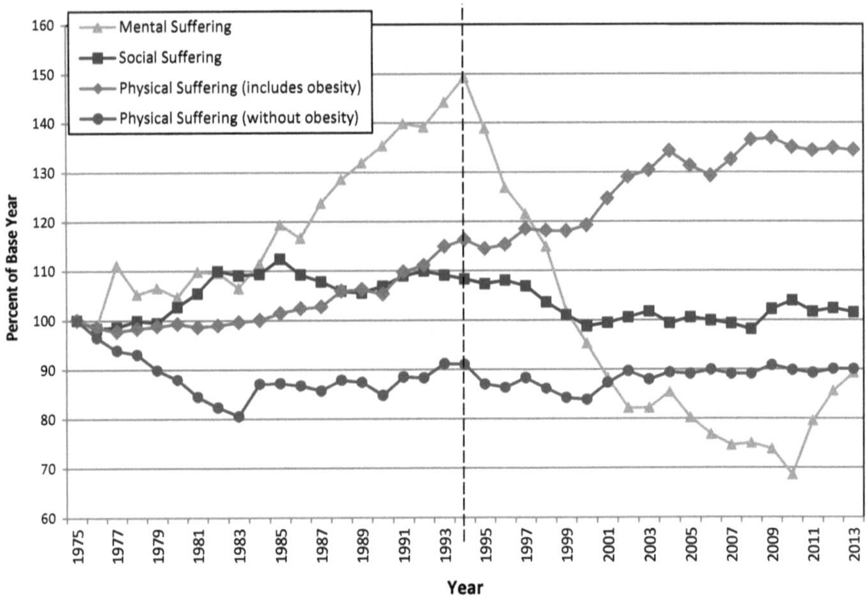

Fig. 2.4 Category-specific child suffering indices, 1975–2013

some years in which overall child and youth well-being increases at the same time that child suffering increases and vice versa. In terms of trends over the 38-year time period, however, both versions of the CSI are consistent with conclusions from the CWI, namely that the years from the mid-1980s to the mid-1990s were years of low overall child and youth well-being and high child and youth suffering.

Analogous to Fig. 2.2 on trends over time in the Domain Indices of the CWI, Fig. 2.4 shows annual percentage changes since 1975 in the three categories of child suffering, with the value of each series in the base year 1975 set equal to 100. These category-specific suffering indices reveal trends that help to interpret the findings from the overall CWI of Fig. 2.1 and the overall CSI of Fig. 2.3.

In Fig. 2.4, it can be seen that the Social Suffering Index, which includes Key Indicators of economic deprivation, fragile family structures, and detachment from mainstream social institutions, begins to increase (which is indicative of increased suffering) in 1980 above its base year 1975 value of 100 and its increase leads the increase of the Mental Suffering Index, which begins in 1984 and includes Key Indicators of Violent Crime Victimization and adolescent/teenage suicide. Both of these Indices show declines (which are indicative of decreased suffering) that begin in the mid-1990s, with the decline of the Mental Suffering Index being much more extensive and continuing through the 2000–2010 decade. By comparison, the Physical Suffering Index with the obesity Key Indicator included begins a long-term rise (indicative of increased suffering) in the mid-1980s that continues through the first decade of the twenty-first century, with stabilization in the years since 2010. If the obesity indicator is not included in the Physical Suffering Index, then the series shows a decline (indicative of decreased suffering) in the first 8 years, bottoming out at 80.51 in 1983. From that point, it increases slightly and varies in the range of 83–90 throughout the remaining years.

In brief, this initial version of a National Child and Youth Suffering Index yields information on trends over time in the status of America's children that focuses on the suffering end of the suffering to well-being/flourishing spectrum. With increasing demographic, social, and economic diversity in American society, it is possible for average levels of child and youth well-being, as measured by the CWI, to increase, while, at the same time, child and youth suffering indices and indicators also are increasing.

Conclusion

Contemporary American parents, similarly to their own parents a generation ago, want the best possible quality-of-life/well-being for their children – they want their children to be secure, to learn how to succeed in contemporary society, and to be happy. Unfortunately, long time series of comparable phenomenological/ethnographic studies with which to make comparisons and inferences about changes in child and youth well-being are not available. Nonetheless, the Child Well-Being Index Project has sought to use empirical findings from subjective well-being studies about domains of well-being to inform the construction of composite/summary quality-of-life/well-being indices from demographic, social, and economic statistical time series. The resulting CWI reveals striking changes in child and youth well-being across the past four decades – with long-term changes in the Index showing a large decline in the 1980s to the mid-1990s followed by a recovery in the late-1990s and fluctuations in the first decade of the twenty-first century and the imprint of the Great Recession of 2008–2009.

Reversing the well-being questions that motivate the CWI to focus on indicators of the physical, social, and mental suffering barriers to the realization of child well-being and happiness produces the Child Suffering Index described above. Trends over time in the CSI corroborate those in the CWI in the sense that when the CWI increases the CSI tends to decrease, thus indicating that improvements in the quality-of-life/well-being of America's children generally are associated with decreases in child suffering. However, American society is highly diverse demographically, socially, and economically and becoming more so. Therefore, monitoring and improving indices of child suffering and trends therein may become highly salient to future child well-being research and social reporting.

References

Anderson, R. E. (2014). *Human suffering and quality of life: Conceptualizing stories and statistics*. New York: Springer.
Andrews, F. M., & Withey, S. B. (1976). *Social indicators of well-being: Americans' perceptions of life quality*. New York: Plenum.
Ben-Arieh, A. (2005). Where are the children? Children's role in measuring and monitoring their well-being. *Social Indicators Research*, 74, 573–596.
Ben-Arieh, A., & Frones, I. (2007). Indicators of children's well-being – concepts, indices and usage. *Social Indicators Research*, 80, 1–4.
Bauer, R. A. (Ed.). (1966). *Social indicators*. Cambridge, Mass.: MIT Press.
Bender, T.A. (1997). Assessment of subjective well-being during childhood and adolescence. In G. Phye (Ed.), *Handbook of Classroom Assessment: Learning, Achievement, and Adjustment* (pp. 199–225). San Diego, CA: Academic Press.
Campbell, A., Converse, P. E., & Rodgers, W. L. (1976). *The quality of American life: Perceptions, evaluations, and satisfactions*. New York: Russell Sage Foundation.
Cummins, R. A. (1996). The domains of life satisfaction: An attempt to order chaos. *Social Indicators Research*, 38, 303–328.
Cummins, R. A. (1997). Assessing quality of life. In R. I. Brown (Ed.), *Quality of Life for Handicapped People*. London: Chapman and Hall.
Diener, E. (1994). Assessing subjective well-being: Progress and opportunities. *Social Indicators Research*, 31, 103–157.
Diener, E., Suh, E. M., Lucas, R. E., & Smith, H. L. (1999). Subjective well-being: three decades of progress. *Psychological Bulletin*, 125, 276–302.
Denzin, N. K., & Lincoln, Y. S. (1998). Introduction: Entering the field of qualitative research. In Denzin, N. K., & Lincoln, Y. S. (Eds.), *Strategies of qualitative inquiry*. Thousand Oaks, CA: Sage.
Erikson, R. (1974). Welfare as a planning goal. Acta Sociologica, 17, 273–288.
Fattore, T., Mason, J., & Watson, E. (2007). Children's conceptualization(s) of their well-being. *Social Indicators Research*, 80, 5–29.
Hagerty, M. R., & Land, K. C. (2007). Constructing summary indices of quality of life: a model for the effect of heterogeneous importance weights. *Sociological Methods and Research*, 35 (May), 455–496.
Hernandez, D. J., Macartney, S., and Cervantes, W. (2012). Measuring social disparities via the CWI: Race-Ethnicity, income, and immigrant status. In Land, K. C. (Ed.), *The well-being of America's children: developing and improving the child and youth well-being index* (pp. 77–120). New York: Springer.
Huebner, E. S. (1991). Correlates of life satisfaction in children. School Psychology Quarterly, 6, 103–111.
Huebner, E. S. (1997). Life satisfaction and happiness. In G. Bear, K. Minke, and A. Thomas (eds.), *Children's Needs II* (pp. 271–278). Silver Springs, MD: National Association of School Psychologists.
Huebner, E. S. (2004). Research on assessment of life satisfaction of children and adolescents. *Social Indicators Research*, 66, 3–33.
Jenicek, M. (2003). *Foundations of Evidence-Based Medicine*. New York: The Parthenon Publishing Group.
Land, K. C. (1983). Social indicators. *Annual Review of Sociology*, 9, 1–26.
Land, K. C. (2012). Introduction. In Land, K. C. (Ed.), *The well-being of America's children: developing and improving the child and youth well-being index* (pp. 1–12). New York: Springer.
Land, K. C. (2014). *Child and Youth Well-Being Index Report: 2014*. Durham, NC: Duke University Center for Child and Family Policy.
Land, K. C., Lamb, V. L., & Fu, Q. (2015). Child well-being and child suffering. In Anderson, R. E. (Ed.) *World Suffering and Quality of Life*. New York: Springer.

Land, K. C., Lamb, V. L., & Meadows, S. (2012). Conceptual and methodological foundations of the child and youth well-being index. In Land, K. C. (Ed.), *The well-being of America's children: developing and improving the child and youth well-being index* (pp. 13–28). New York: Springer.

Land, K. C., Lamb, V. L., & Mustillo, S. K. (2001). Child and youth well-being in the United States, 1975–1998: Some findings from a new index. *Social Indicators Research*, 56, (December):241–320.

Land, K. C., Lamb, V. L., Meadows, S. O., & Taylor, A. (2007). Measuring trends in child well-being: An evidence-based approach. *Social Indicators Research*, 80, 105–132.

Lazarus, R.S. 1991. *Emotion and Adaptation*. New York: Oxford University Press.

Lee, J., Lamb, V. L., & Land, K. C. (2009). Composite indices of changes in child and youth well-being in the San Francisco Bay Area and the State of California, 1995–2005. *Child Indicators Research*, 2(December), 353–374.

Moore, K. A. (1999). Indicators of child and family well-being: the good, the bad, and the ugly. Bethesda, MD: National Institutes of Health, Office of Behavioral and Social Sciences, 1999 Seminar Series.

McCullough, M.E., & Snyder, C. R. (2000). Classical sources of human strength: Revisiting an old home and building a new one. *Journal of Social and Clinical Psychology*, 19, 1–10.

Noll, H.-H. (2002). Social indicators and quality of life research: Background, achievements and current trends. In N. Genov (Ed.) *Advances in sociological knowledge over half a century* (pp. 168–206). Paris: ISSC.

O'Hare, W. P., Mather, M., Dupuis, G., Land, K. C., Lamb, V. L., & Fu, Q. (2013). Analyzing differences in child well-being among U.S. states. *Child Indicators Research*, 6(June), 401–413).

Noll, H.-H., & Zapf, W. (1994). Social indicators research: Societal monitoring and social reporting. In I. Borg & P. P. Mohler (Eds.), *Trends and perspectives in empirical social research*. New York: Walter de Gruyter.

Seligman, M.E.P., & Csikszentmihalyi, M. (2000). Positive psychology: An introduction. *American Psychologist*, 55, 5–14.

Sheldon, E. B., & Moore, W. E. (Eds.). (1968). *Indicators of social change: Concepts and measurements*. New York: Russell Sage Foundation.

Shin, D., & Johnson, D. M. (1978). Avowed happiness as an overall assessment of the quality of life. *Social Indicators Research*, 5, 475–492.

U. S. Department of Health and Human Services. 2000. *Healthy People 2010*. Washington, DC: U.S. Government Printing Office.

Chapter 3
The Role of Positive Youth Development and Family Functioning in Chinese Adolescent Well-Being: Theoretical Considerations and Empirical Evidence

Daniel T.L. Shek

Introduction

There is an upsurge of adolescent problem behaviors (e.g., substance abuse) in the global contexts, resulting in the claim that 'youth are broken and in need of fixing' (Theokas et al. 2005, p. 114). However, before we can "fix" adolescent problems and promote their well-being, we have to search for explanations for adolescent problem behavior and identify factors that contribute to adolescent well-being. In social science disciplines adopting the ecological perspective, a central belief is that personal factors such as resilience and environmental factors such as family factors shape adolescent development. In this chapter, two important personal and family factors influencing adolescent wellness are focused upon. These are positive youth development (PYD) attributes and family functioning. While the former can be regarded as an indicator of personal well-being, the latter has been treated as a form of family well-being.

Historically, the prevention approach and the deficit-oriented approach have been used to understand problems related to adolescent well-being and to keep adolescents from engaging in risk behavior and reduce incidences of risk behavior. While these approaches have generated successful adolescent prevention programs, they are commonly criticized as focusing too much on the problems and deficiencies of adolescents (Catalano et al. 2002). As such, there are views arguing that researchers should put more attention on adolescent developmental assets (i.e., asset-oriented approaches) or positive youth development. In other words, instead

This paper and the Project P.A.T.H.S. are financially supported by the Hong Kong Jockey Club Charities Trust. Address all correspondence to Daniel T.L. Shek, Department of Applied Social Sciences, The Hong Kong Polytechnic University (daniel.shek@polyu.edu.hk).

D.T.L. Shek (✉)
Department of Applied Social Sciences, The Hong Kong Polytechnic University,
Hung Hom, Hong Kong
e-mail: daniel.shek@polyu.edu.hk

F. Maggino (ed.), *A Life Devoted to Quality of Life*, Social Indicators Research Series 60, DOI 10.1007/978-3-319-20568-7_3

of focusing on "problems" of young people, greater attention should be put on "potentials and abilities" of young people. As pointed out by Schulman and Davies (2007), 'positive youth development requires more than the absence of negative behaviors: it is the acquisition of all the knowledge, skills, competencies, and experiences required to successfully transition from adolescence to adulthood' (p. 4).

There are several distinct features of the positive youth development approach. The first feature is its ecological emphasis. The ecological model of human development is an important theoretical perspective influencing PYD theory. According to Bronfenbrenner (1994), the environment within which an individual lives and the interaction between a person and his/her environment influences and shapes human development. Advocates of the positive youth development approach commonly adopt the ecological perspective as the lens to explore the reciprocal interactions between adolescents and different contexts such as family, school and community (Silbereisen and Lerner 2007). As pointed out by Lerner (2005), 'if the strengths of adolescents are aligned with resources for healthy growth present in the key contexts of adolescent development – the home, the school, and the community – then enhancements in positive functioning at any one point in time (i.e., well-being) may occur; in turn, the systematic promotion of positive development will occur across time (i.e., thriving)' (p. 28). Besides, different contexts provide different levels of either risk or protection.

The second component of the PYD approach is developmental asset which is closely related to resources in different ecological systems. As Benson (2003) noted, developmental assets are resources which constitute the social and ecological 'nutrients' for youth development. According to Benson (1997), PYD was promoted when actions are taken to enhance the strengths of an individual (e.g., spirituality), a family (e.g., positive parenting which both empower children and set boundaries) and a community (e.g., social support). Benson (2007) further defined the concept of developmental asset as 'a theoretical construct identifying a wide range of environmental and interpersonal strengths known to enhance educational and health outcomes for children and adolescents' (p. 33). Termed 'youth assets' (MacKay 2007), these resources are similar to protective factors in the resilience literature and their presence reduces risk behavior and increases positive outcomes.

According to the Search Institute, there are 40 developmental assets which adolescents need to grow into healthy, caring and responsible adults. The assets comprise both internal assets, which include 'qualities that guide the choices youth make and give them a sense of centeredness, purpose and focus' (Grantmakers in Health 2002, p. 5) and external assets which include 'positive experiences that youth receive from the people and institutions in their lives' (Grantmakers in Health 2002, p. 5). The 40 developmental assets are grouped into eight categories, with external assets including support, empowerment, boundaries and expectations, constructive use of time, and internal assets including commitment to learning, positive values, social competencies, and positive identity (Benson and Leffert 2001).

While it is believed that adolescents would be nurtured to have positive development, the question remained to be resolved is whether accumulation of assets could promote positive youth development (Lerner 2005). Empirically, there are research showing that the effect of developmental assets on adolescent development was addictive in nature (i.e., more assets the better). These studies showed that adolescents with more developmental assets were less likely to engage in risky behaviors such as sexual behavior (e.g., Vesely et al. 2004) and violent behaviors (e.g., Scales et al. 2000). Besides, they were more likely to achieve positive outcomes such as academic achievement (Theokas and Lerner 2005).

The third concept closely related to the PYD approach is the concept of psychosocial competence. The World Health Organization (1997) defined psychosocial competence as 'a person's ability to deal effectively with the demands and challenges of everyday life. It is a person's ability to maintain a state of mental well-being and to demonstrate this in adaptive and positive behavior while interacting with others, in his/her culture and environment' (p. 1). Although different PYD frameworks exist, the psychosocial competence of young people is a common feature in these frameworks (Shek 2013). Generally speaking, psychosocial competence is comprised of five domains: self-awareness (i.e., recognizing one's strengths and weaknesses and one's own feelings as well as emotions); social awareness (i.e., showing empathy, taking other people's perspectives); self-management (i.e., managing one's emotions and coping with one's negative emotions); responsible decision making (i.e., analyzing situations, solving problem, taking up personal responsibilities); and relationship skills (i.e., encompassing communication, relationship building and negotiation skills). It has been found that if young people have psychosocial competencies, the risks to engage in problem behavior will be largely reduced (Shek et al. 2011).

The fourth attribute of the PYD approach is its distinct challenge to the traditional deficit-based perspectives. In contrast to deficit-based perspectives, the PYD approach perceives adolescents not as problems to be managed but rather as resources to be developed (Roth and Brooks-Gunn 2003a, b). The core belief in PYD approach is that all adolescents have strengths and resources; through appropriate nurturance, adolescents will thrive and experience a successful transition to adulthood. Besides simply "deficit-free", it is also important to nurture young people to grow up happily, healthily, be fully engaged in life and contribute to society (Peterson 2004). The belief is clearly revealed in the motto that "problem-free is not fully prepared" (Pittman 1991). As argued by Lerner and Benson (2003), 'preventing a problem from occurring does not guarantee that adolescents are being provided with the assets they need to develop in a positive manner. Even assuming that prevention efforts could be completely successful, preventing problems among young people does not mean that they would be capable of making positive, healthy contributions to family community, and civil society' (Lerner and Benson 2003, p. 7). The notion that sheer absence of symptoms is not enough is reflected in the "ideal" developmental outcomes in the PYD approach. According to Lerner (2004), there are six Cs in the developmental ideals, including competence, confidence, connection, character, caring and contribution. These developmental outcomes are linked to the positive outcomes of adolescent development programs (e.g., Roth and Brooks-Gunn 2003a). Dukakis and colleagues (2009) noted that these domains are interactive and adolescents need healthy development in all of them.

Positive Youth Development Programs

According to developmental systems theories (Leffert et al. 1998), the idea of plasticity in human development maintains that individual's development is shaped by changes in the individual or the environment. Hence, if researchers can appropriately apply positive youth development in different systems, promotion of positive development and reduction of adolescent risky behavior would be possible. In addition, Benson et al. (2006) proposed three directions for potential intervention. First, it is helpful to increase the caring capacity of contexts such as having mentors and healthy adults. For example, Scales and colleagues (2006) showed that caring adults outside of a young person's own family played significant roles in providing developmental assets and in the promotion of adolescent well-being. Second, it is important to enhance adolescents' psychosocial skills (i.e., competencies which can further enable adolescents' ability to engage with, connect, change, and learn from their social contexts). Finally, providing an opportunity for adolescents to use their talents and competencies promotes positive youth development.

There are research studies showing that PYD programs were effective in promoting youth development. For example, Catalano and colleagues (1998) analyzed 25 youth programs (e.g., Big Brothers) which adopted the PYD approach and found that 19 programs successfully showed positive changes in behavior among the participants such as improved interpersonal skills, self-control, better peer and adult relationships, improved cognitive competencies, self-efficacy, and increased commitment to school and academic achievement. In addition, among the 25 programs, 24 showed reduction in problem behaviors such as substance use and aggressive behavior. Similarly, Roth and Brooks-Gunn (2003a) compared programs promoting the 5Cs of PYD (i.e., competence, confidence, connection, character and caring) with programs that only have youth focus but did not aim at promoting youth development. Results showed that positive youth development programs were more successful at improving the competence, confidence and connections among participants than programs with youth focus but which did not specifically aim at promoting youth development. Catalano et al. (2004) showed that PYD programs could be effective at promoting youth development if they could promote attributes of confidence (e.g., self-determination and a clear and positive identity), social connection (e.g., bonding), character (e.g., belief in the future), and competence (e.g., emotional, social, cognitive, behavioral and moral competence). Besides, programs that are effective at promoting PYD also included ecological assets such as the provision of opportunities for prosocial involvement and the support of prosocial norms or standards for healthy behavior (Catalano et al. 2004).

Catalano and colleagues (2004) reported that about 75 % of the effective PYD programs possessed three specific design features that researchers called the 'Big Three' design features of effective PYD programs (Roth and Brooks-Gunn 2003a, b), as follows: (1) the program provides opportunities for youth participation; (2) the program lays emphasis on the development of life skills; (3) the program is held within the context of a sustained and caring adult-youth relationship (Lerner et al.

2006). Catalano et al. (2004) emphasized that effective PYD programs 'targeted healthy bonds between youth and adults, increased opportunities for youth participation in positive social activities, ... [involved] recognition and reinforcement for that participation' (p. vi), and often used skills training as a youth competency strategy. Similarly, Roth and Brooks-Gunn (2003b) noted that PYD programs promoted youth competencies through 'increasing participants' exposure to supportive and empowering environments where activities create multiple opportunities for a range of skill-building and horizon-broadening experiences' (p. 94). Roth and Brooks-Gunn (2003a) further emphasized that no matter what the specific activity is, the emphasis lies in providing real challenges and active participation. In particular, they argued that when the program activities clearly convey the belief that young people should be viewed as resources to be developed rather than problems to be managed which instill in young people a feeling of hope in the future, then the goals of promoting PYD are likely to be fulfilled. Lerner et al. (2006) pointed out that there are four conditions which are conducive to positive youth development, including skill-building opportunities, active participation of young people, presence of positive and supportive adult, and positive youth relations).

Positive Youth Development and Chinese Adolescents

Existing research studies on the link between positive youth development and adolescent development have mainly been conducted in Western contexts. As Chinese adolescents constitute roughly one-fifth of all adolescents in the world, it is legitimate to ask how positive youth development influences development in Chinese adolescents. A review of major scientific databases such as PsycINFO and Medline shows that there are very few studies in this area, possibly with the exception of the Project P.A.T.H.S. in Hong Kong. The Project P.A.T.H.S. is a large-scale positive youth development program designed to promote holistic development in Chinese adolescents in Hong Kong. In the programs developed, positive youth development constructs identified in the successful positive youth development programs (Catalano et al. 2012), including resilience, bonding, psychosocial competencies (social, emotional, cognitive, behavioral and moral competencies), self-determination, self-efficacy, positive identity, spirituality, beliefs in the future, promotion of prosocial norms, provision of opportunities for prosocial involvement, and recognition for positive behavior (Shek and Sun 2013a, b).

To examine the effectiveness of the program, a 5-year longitudinal study with eight waves of data was conducted (Shek and Ma 2012; Shek and Yu 2012). There were 24 pairs of schools which were randomly drawn from the participating schools at the beginning of the project. In each pair of school, one school was randomized to the experimental group and another one to the control group. In the first 3 years during which the program was implemented, pretest and posttest data were collected. In Year 4 and Year 5, posttest data were collected at the end of each school year. In each wave of data collection, instruments assessing positive youth development, life satisfaction and problem behavior, were used. The Chinese Positive Youth Development Scale was used to assess positive youth development in Chinese adolescents.

Using Wave 1 data of the study (N = 7975), Sun and Shek (2010) examined the linkages amongst life satisfaction, positive youth development, and problem behavior. Results showed that a higher level of positive youth development was negatively related to adolescent problem behavior. Structural equation modeling analyses suggest that positive youth development positively predicted life satisfaction and negatively predicted problem behavior, with life satisfaction and problem behavior are mutually influencing each other. Sun and Shek (2012) conducted a replication study to examine the relationship between positive youth development and adolescent problem behavior using data collected from Secondary 2 students (N = 7151). Consistent with our prediction, there was negative relationships between positive youth development measures and adolescent problem behavior. Similarly, while positive youth development negatively predicted adolescent problem behavior, it positively predicted life satisfaction. Sun and Shek (2013) further examined both the cross-sectional and longitudinal impact of positive youth development on adolescent problem behavior using data collected at Secondary 1, Secondary 3 and Secondary 5 levels. Results showed that positive youth development at Secondary 1 was negatively related to adolescent problem behavior at Secondary 1 and Secondary 3, with the relationship mediated by life satisfaction.

Besides the above-mentioned 5-year longitudinal study, a 6-year longitudinal study (2009–2010 to 2014–2015 academic years) was also conducted in the extension phase of the project (Shek 2013). There were 28 schools joining the Wave 1 data collection, with 3325 Secondary 1 students participating in the project. Besides measures on family quality of life, such as systemic family functioning and parent-child relational qualities (e.g., behavioral control and psychological control), different measures of personal well-being were used, including measures of positive youth development, life satisfaction and adolescent risk behavior such as delinquency and substance abuse. Findings based on this longitudinal study showed that positive youth development attributes were negatively related to adolescent risk behavior: Shek and Leung (in press) reported that positive youth development attributes were negatively related to adolescent substance abuse in the junior secondary school years; Shek and Lin (in press) showed that positive youth development attributes were negatively related to juvenile delinquent behavior in the junior secondary school years. Besides, Law and Shek (2013) showed that positive youth development attributes were negatively related to self-harm and suicide; Yu and Shek (2013) reported that positive youth development negatively predicted Internet addiction in adolescents over time. There are also findings showing that positive youth development negatively predicted problem adolescent sexual behavior over time, including consumption of pornographic materials, sexual behavior and compensated dating (Lee and Shek 2013; Ma and Shek 2013; Shek 2013).

Besides research on the positive relationship between positive youth development and adolescent development, findings showed that positive youth development programs are beneficial to the development of Chinese adolescents. In the Project

P.A.T.H.S., positive youth development constructs were incorporated in the curricula-based materials which were taught in classroom settings. For each grade, 10–20 h were used to promote psychosocial competencies in students. To gain an in-depth evaluation of the program, different evaluation strategies were used, including objective outcome evaluation (e.g., pretest-posttest analyses plus a longitudinal randomized group trial), subjective outcome evaluation data collected from the program implementers and program participants, qualitative evaluation involving focus groups for program implementers and participants, interviews, and weekly diaries, as well as repertory grid test evaluation. Overall, the evaluation findings are very consistent in providing confirmation that the program was positively perceived by different stakeholders and that the program was effective in promoting holistic development in Chinese adolescents in Hong Kong (Shek and Sun 2013a, b). With particular reference to the randomized group trial, results showed three observations. First, compared with the control students, students in the experimental group did better in positive youth development attributes. Second, compared with experimental students, control group students showed faster and greater increase in substance abuse behavior. Third, compared with control subjects, experimental group students showed slower and less increase in delinquent behavior and intention to engage in delinquency behavior. In short, evaluation findings showed that the Project P.A.T.H.S. is able to delay the onset of adolescent risk behavior and promote positive behavior in Chinese adolescents.

Family Functioning as a Form of Family Well-Being

Family functioning can be conceived as a family's ability to carry out its functions such as satisfying the physical and emotional needs of family members (Dickstein 2002; Eichelsheim 2010). In different models of family functioning, different dimensions of family functioning, such as adaptability, family health, and emotional involvement have been proposed. According to Eichelsheim et al. (2010), family functioning has both affective aspect (e.g., family conflict) and instrumental aspect (e.g., family communication and family rules). As family functioning addresses the question of how well a family functions, it can be regarded as a measure of quality of family life. In many models of family functioning, it is commonly proposed that family functioning affects the functioning of individual family members, including that of adolescents.

In the field of family functioning, there are three models of family functioning proposed for the "normal" population (Walsh 1993). The first one is Beavers Systems Model of Family Functioning (Beavers and Hampson 1993, 2000; Sutphin et al. 2013) in which two dimensions (i.e., family competence and family style) are proposed. Regarding family competence, it refers to skills of the family in handling tensions between individual freedom and group belonging "ranging from optimal through adequate, midrange and borderline to severely dysfunctional" (Beavers and Hampson 2000, p. 128). Besides, family competence is conceived as "how well the family, as an interactional unit, performs the necessary and nurturing tasks of organizing and managing itself" (Beavers and Hampson 1993, p. 74). Generally speaking, "competent" families having open communication and conflict resolution skills usually display optimistic feelings whereas "dysfunctional" families generally show pessimistic perspective to life (Beavers and Hampson 1993). Concerning family style, it refers to the interaction quality of family members, which "bears a curvilinear relationship to healthy functioning and ranges from centripetal to centrifugal" (Beavers and Hampson 2000, p. 130).

The second commonly used model to conceive family functioning is the McMaster Model of Family Functioning which is based on a systems theory (Miller et al. 2000) rather than merely focusing on a single dimension of the family (Epstein et al. 1993). There are six dimensions of family functioning in the McMaster Model, including problem solving, communication, roles, affective responsiveness, affective involvement and behavior control, all of which can have an influence on family members' physical and emotional health or problems (Epstein et al. 1993). For "problem solving", it refers to the family's ability to deal with instrumental and affective problems and maintain effective family functioning in an appropriate way. Regarding "communication", it includes instrumental and affective communication among family members. For "family role", it refers to family members' ability in fulfilling family functions such as maintaining family routines. There are two dimensions of family functioning related to affect, including "affective responsiveness" (the ability to feel and respond by expressing appropriate feelings across different situations) and "affective involvement" (family members' share feelings of family members not in an enmeshed way). Finally, "behavior control" refers to family members' ability to handle their behavior in situations of physical danger, situations of psychobiological needs, and social situations.

The third model commonly using the family functioning model is the Circumplex Model of Marital and Family Systems which was developed based on the research, theory and practice of system theory and family development theory (Olson 2000). There are three central dimensions including "family cohesion", "flexibility" and "communication", which are generated from over 50 concepts used to describe the dynamic similarity of balanced, midrange and extreme family types (Olson 1993, 2000).

Regarding family cohesion, it is "the emotional bonding that family members have toward one another" (Olson 2000, p. 145). It was proposed that there are four possible levels of cohesion, ranging from disengaged relationship (extreme emotional separateness), separated relationship (some emotional separateness which is not so extreme), connected relationship (emotional closeness and loyalty to the relationship) to enmeshed relationship (a remarkable amount of emotional closeness and loyalty are demanded). Olson (2000) argued that cohesion has a curvilinear relationship with healthy family functioning (i.e., too much or too little family cohesion is problematic) and families with balanced cohesion allow their members to be both connected to but independent from their families.

Concerning family flexibility, it is defined as "the amount of change in its leadership, role relationships and relationship rules" (Olson 2000, p. 147). Flexibility in family functioning can be related to family processes such as leadership, roles and rules, and family different levels of flexibility are possible, ranging from rigid, structured, flexible to chaotic. Olson (2000) argued that while structured and flexible functioning types are beneficial to healthy marital and family functioning, rigid and chaotic levels are problematic for families. Olson (2000) further reasoned that as keeping stable and making changes are important for family functioning, structured and flexible family types are more likely to be functional. In short, flexibility has a curvilinear relationship with healthy family functioning where too little (i.e., rigid family structure) or too much flexibility (i.e., chaotic family structure) is problematic for a family.

Finally, family communication refers to "listening skills, speaking skills, self-disclosure, clarity, continuity-tracking, and respect and regard" of families (Olson 2000, p. 149). It was proposed that family communication facilitates cohesion and flexibility in a family and balanced family systems generally are good at communication while unbalanced family systems usually have poor communication (Olson 2000).

Based on the above dimensions, different family types with different levels of family functioning could be identified, including "balanced", "rigidly balanced", "midrange", "flexibly unbalanced", "chaotically disengaged" and "unbalanced" types, which represent the healthiest to the most problematic family types (Olson and Gorall 2006). For example, balanced families could maintain stability in a system and they can adapt for the needs of family development at the same time (Olson 2000).

Besides the above models proposed for family functioning in the general population, there are many clinical models on family functioning in the clinical literature such as family therapies. Two examples are presented below. The first example is the Satir model which was recognized as a pioneer of family therapy. With its root in the humanistic/transpersonal psychological thoughts, the Satir model emphasizes the importance of well-being on family functioning, with the belief that "on change towards greater wholeness, more harmony, greater responsibility and, ultimately, a fuller life" (Banmen 2002, p. 22).

The Satir model focuses on the three areas of therapeutic intervention including "the intrapsychic", "the interactive" and "the family of origin" (Banmen 2002). As far as the intrapsychic focus, Satir (1964) said that "for too long we have been caught in the morass of 'pathology' and have forgotten that growth is possible at any age, given the proper context" (Lewis and Banmen 2008, p. 17). Based on positive attitudes towards human beings, the four meta-goals set by the Satir model promoting positively directional and change focused therapy include "raising the self-esteem of the clients", "helping clients to be their own choice makers", "helping clients to be more responsible" and "helping clients become congruent" (Banmen 2002, p. 11). These assertions are in line with the basic tenets of positive youth development approach.

Another clinical model of family functioning is Bowen Family Systems Theory (Bowen 1976; Kerr and Bowen 1988) which is a well-known and widely used marriage and family therapy theory. Kerr and Bowen (1988) argued that family is an emotional unit that governs individual behavior and development where family members function in the reciprocal relationship to each other. Bowen (1974) argued that helping family members reach a better "differentiation of self" is one of the most important goals of family systems therapy. Differentiation of self "describes the process by which individuality and togetherness are managed by a person and within a relationship system" (Kerr and Bowen 1988, p. 95). According to Bowen (1974), people have higher levels of differentiation would have healthier family functioning. Differentiation family functioning in turn shapes psychosocial competences.

Impacts of Family Functioning on Adolescent Development

Generally speaking, research findings indicated that family functioning is positively related to adolescent development. For example, there are studies showing that family functioning influences adolescent self-efficacy and personality (Gontang and Erickson 1996; Jaggers et al. 2014; Reitz et al. 2014; Swenson and Prelow 2005) as well as academic and behavioral development (Cavendish et al. 2014).

Besides, negative relationship between family functioning and adolescent problem behavior has been reported. While good family functioning showed protective effects on adolescents (Gorman-Smith et al. 2000), Eichelsheim and colleagues (2010) found that a higher level of family negativity was associated with a higher level of adolescent delinquent behavior. In addition, Young et al. (2013) found that adolescents with bipolar disorder or attention-deficit/hyperactivity disorder had worse general family functioning than did adolescents from typically developing controls families. Abu-Rayya and Yang (2012) reported that unhealthy family functioning would make adolescents at risk through increasing their emotional problems, peer problems and behavioral problems.

In the study of Tafà and Baiocco (2009), researchers found that family relationship is a contributor of adolescents' well-being and a protector of their risky and addictive behaviors (e.g., drinking, drug use and gambling). Youngblade et al. (2007) indicated that a series of family characteristics such as family closeness and communication were linked to both positive outcomes and negative outcomes of adolescent development. As Gorman-Smith and colleagues (2000) and Gorman-Smith et al. (2004) argued, family functioning was not only related to the areas such as internalizing and externalizing disorders, attitudes toward education and personal aspirations, but it was also an effective way of promoting the positive functioning in these areas.

Although family functioning may not have direct effects on some variables of adolescent development, it has indirect and moderating effects on these variables (e.g., Greenley et al. 2007). For example, family functioning could influence boys' delinquent behaviors through influencing their self-restraint (Feldman and Weinberger 1994). Church et al. (2009) found that poor family cohesion would make adolescents commit delinquent acts by lowering their self-images and increasing their interaction with delinquent peers. In addition, family functioning has the moderating effects under some circumstances. Henneberger et al. (2013) reported that both parental monitoring and family cohesion in the early adolescence would moderate the relationship between peer violence in the early adolescence and delinquency in the middle adolescence; and parental monitoring would moderate the relationship between peer popularity in the early adolescence and future delinquent behaviors.

With particular reference to Chinese adolescents, two observations can be highlighted from the literature on family functioning on Chinese adolescents. First, there are few studies in this area, particularly studies using longitudinal design. Second, there is support for the general thesis that family functioning is positively related to adolescent development (e.g., Shek 2005). In a 2-year longitudinal study, research findings showed that family functioning based on ratings obtained from different sources were positively related to adolescent psychological well-being and school adjustment but negatively related to problem behavior (Shek 1998a, b). In the 5-year longitudinal study, perceptions of the family environment were positively related to personal well-being but negatively related to indices of risk behavior (Shek and Ma 2012; Shek and Yu 2012). Similarly, in the 6-year longitudinal study, family functioning was found to be positively related to life satisfaction and positive youth development (Shek and Liu 2014). On the other hand, family functioning was negatively related to Internet addiction (Yu and Shek 2013), consumption of pornographic materials (Ma and Shek 2013), intention to engage in risk behavior (Shek and Yu in press), self-harm and suicidal behavior (Law and Shek 2013, in press) and compensated dating (Lee and Shek 2013, in press).

Conclusion

According to the ecological perspective, human behavior is governed by personal and environmental factors. In this chapter, two factors which influence adolescent adjustment including positive youth development attributes and family functioning are discussed. While positive youth development attributes can be regarded as measures of personal well-being, family functioning can be regarded as an index of family quality of life. Concerning positive youth development, different PYD models and programs are presented. With specific reference to the Chinese context, the Project P.A.T.H.S. as a PYD program and research findings on the influence of positive youth development attributes on adolescent development are discussed. Regarding family functioning, different models of family functioning and the role of family functioning in adolescent development are outlined. The review in this chapter suggests that positive youth development attributes and family functioning shape the development of Chinese adolescents. The findings are consistent with the Confucian emphasis of self-cultivation and family regulation "xiu shen, qu jia" as the desired goals of human development.

References

Abu-Rayya, H. M., & Yang, B. (2012). Unhealthy family functioning as a psychological context underlying Australian children's emotional and behavioural problems. *Internet Journal of Mental Health, 8*(1).

Banmen, J. (2002). The Satir model: Yesterday and today. *Contemporary Family Therapy, 24*(1), 7–22.

Beavers, W. R., & Hampson, R. B. (1993). Measuring family competence: The Beavers Systems Model. In F. Walsh (Ed.), *Normal family processes* (2nd, pp. 73–103). New York, NY: The Guilford Press.

Beavers, R., & Hampson, R. B. (2000). The Beavers systems model of family functioning. *Journal of Family Therapy, 22*(2), 128–143.

Benson, P. L. (1997). *All kids are our kids: What communities must do to raise caring and responsible children and adolescents*. San Francisco: Jossey-Bass.

Benson, P. L. (2003). Developmental assets and asset-building community: Conceptual and empirical foundations. In R. M. Lerner & P. Benson (Eds.), *Developmental assets and asset-building communities: Implications for research, policy, and practice* (pp. 19–43). Norwell, MA: Kluwer Academic.

Benson, P. L. (2007). Developmental assets: An overview of theory, research and practice. In R. K. Silbereisen & R. M. Lerner (Eds.), *Approaches to positive youth development* (pp. 33–58). London: Sage Publications Ltd.

Benson, P. L., & Leffert, N. (2001). Childhood and adolescence: Developmental assets. In N. J. Smelser & P. G. Baltes (Eds.), *International Encyclopedia of the social and behavioral sciences* (pp. 1690–1697). Oxford: Pergamon.

Benson, P. L., Scales, P. C., Hamilton, S. F., & Sesma, A. Jr. (2006). Positive youth development: Theory, research and applications. In R. M. Lerner, W. Damon, & R. M. Lerner (Eds.), *Handbook of child psychology* (6th, pp. 894–942). John Wiley & Sons, Inc.

Bowen, M. (1974). Toward the differentiation of self in one's family of origin. In M. Bowen (Ed.), *Family therapy in clinical practice* (pp. 529–553). Rowman & Littlefield Publishers, Inc.

Bowen, M. (1976). Theory in the practice of psychotherapy. In M. Bowen. (Ed.), *Family therapy in clinical practice* (pp. 337–388). Rowman & Littlefield Publishers, Inc.

Bronfenbrenner, U. (1994). Ecological models of human development. In M. Gauvain & M. Cole (Eds.), *Readings on the development of children* (pp. 37–43). New York: Freeman.

Catalano, R. F., Berglund, L. M., Ryan, J. A., Lonczak, H. S., & Hawkins, J. D. (1998). *Positive youth development in the United States: Research findings on evaluations of positive youth development programs*. Social Development Research Group, University of Washington, WA.

Catalano, R. F., Berglund, M. L., Ryan, J. A. M., Lonczak, H. S., & Hawkins, J. D. (2002). Positive youth development in the United States: Research findings on evaluations of the positive youth development programs. *Prevention & Treatment. 5*(15), 1–111.

Catalano, R. F., Berglund, M. L., Ryan, J. A. M., Lonczak, H. S., & Hawkins, J. D. (2004). Positive youth development in the United States: Research findings on evaluations of positive youth development programs. *The Annals of the American Academy of Political and Social Science, 591*, 98–124. DOI: 10.1177/0002716203260102.

Catalano, R. F., Fagan, A. A., Gavin, L. E., Greenberg, M. T., Irwin, C. E., Ross, D. A., & Shek, D. T. L. (2012). Worldwide application of prevention science in adolescent health. *Lancet, 379*(9826), 1653–1664.

Cavendish, W., Montague, M., Enders, C., & Dietz, S. (2014). Mothers' and adolescents' perceptions of family environment and adolescent social-emotional functioning. *Journal of Child and Family Studies, 23*(1), 52–66.

Church, W. T., Wharton, T., & Taylor, J. K. (2009). An examination of differential association and social control theory: Family systems and delinquency. *Youth Violence and Juvenile Justice, 7*(1), 3–15.

Dickstein, S. (2002). Family routines and rituals – The importance of family functioning: Comment on the special section. *Journal of Family Psychology, 16*(4), 441–444.

Dukakis, K., London, R. A., McLaughlin, M., & Williamson, D. (2009). *Positive youth development: Individual, setting and system level indicators* (Issue brief: Positive youth development indicators). Stanford, CA: John W. Gardner Center for Youth and Their Communities.

Eichelsheim, V. I. (2010). General introduction. In V. I. Eichelsheim (Ed.), *The complexity of families: Assessing family relationships and their association with externalizing problems* (pp. 7–18). Labor Grafimedia BV, Utrecht.

Eichelsheim, V. I., Dekovic, M., Buist, K. L., Prinzie, P., & Hoeve, M. (2010). Family functioning and child externalizing behavior: A meta-analysis. In V. I. Eichelsheim (Ed.), *The complexity of families: Assessing family relationships and their association with externalizing problems* (pp. 57–80). Labor Grafimedia BV, Utrecht.

Epstein, N. B., Bishop, D., Ryan, C., Miller, I., & Keitner, G. (1993). The McMaster model view of healthy family functioning. In F. Walsh (Ed.), *Normal family processes* (pp. 138–160). New York, NY: The Guilford Press.

Feldman, S. S., & Weinberger, D. A. (1994). Self-restraint as a mediator of family influences on boys' delinquent behavior: A longitudinal study. *Child Development, 65*(1), 195–211.

Gontang, R., & Erickson, M. T. (1996). The relationship between Millon's personality types and family system functioning. *American Journal of Family Therapy, 24*(3), 215–226.

Gorman-Smith, D., Henry, D. B., & Tolan, P. H. (2004). Exposure to community violence and violence perpetration: The protective effects of family functioning. *Journal of Clinical Child and Adolescent Psychology, 33*(3), 439–449.

Gorman-Smith, D., Tolan, P. H., Henry, D. B., & Florsheim, P. (2000). Patterns of family functioning and adolescent outcomes among urban African American and Mexican American families. *Journal of Family Psychology, 14*(3), 436–457.

Grantmakers in Health (2002). *Positive youth development: A pathway to healthy teens* (Issue brief No. 15). Washington, DC.

Greenley, R. N., Taylor, H. G., Drotar, D., & Minich, N. M. (2007). Longitudinal relationships between early adolescent family functioning and youth adjustment: An examination of the moderating role of very low birth weight. *Journal of Pediatric Psychology, 32*(4), 453–462.

Henneberger, A. K., Durkee, M. I., Truong, N., Atkins, A., & Tolan, P. H. (2013). The longitudinal relationship between peer violence and popularity and delinquency in adolescent boys: Examining effects by family functioning. *Journal of Youth and Adolescence, 42*(11), 1651–1660.

Jaggers, J. W., Church II, W. T., Tomek, S., Hooper, L. M., Bolland, K. A., & Bolland, J. M. (2014). Adolescent development as a determinant of family cohesion: A longitudinal analysis of adolescents in the mobile youth survey. *Journal of Child and Family Studies*. Retrieved from http://download.springer.com/static/pdf/513/art%253A10.1007%252Fs10826-014-9966-8.pdf?auth66=1405575772_a7910f6ff7e6d1ea832aeb5e0d02380a&ext=.pdf

Kerr, M. E. & Bowen, M (1988). *Family evaluation: An approach based on Bowen theory.* New York: Norton.

Law, B. M. F., & Shek, D. T. L. (2013). Self-harm and suicide attempts among young Chinese adolescents in Hong Kong: Prevalence, correlates, and changes. *Journal of Pediatric and Adolescent Gynecology, 26*(3S), S26–S32.

Law, B. M. F. & Shek, D. T. L. (in press). A longitudinal study on deliberate self-harm and suicidal behaviors among Chinese adolescents. In D. T. L. Shek, R. C. F. Sun, & C. M. S. Ma (Eds.), *Chinese adolescents in Hong Kong – Family life, psychological well-being and risk behavior.* Singapore: Springer.

Lee, T. Y., & Shek, D. T. L. (2013). Compensated dating in Hong Kong: Prevalence, psychosocial correlates, and relationships with other risky behaviors. *Journal of Pediatric and Adolescent Gynecology, 26*(3S), S42–S48.

Lee, T. Y., & Shek, D. T. L. (in press). Compensated Dating and Juvenile Prostitution in Early Adolescents in Hong Kong. In D. T. L. Shek, R. C. F. Sun, & C. M. S. Ma (Eds.), *Chinese adolescents in Hong Kong - Family life, psychological well-being and risk behavior*. Singapore: Springer.

Leffert, N., Benson, P. L., Scales, P. C., Sharma, A. R., Drake, D. R., & Blyth, D. A. (1998). Developmental assets: Measurement and prediction of risk behaviors among adolescents. *Applied Developmental Science*, *2*(4), 209–230.

Lerner, R. M. (2004). *Liberty: Thriving and civic engagement among America's youth*. Thousand Oaks, CA: Sage Publications.

Lerner, R. M. (2005). *Promoting positive youth development: Theoretical and empirical bases*. Retrieved from http://ase.tufts.edu/iaryd/documents/pubpromotingpositive.pdf

Lerner, R. M., Alberts, A. E., Jelicic, H., & Smith, L. M. (2006). Young people are resources to be developed: Promoting positive youth development through adult-youth relations and community assets. In E. G. Clary & J. E. Rhodes (Eds.), *Mobilizing adults for positive youth development: Strategies for closing the gaps between beliefs and behaviors series* (pp. 19–39). US: Springer. DOI: 10.1007/0-387-29340-x_2. Retrieved from http://www.google.com.hk/url?sa=t&rct=j&q=&esrc=s&source=web&cd=1&ved=0CB8QFjAA&url=http%3A%2F%2Fwww.springer.com%2Fcda%2Fcontent%2Fdocument%2Fcda_downloaddocument%2F9780387291734-c2.pdf%3FSGWID%3D0-0-45-326600-p107023666&ei=-V6lU5e_BsH48QX70oDQDg&usg=AFQjCNEhw3VT5puNlZyUgsHxWqYcrot9Aw&bvm=bv.69411363,d.dGc

Lerner, R. M., & Benson, P. I. (2003). *Developmental assets and asset-building communities: Implications for research, policy, and practice*. New York: Kluwer Academic/Plenum.

Lewis, L., & Banmen, J. (2008). The positive psychology of Virginia Satir. In J. Banmen (Ed.), *Satir transformational systemic therapy* (pp. 17–39). Palo Alto, CA: Science & Behavior Books.

Ma, C. M. S., & Shek, D. T. L. (2013). Consumption of pornographic materials in early adolescents in Hong Kong. *Journal of Pediatric and Adolescent Gynecology*, *26*(3S), S18–S25.

MacKay, L. J. (2007). *Healthy youth development: The role of youth assets* (Doctoral dissertation). Simon Fraser University, Canada.

Miller, I. W., Ryan, C. E., Keitner, G. I., Bishop, D. S., & Epstein, N. B. (2000). The McMaster approach to families: Theory, assessment, treatment and research. *Journal of Family Therapy, 22*(2), 168–189.

Olson, D. H. (1993). Circumplex model of marital and family systems: Assessing family functioning. In F. Walsh (Ed.), *Normal family processes* (1st, pp. 104–137). New York, NY: The Guilford Press.

Olson, D. H. (2000). Circumplex model of marital and family systems. *Journal of Family Therapy, 22*(2), 144–167.

Olson, D. H., & Gorall, D. M. (2006). *FACES IV & the Circumplex model*. Minneapolis, MN: Life Innovations, Inc.

Peterson, C. (2004). Positive social science. *The Annals of the American Academy of Political and Social Science*, *591*, 186–201.

Pittman, K. (1991). *Promoting youth development: Strengthening the role of youth serving and community organizations*. Washington, DC: Academy for Educational Development.

Reitz, A. K., Motti-Stefanidi, F., & Asendorpf, J. B. (2014). Mastering developmental transitions in immigrant adolescents: The longitudinal interplay of family functioning, developmental and acculturative tasks. *Developmental Psychology, 50*(3), 754–765.

Roth, J. L., & Brooks-Gunn, J. (2003a). What is a youth development program? Identifying and defining principles. In F. Jacobs, D. Wertlieb, & R. M. Lerner (Eds.), Enhancing the life chances of youth and families: Public service systems and public policy perspectives: Vol. 2. *Handbook of applied developmental science: Promoting positive child, adolescent, and family development through research, policies, and programs* (pp. 197–223). Thousand Oaks, CA: Sage.

Roth, J. L., & Brooks-Gunn, J. (2003b). What exactly is a youth development program? Answers from research and practice. *Applied Developmental Science*, *7*(2), 94–111.

Satir, V. (1964). *Conjoint family therapy*. Palo Alto, CA: Science and Behavior Books.

Scales, P. C., Benson, P. L., Leffert, N., & Blyth, D. A. (2000). Contribution of developmental assets to the prediction of thriving among adolescents. *Applied Developmental Science, 4*(1), 27–46.

Scales, P. C., Benson, P. L., & Mannes, M. (2006). The contribution to adolescent well-being made by nonfamily adults: An examination of developmental assets as contexts and processes. *Journal of Community Psychology, 34*(4), 401–413.

Schulman, S., & Davies, T. (2007). Evidence of the impact of the 'Youth development model' on outcomes for young people – a literature review. Retrieved from http://blog.practicalparticipation.co.uk/wp-content/uploads/2009/08/V1-2-EVIDENCE-OF-THE-IMPACT-OF-THE-YOUTH-DEVELOPMENT-MODEL-ON-OUTCOMES-FOR-YOUNG-PEOPLE-%E2%80%93-A-LITERATURE-REVIEW.pdf

Shek, D. T. L. (1998a). A longitudinal study of Hong Kong adolescents' and parents' perceptions of family functioning and well-being. *Journal of Genetic Psychology, 159*(4), 389–403.

Shek, D. T. L. (1998b). A longitudinal study of the relationship between family functioning and adolescent psychological well-being. *Journal of Youth Studies, 1*(2), 195–209.

Shek, D. T. L. (2005). A longitudinal study of perceived family functioning and adolescent adjustment in Chinese adolescents with economic disadvantage. *Journal of Family Issues, 26*(4), 518–543.

Shek, D. T. L. (2013). Sexual behavior and intention to engage in sexual behavior in junior secondary school students in Hong Kong. *Journal of Pediatric and Adolescent Gynecology, 26*(3S), S33–S41.

Shek, D. T. L., & Leung, J. (in press). Substance Abuse in Junior Secondary School Students in Hong Kong. In D. T. L. Shek, R. C. F. Sun & C. M. S. Ma (Eds.), *Chinese Adolescents in Hong Kong - Family life, psychological well-being and risk behavior*. Singapore: Springer.

Shek, D. T. L., & Lin, L. (in press). Development of Delinquent Behavior in Early Adolescents in Hong Kong. In D. T. L. Shek, R. C. F. Sun & C. M. S. Ma (Eds.), *Chinese Adolescents in Hong Kong - Family life, psychological well-being and risk behavior*. Singapore: Springer.

Shek, D. T. L., & Liu, T. T. (2014). Life satisfaction in junior secondary school students in Hong Kong: A 3-year longitudinal study. *Social Indicators Research, 117*(3), 777–794.

Shek, D. T. L., & Ma, C. M. S. (2012). Impact of the Project P.A.T.H.S. in the junior secondary school years: Objective outcome evaluation based on eight waves of longitudinal data. *The Scientific World Journal*, 2012, Article ID 170345, 12 pages. doi:10.1100/2012/170345.

Shek, D. T. L., Ma, H. K., & Sun, R. C. F. (2011). A brief overview of adolescent developmental problems in Hong Kong. *The Scientific World Journal, 11*, 2243–2256. doi: 10.1100/2011/896835.

Shek, D. T. L., & Sun R. C. F. (Eds.) (2013a). *Development and evaluation of positive adolescent training through holistic social programs* (P.A.T.H.S.). Singapore: Springer Science Business Media.

Shek, D. T. L., & Sun, R. C. F. (2013b). The Project P.A.T.H.S. in Hong Kong: Development, training, implementation, and evaluation. *Journal of Pediatric and Adolescent Gynecology, 26*(3), S2–S9. doi: 10.1016/j.jpag.2013.03.009.

Shek, D. T. L., & Yu, L. (2012). Longitudinal impact of the Project P.A.T.H.S. on adolescent risk behavior: What happened after five years? *The Scientific World Journal, 2012*, Article ID 316029, 13 pages. doi:10.1100/2012/316029.

Shek, D. T. L., & Yu, L. (in press). Intention to gamble amongst junior secondary school students In Hong Kong: Changes and predictors. In D. T. L. Shek, R. C. F. Sun, & C. M. S. Ma (Eds.), *Chinese adolescents in Hong Kong – Family life, psychological well-being and risk behavior*. Singapore: Springer.

Silbereisen, R. K., & Lerner, R. M. (2007). Approaches to positive youth development: A view of the issues. In R. K. Silbereisen & R. M. Lerner (ERds.), *Approaches to positive youth development* (pp. 3–30). Sage Publications Ltd.

Sun, R. C. F., & Shek, D. T. L. (2010). Life satisfaction, positive youth development and problem behavior among Chinese adolescents in Hong Kong. *Social Indicators Research, 95*(2), 455–474.

Sun, R. C. F., & Shek, D. T. L. (2012). Positive youth development, life satisfaction and problem behavior among Chinese adolescents in Hong Kong: A replication. *Social Indicators Research, 105*(3), 541–559.
Sun, R. C. F., & Shek, D. T. L. (2013). Longitudinal influences of positive youth development and life satisfaction on problem behavior among adolescents in Hong Kong. *Social Indicators Research, 114*(3), 1171–1197.
Sutphin, S. T., McDonough, S., & Schrenkel, A. (2013). The role of formal theory in social work research: Formalizing family systems theory. *Advances in Social Work, 14*(2), 501–517.
Swenson, R. R., & Prelow, H. M. (2005). Ethnic identity, self-esteem, and perceived efficacy as mediators of the relation of supportive parenting to psychosocial outcomes among urban adolescents. *Journal of Adolescence, 28*(4), 465–477.
Tafà, M., & Baiocco, R. (2009). Addictive behavior and family functioning during adolescence. *The American Journal of Family Therapy, 37*(5), 388–395.
Theokas, C., Almerigi, J. B., Lerner, R. M., Dowling, E. M., Benson, P. L., Scales, P. C., & von Eye, A. (2005). Conceptualizing and modeling individual and ecological asset components of thriving in early adolescence. *Journal of Early Adolescence, 25*(1), 113–143.
Theokas, C., & Lerner R. M. (2005). Promoting positive youth development across variations in socioeconomic status: Framing the structural equation modeling approach within a developmental systems perspective. In V. L. Bengtson, A. C. Acock, K. R. Allen, P. Dilworth-Anderson, & D. M. Klein (Eds.), *Sourcebook of family theory and research* (pp. 488–492). Sage Publications, Inc.
Vesely, S. K., Wyatt, V. H., Oman, R. Y., Aspy, C. B., Kegler, M. C., Rodline, S., … & McLeroy, K. R. (2004). The potential protective effects of youth assets from adolescent sexual risk behaviors. *Journal of Adolescent Health, 34*(5), 356–365.
Walsh, F. (Ed.) (1993). *Normal family processes*. New York, The Guilford Press.
World Health Organization. (1997). *Life skills education for children and adolescents in schools*. Programme on Mental Health Organization. Geneva: WHO.
Young, M. E., Galvan, T., Reidy, B. L., Pescosolido, M. F., Kim, K. L., Seymour, K., & Dickstein, D. P. (2013). Family functioning deficits in bipolar disorder and ADHD in youth. *Journal of Affective Disorders, 150*(3), 1096–1102.
Youngblade, L. M., Theokas, C., Schulenberg, J., Curry, L., Huang, I. C., & Novak, M. (2007). Risk and promotive factors in families, schools, and communities: A contextual model of positive youth development in adolescence. *Pediatrics, 119* (Suppl 1), S47–S53.
Yu, L., & Shek, D. T. L. (2013). Internet addiction in Hong Kong adolescents: A three-year longitudinal study. *Journal of Pediatric & Adolescent Gynecology*, *26*(3S), S10–17. doi: 10.1016/j.jpag.2013.03.010.

Part II
Theoretical Issues

Chapter 4
The Theory of Subjective Wellbeing Homeostasis: A Contribution to Understanding Life Quality

Robert A. Cummins

Introduction

The Theory of Subjective Wellbeing Homeostasis originated through the convergence of three facilitating factors. The idea of homeostasis was familiar to me as a student of both physiology and psychology. Second, a fortuitous collaboration with Bruce Headey and Alex Wearing in the late 1980s, through a grant to investigate 'quality of life', introduced me to their ground-breaking work on subjective wellbeing (SWB). The third factor was Alex Michalos, as Editor of Social Indicators Research.

I had submitted an empirical review. This reported remarkable consistency in SWB when population mean scores from Western countries were standardized and used as data. So my manuscript concluded with the proposition that this consistency could, perhaps, be accounted for by a 'psychological homeostatic mechanism'. The reviewers were underwhelmed by my brash suggestion and recommended, inter alia, that I collect more data. But Alex recognised that the manuscript represented a novel, if undercooked idea, and it was accepted for publication on 7th February 1995. This paper (Cummins 1995) has since received around 300 citations, the later companion paper (Cummins 1998) over 400, and developing the theory of SWB homeostasis became my major life's work.

This theory is but one of many schemes proposed to account for the characteristics of SWB. However, within this family of ideas, SWB homeostasis is unique in incorporating the idea of a positive construct managed by an open- system, which displays the characteristics of attractors, resilience, stability, and nonlinear relationships. The use of homeostasis in this context, is consistent with the definition

R.A. Cummins (✉)
School of Psychology, Deakin University,
221 Burwood Highway, Burwood, VIC 3125, Australia
e-mail: robert.cummins@deakin.edu.au

F. Maggino (ed.), *A Life Devoted to Quality of Life*, Social Indicators Research Series 60, DOI 10.1007/978-3-319-20568-7_4

provided by McEwen and Wingfield (2003), as the 'management of an essential variable to a set-point, representing an optimal level for the operation for each individual'.

The remainder of this chapter describes current status. It presents a contemporary version of the theory and examines evidence for and against. Irrespective of whether this theory survives future scrutiny, the research it has stimulated represents one small part of the Michalos scientific legacy.

The Character of SWB

Underpinning the theory of SWB homeostasis is the metric used to standardize SWB results to a 0–100 point range called "percentage of Scale Maximum" (%SM). The formula for this conversion is presented in the manual for the Personal Wellbeing Index (International Wellbeing Group 2013). This standardization allows results from disparate measurement scales to be compared, and the application of this procedure has facilitated understanding that SWB is normally positive, stable, and that its content is dominated by mood.

SWB Is Positive

The most basic property of SWB is that it is normally positive. On a rating scale from 'feeling very bad' to 'feeling very good', when reasonably benign living conditions are the norm within population samples, only a very small proportion of people lie below the scale mid-point. For example, using general population data from over 60,000 people gathered over 13 years by the Australian Unity Wellbeing Index surveys (Cummins et al. 2013) only around 4 % of scores lie below 50 percentage points. It is, thus, normal for people to feel good about themselves.

SWB Mainly Comprises Mood

The most contentious issue involving SWB concerns its composition. Since the early work of Campbell et al. (1976), it has been generally agreed that SWB comprises some mixture of affect and cognition. However, whether as claimed by Diener et al. (2004), SWB represents a dominantly cognitive evaluation, is certainly moot. To the contrary, a substantial body of more recent research now attests to the essence of SWB being affect (Blore et al. 2011; Davern et al. 2007; Longo 2014; Tomyn and Cummins 2011).

The first systematic challenge to the cognition hypothesis came from Davern et al. (2007) who, using a circumplex model of affect and structural equation modelling, concluded the essence of SWB to be a construct they called 'Core Affect.' This term had been coined by Russell (2003) to describe a neurophysiological state experienced as a feeling, and which may be conceptualized as a deep form of trait affect or mood. He considers it analogous to felt body temperature in that it is always there, it can be accessed when attention is drawn to it, extremes are most obvious, and it exists without words to describe it. Russell described Core Affect in conformity with his circumplex model of affect, comprising a blend of hedonic (pleasant–unpleasant) and arousal values (activation–deactivation).

The reason Davern et al. were attracted to adopt this term was Russell's description of Core Affect as a biologically influenced mood, rather than an emotion. If the perception of affect becomes linked to a cause then, Russell (2003) claimed, the feeling state transitions from mood to an emotion.

Some 6 years later, however, Russell (2009) changed his mind, and now considers Core Affect to be involved in both moods and emotions. Thus, he proposes that Core Affect may become directed at something and, indeed, that Core Affect is not stable, being subject to change by a variety of influences. Because of this reconceptualization, a new term was required to describe the stable mood affect associated with homeostasis. Homeostatically Protected Mood (HPMood) now describes this most basic feeling state (Cummins 2010) and it has the following characteristics:

1. It is a neuro-physiologically generated mood that comprises the simplest, constant, non-reflective feeling. It is hardwired for each individual, representing the tonic state of affect that provides the underlying activation energy, or motivation, for routine behavior.
2. It is not modifiable by conscious experience, yet it is a ubiquitous, background component of conscious experience. It is best reflected as a general feeling of contentment, but also comprises aspects of related affects including happy and alert.
3. When SWB is measured using either the Satisfaction With Life Scale (Diener et al. 1985) or the Personal Wellbeing Index (International Wellbeing Group 2013), HPMood accounts for over 60 % of the variance. This challenges the conventional view that SWB is dominated by either personality or cognition, as has been commonly reported (Emmons and Diener 1985).
4. Under normal resting conditions, the average level of HPMood for each person represents their 'set-point', which is a genetically-determined, individual difference. Within the general Australian population, these set-points are normally distributed between 70 and 90 percentage points, referenced to the 0–100 point scale (Cummins et al. 2014).
5. Each set-point has a 'set-point-range'. This describes the limits within which homeostatic processes strive to maintain HPMood for each individual.
6. HPMood perfuses all cognitive processes to some degree, but most strongly the rather abstract notions of self (e.g., I am a lucky person). Because of this, these self-referent perceptions are normally held at a level that approximates each set-point-range. The individual difference of HPMood accounts for much of the typical correlational variance between self-report variables (see, Lai and Cummins 2013).

7. Under resting conditions, SWB is a reasonable proxy for HPMood. However, SWB can vary outside the set-point-range for HPMood when a strong emotion is generated by momentary experience. The emotional affect then dominates conscious awareness, infiltrates the experience of SWB, and causes the reported level of SWB to be different from set-point. When this occurs, homeostatic forces are activated, which attempt to return experienced affect to set-point-range. Thus, daily affective experience normally oscillates around its set-point.

SWB Is Normally Stable

Perhaps the most compelling feature of SWB is its stability over time, which has been in evidence since Hartmann (1934) reported a 1-month test–retest reliability of .70. By the 1970s, many significant retest correlations had been reported over periods of years (Andrews and Withey 1976; Palmore and Kivett 1977).

Further insight into this stability came through the use of population mean scores as data Cummins (1995). This paper combines the means from population surveys conducted in various Western countries over the decades 1970–1990. Following conversion to %SM, and using these standardised population mean scores as data, the grand mean averages 75 points, with a standard deviation of just 2.5. Thus, within the range 70–80 points, there is a 95 % probability of including any particular survey mean. This represents the first estimation of a normal range for SWB population mean scores.

Clearly, however, this estimation is heavily contaminated with error variance resulting from the many methodological differences between studies. Much greater stability has been revealed by the 30 surveys conducted over the period 2001–2013 using the Australian Unity Wellbeing Index (Cummins et al. 2013) supplying SWB data from the Personal Wellbeing Index (International Wellbeing Group 2013).

Using the mean scores of these 30 surveys as data, the grand mean is 75.3 points and the standard deviation 0.72. This yields a normative range of 73.8–76.7 points. In other words, over a 13 year period, the mean score of a random survey of people in Australia could be predicted, with 95 % certainty, to lie within a 2.9 percentage point range. There is no precedent for such extraordinary stability in measures of SWB.

This does not mean, however, that SWB is entirely stable. There are two further considerations. First, there is substantial variation due to adverse living circumstances, as has been widely reported and as predicted by homeostatic failure. Second, it remains uncertain how much of the measured SWB variance is, actually, stable. In a recent review of longitudinal state-trait model analyses, Yap et al. (2014) estimate that about a third of the measured variance in life satisfaction is stable even over very long time periods, another third changes slowly over time, and the remaining third is occasion specific. This seems like the best approximation we have to date.

The Cause of Chronic SWB Stability

Personality

In the 1980s, researchers started to ask what might be the cause of SWB stability, and personality seemed an obvious choice. After all, extraversion and neuroticism were known to have strong links to SWB (Costa and McCrae 1980) and there was a conventional view that personality was largely genetically determined (for a review see Block 1981). So, it was believed, these linkages caused SWB to be stable.

The next conceptual step toward understanding was provided by Headey and Wearing (1989). Using longitudinal data, they reported that, when the level of SWB changed following some major event, it tended to return to its previous level over time. To account for this, the authors propose that each person has an 'equilibrium level' of SWB, and that personality causes the restoration of equilibrium after change by making certain kinds of events more likely. Thus, personality, life events, and SWB are in dynamic equilibrium with one another, they claimed.

However, the idea that SWB stability was vested in personality did not fit happily with the view that SWB was dominated by cognition (Diener et al. 2004). Elucidation came from linking SWB stability directly with genetics, rather than indirectly through personality.

Genetics

The idea that emotionality has a strong genetic basis has been known to animal breeders since time immemorial (see, Smith 1961, Chapter 6). So it did not take long for researchers to study the relative influence of genetics and environment on the SWB stability of twins. An early study (Tellegen et al. 1988) concerned both monozygotic (MZ) and dizygotic (DZ) pairs of middle-aged twins either reared together, or separated in infancy and reared apart. Their estimate of wellbeing heritability was .48 (SD .08) and the contribution of common family environment was negligible.

Further clarification came from Lykken and Tellegen (1996) who reported a retest correlation for DZ of .07 and for MZ .40. They state this latter figure represents "80 % of the retest correlation of .50" which they argue "suggests that the stable component of well-being (i.e., trait happiness) is largely determined genetically" (p. 188).

Since this ground-breaking work, great strides in understanding the link between SWB and genetics have been made. In their review, Røysamb et al. (2014) conclude: (a) As much as 80 % of the stable level of SWB is attributable to genes. (b) Correlations among quality of life in general, satisfaction with life, quality of life at present, and subjective happiness, are largely attributable to shared genes, "suggesting that these four indicators do not differ at the genetic level" (p. 18).

These conclusions are consistent with the idea of a genetically determined 'set-point' for SWB, as first suggested by McGue et al. (1993), with the set-point actually being for HPMood (Cummins 2010). More recently, set-points for SWB have been demonstrated (Cummins et al. 2014) and the returning mechanism following perturbation from set-point has been formalized as the theory of subjective wellbeing homeostasis.

The Theory of SWB Homeostasis

The term 'homeostasis' was coined by Cannon (1932) to assist his understanding of the physiological response to stress. The term is now more generally employed to describe the process by which separate systems can work together under challenging conditions to re-establish stability in a managed variable.

Homeostatic systems are commonplace. Wherever a variable needs to be maintained within a narrow range, around some specific average value for normal functioning, the universal solution has been to evolve a homeostatic system of management (Bernard and Cannon 1998). The best-known example is the maintenance of core body temperature at 37 °C in mammals.

In their chapter 'Psychological functioning: a homeostatic perspective', Williams and Thompson (1993) describe the idea of psychological functioning being managed around a set-point, which they envisage as designating a particular level of an individual's psychological functioning. Moreover, surrounding this set-point they imagined a bandwidth of functioning in which the individual would be most comfortable operating.

This conception of theoretical boundaries leads naturally to the idea that some force is operating to 'attract' or limit the operation of relevant variables. This conception is included within Dynamic Systems Theory (e.g., Vallacher and Nowak 1997), however the actual operational mechanisms are not described.

Building on the information that SWB is generally quite stable and that each person has a set-point for their resting level of SWB, the idea that SWB could be managed by a homeostatic system was first mooted by Cummins (1995). Such management is considered to be the product of dispositional, genetically pre-wired, neurological systems.

The theory of subjective wellbeing homeostasis concerns the theoretical relationship between experience and levels of SWB. The model depicting this relationship is shown in Fig. 4.1.

This figure is described as follows:

1. The vertical axis shows the 0–100 scale of SWB and includes the average set-point range of 70–90 points. It also shows an illustrative set-point at 80 points (Cummins et al. 2014).
2. The lower horizontal axis shows the two opposing forces as:

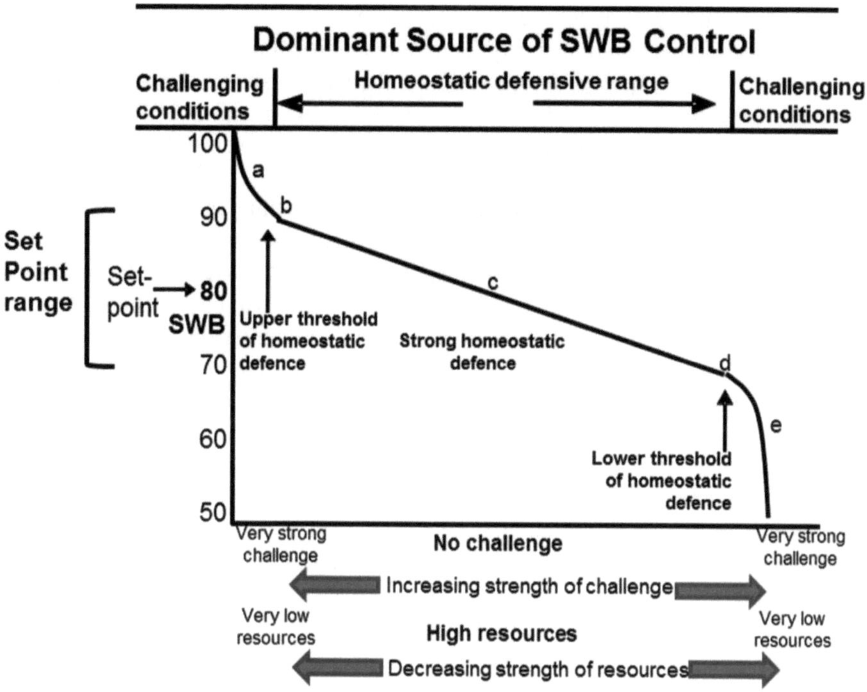

Fig. 4.1 Changing levels of SWB as homeostasis is challenged

(i) The strength of the combined challenges to homeostatic control, either positive or negative, such as might be caused by gaining a sought-after promotion or being retrenched.
(ii) The strength of the combined resources aiding homeostatic control, such as might come from an intimate relationship or money.

3. The upper horizontal axis shows the dominant source of control over SWB. This source changes depending on whether SWB is under homeostatic control, or whether the level of SWB is being determined by the challenging conditions, be they either positive or negative.
4. The curving "response line" depicts the changing level of SWB as it moves from:

(a) Homeostatic defeat due to a powerful positive challenge.
(b) The upper margin of the set-point range at 90 points.
(c) Homeostatic control
(d) The lower margin of the set-point range at 70 points.
(e) Homeostatic defeat due to a powerful negative challenge.

5. The depiction of a set-point at 80 points is illustrative only. Other set-points will cause the vertical positioning of markers b–e to vary accordingly. Thus, for a set point of 70, the response line will be 10 points lower.

Figure 4.1 shows the theoretical outcome of combined supportive and challenging influences acting simultaneously. Thus, any empirical investigation to verify the model can only be expected to approximate the pattern shown. However, specific aspects of the model would be more easily falsified. In order to facilitate such empirical examination, the proposed relationship between levels of SWB, resources, and challenges can be elaborated as follows:

In a normal resting state, where the person is not feeling anxious, depressed or distressed, their level of SWB will approximate their set-point (level c).

As mild sources of threat are experienced, the level of SWB will vary within its set-point range (b–d). Its actual position within the range will be a probability statement determined by the balance of good and bad momentary experience and the resilience of the homeostatic system. Thus, a sustained environment where good experience dominates will cause SWB to average higher than the set point, while a chronic bad experience will cause SWB to average lower than the set point. However, the extent of such fluctuations is predicted to be quite modest. Since the magnitude of the set-point range is calculated to be around ten percentage points on either side of the set-point (Cummins et al. 2014), and since this represents just one unit on a 0–10 response scale, the overall impression from a measurement perspective will be one of stability.

As the strength of emotional threat intensifies, the strength of the homeostatic defence also increases in an attempt to maintain stable levels of SWB. This is depicted by the threshold lines at (b) and (d). Here, homeostasis manages to hold the line and prevents SWB from moving either above or below its set-point-range. Importantly, within phase (c) the value of SWB is pretty insensitive to the challenging agent. That is, despite the strength of the challenge increasing, SWB will remain within the range (b)–(d). This will continue as long as the homeostatic system is effective.

At some higher strength of challenge, homeostasis will be overwhelmed. The strength of the challenging agent has now become too strong for homeostatic management. Now the value of SWB enters phases (a) or (e). In these phases, control over the level of SWB has shifted from homeostasis to the challenging agent. Now, the value of SWB is sensitive to the strength of the challenging agent, and as the strength of the challenge increases, the value of SWB will sharply rise or fall. The resulting higher or lower level of SWB will persist until homeostasis regains control.

This description of homeostasis from Fig. 4.1 is in outline only. The next section elaborates some of the mechanisms involved.

Homeostatic Processes

The affect produced by HPMood provides a steady background to consciousness, which influences general feeling about the self. This background normally approximates the set-point and so provides the target level for homeostatic management. When average levels of felt affect deviate from this background, homeostatic processes are activated for the purpose of restoring the level of felt affect to set-point.

There are, thus, two types of processes involved in homeostatic management. One is to establish conditions for the self which minimize the probability of homeostatic failure. The other is to use resources to facilitate recovery after homeostatic failure. Both of these processes are normally under the primary control of behavior.

Behavior

It is intuitive that behavior can be used to either engage or disengage from an emotionally intense situation. In the case of a positive experience, a desire for prolonged engagement is potentially threatening to homeostasis. It is not generally adaptive to hold positive affect above the set-point-range for a protracted period since it alters cognitive processing to 'good times' processing, reducing critical thinking and error-checking (Lyubomirsky et al. 2005). In practice, however, strong positive experience cannot be naturally maintained for long. The operational behavior becomes limited in variety, and decreasing variety causes enhanced habituation and adaptation. This is one reason the techniques of positive psychology have such weak long-term effectiveness to raise SWB in normally functioning people (Cummins 2013).

On the reverse side of the affective coin, behavior is also a first line of defence following experience of negative affect (Schulz and Heckhausen 1996). People generally disengage from unpleasant situations. They also reduce the probability of encountering unsought challenges by establishing life routines that make daily experiences predictable and manageable. Other behavioral responses to negative threats require the support of suitable resources. The first of these to be described are the 'external buffers', which protect HPMood by facilitating adaptive behaviors (Ensel and Lin 1991).

External Buffers

The resources external to the person, which can be used to facilitate homeostasis, are referred to as the external buffers. While their primary function is to defend against homeostatic failure, they can also assist homeostatic recovery. There are three primary external buffers, the 'Triumvirate' (TriVs), as follows:

Money

There are serious misconceptions as to what money can and cannot do in relation to SWB. People who are rich experience rapid adaptation to high living standards, so living in a mansion with servants may feel luxurious in the short term, but over time it will just feel 'normal'. Moreover, high wealth cannot shift the set point to create a perpetually happier person. So, in this sense, money cannot buy happiness.

No matter how rich someone becomes, once their level of income saturates the wealth-dependent buffering capacity of the homeostatic system, additional wealth will not raise SWB further.

The real power of wealth is to protect wellbeing through its capacity as a flexible resource to assist homeostasis (Cummins 2000). It does this by allowing people to minimize the unwanted challenges they experience in their daily life. Wealthy people pay others to perform tasks they do not wish to do themselves. Thus, SWB rises with income in an asymptotic curve.

Relationships

The second external buffer is a relationship with another person that involves mutual sharing of intimacies and support. Almost universally, the research literature attests to the power of such relationships to moderate the influence of potential stressors on SWB (for a review see, Sarason et al. 1990)

Achieving in Life

The process of active engagement, providing purpose in life, is the third external buffer. A voluminous literature attests to the fact that when people lose this buffer through, for example, unemployment, their SWB is severely threatened (Clark et al. 2008).

Two additional sets of buffers assisting homeostasis are internal to each person. These are the automatic-subconscious and the cognitive buffers.

Automatic: Subconscious Buffers

The automatic-subconscious buffers are activated by any percept causing an affective response where the generated emotion is at a different level from HPMood. These buffers function to return felt emotion towards the set-point and are as follows:

Access to Positive Affect

Immediately after SWB is threatened by a negative threat, the counteractive response is to increase nonconscious positive emotions (DeWall et al. 2011). This includes increased access to positive memories and greater attention to positive cues.

Habituation

This is a general term meaning decreasing responsiveness to a repeated stimulus (Thompson 2009). It is an adaptive behavior involving primitive learning. Its purpose is to conserve resources by reducing the response to stimuli that are predictable.

So, for example, the delight of being hoisted in a ferris-wheel disappears with repeated revolutions as habituation takes control.

Adaptation

The automatic process of adaptation also works over time to diminish awareness of an emotionally challenging experience. Activated by either positive or negative emotion, adaptation is a form of contrast which is best understood through Adaptation Level (AL) Theory (Helson 1964). The general principle is that, under regular circumstances of living, people naturally adapt to a point of felt affective neutrality, which, in benign living circumstances is their HPMood set-point. This is the benchmark against which people judge the strength of current positive or negative experience. However, AL can be raised or lowered by past experience (Eiser and Stroebe 1972) and this moderates the affective impact of current circumstances. For example, an extremely positive event, such as winning a million dollars, initially causes intense positive feelings because the emotion is so much more positive than AL. However, over time, AL shifts upwards, thereby dampening the pleasure. The same process works in reverse to assist recovery from misfortune.

Domain Compensation

This occurs when the homeostatic threat is chronic (Best et al. 2000; Heidemeier and Göritz 2013). It involves an adjustment in the relative extent to which particular domains contribute to SWB. For example, unemployment may cause a weaker contribution from the domain of 'achieving in life', compensated by an enhanced contribution from the domain of 'relationships'. This adjustment assists stability in the average level of domains, and therefore SWB.

Automatic: Conscious: The Cognitive Buffers

The cognitive buffers are used to consciously defend the emotional self against negative challenges (Cummins and Nistico 2002). They correspond with the same three constructs used by Taylor and Brown (1988) as evidence of positive distortion in self-evaluation, as self-esteem, perceived control, and optimism.

As self-referential constructs, all three cognitive buffers are strongly perfused with HPMood (Lai and Cummins 2013). Thus, under resting conditions, people feel worthy, in control, and optimistic, all at the level of their set-point. Their mechanism of defence in the face of a homeostatic challenge, is to reconstruct negative experience in a way to minimize the adversity and maximize advantage to self. Thus, for example, a failure of perceived control that causes SWB to fall may be counteracted by thinking that the failure experience will provide long-term benefit (Affleck and Tennen 1996).

In summary, there are numerous behavioural, conscious, and unconscious processes acting to defend set-point levels of HPMood. Whether, and for how long, a particular challenge will move experienced affect outside a set-point-range will depend on the strength of the challenge matched against resilience (Kennedy et al. 2000).

Resilience

The most sophisticated definition of resilience is also the simplest. This is offered by Merriam-Webster as 'an ability to recover from or adjust easily to misfortune or change'. The advantage of this definition is its general applicability. It does not specify the process of recovery or adjustment, the nature of the misfortune or change, or the temporal dimension. This allows it to be equally applicable to both children and adults under all relevant conditions.

In empirical terms, resilience has been described as the sum of the protective resources (Rutter 1985). However, in the context of homeostasis, resilience is the capacity to utilise such protective resources to defend against the threat. Two unifying observations can be made to round-out this description. The first is that, while the relative strength of each resource is likely specific to the nature of the challenge and situation, the triumvirate buffers of money, relationships, and achieving in life, are commonly preeminent. For example, they dominate the extensive list of positive psychological resources provided by Masten (2007). The reason for this domination is that each TriV buffer has a double benefit. They provide both a defence and a recovery resource with respect to homeostatic failure. This double-benefit has been observed by many authors in relation to money (Cummins 2000), belonging [relationships] (Conger and Conger 2002), and of being in control [achieving] (Carver 1998). Moreover, the relative importance of these three key resources crosses cultural and age demographics (e.g., Werner 1995).

The second observation is that resilience is commonly proposed to be enhanced by higher SWB (e.g., Graham and Oswald 2010). It is, indeed, logical that high set-points and their associated high levels of HPMood cause people to be more resilient. That is, high levels of HPMood organize a 'resilience package' that includes higher levels of extraversion, higher levels of the TriVs, and higher levels of the cognitive buffers. Thus, it is proposed, the strength of resilience is predicted by the HPMood set-point.

Principles for Strengthening Homeostatic Resilience

Homeostatic resilience is strengthened by the behavioral, external, and internal resources described above. However, increasing each of these resources has adaptive limitations. The overarching principle is that each form of resource has an optimal level that is both enhancing of resilience and also generally adaptive. Beyond an optimal level, more of a particular resource may harm adaptation, as will now be described.

(a) The effect of using a simple behavior as a resilience resource, such as disengaging from the source of challenge, is effective only if disengagement is adaptive (Lowenthal and Boler 1965). It may be so when faced with a verbally abusive stranger. However, an overuse of disengagement may cause ineffective engagement with the normal world of interpersonal relationships. A similar argument can be made in relation to the use of any other single behavioral strategy, such as active confrontation, physical submission, friendly demeanour, etc. For all of these, the strategy needs to be used with discretion in order to be optimally useful as a resilience resource.
(b) In relation to the TriV resources of income, relationships and achieving, the adaptive value of increasing each resource will depend on the degree to which homeostatic resilience is already saturated with that resource. If someone does not have an intimate relationship, then acquiring one will almost certainly strengthen resilience (Gutheil 1991). However, for someone who already has such a relationship, while acquiring another may marginally increase resilience, it will be at the cost of additional interpersonal demands.
(c) Increasing the strength of the cognitive buffers may, or may not, be an adaptive strategy. People normally have a robust level of optimism which is generally adaptive. However, very high levels can give rise to unrealistic expectations (Ruthig et al. 2004) and impulsive choices in complex situations. Moreover, the optimal level of impulsivity will change according to circumstances. Deciding when to sow a crop is advantaged by a slow and deliberate choice. Deciding which parry or thrust is advantageous in the heat of battle requires instantaneous judgment. A similar argument applies to the other cognitive buffers of self-esteem and perceived control (Robins and Beer 2001).

In summary, for each person there is an optimal level of each resilience resource, and that level is situation-specific.

Dangers of Resilience That Is Too Strong

Because the buffers create perceptions that are not consistent with external reality, these positive biases must be held in check and not allowed to rise so high that they lose touch with reality all together. The thought "I do not need either my income or my friends" is rarely likely to be adaptive. Even normal levels of optimism can be a risk factor. For example, their personal optimism causes physicians to prefer a less effective, less invasive and more risky treatment option for themselves (i.e. watchful waiting) than they will recommend for their patients (Mendel et al. 2010).

Dangers of Resilience That Is Too Weak

While an over-abundance of resilience resources may be either of little value, or even pose a mild danger to a normal functioning system, by far the greatest threat to homeostasis is paucity of resources. While a deficit in any of the specific resources can create this potential danger, reduced levels of the TriVs stand out as being the most damaging.

Homeostatic Theory: Critiques and Implications

Critiques

The only critiques of SWB homeostasis theory known to me are those against the existence of set-points. These critiques are based on the fact that, when tracking large samples over time, a sub-group can be identified that has evidenced substantial change in levels of SWB (e.g., Headey et al. 2010). The valid explanation for such chronic change is either the occurrence of homeostatic defeat due to some long-acting negative event, such as unemployment, or the recovery from homeostatic defeat due to either adaptation or the provision of appropriate resources. It is not, as the authors tend to claim, evidence of changing set points. This counter-argument has been made in detail (Cummins 2014; Cummins et al. 2014) and no rebuttals to these counters are known.

Implications for Researchers

Three diagnostic ranges for SWB can be calculated, based on the findings (Cummins et al. 2014) that set-points exist between the levels of 70 and 90 points and have a normal operating range (set-point-range) of around 18–20 points. From these results it can be calculated that for individual respondents:

1. SWB at or above 70 points reflects a normally-functioning homeostatic system.
2. SWB at or below 50 points represents homeostatic failure and a high risk of depression.
3. SWB between 51 and 69 points cannot be unequivocally interpreted. Any score within this range may represent the homeostatic failure of a high set-point or the homeostatic normality of a low set-point.

Knowledge of these ranges is highly relevant for research into SWB. This is most particularly evident in terms of what constitutes a 'normal' sample of participants.

Implications for Normative Samples

Almost all SWB researchers assume that a sample conforming to the national demographic profile is 'normal'. In statistical terms this is correct. However, more important for most psychological research is that the sample comprises normally functioning people. It is therefore instructive that normal population samples, so formed, always contain a proportion of people who have SWB below 50. Confirming psychometric pathology within this group, Richardson et al. (2015) applied multiple regression analysis, multiple group confirmatory factor analysis, and Rasch modelling. They found that while the Personal Wellbeing Index functioned as intended for the normal group, SWB in the <50 group was lower across all PWI domains, more variable, and domain scores lacked the normal strength of inter-correlation. The implications are clear. Including people with pathologically low SWB in a sample will damage data validity and reliability.

Implications for Health Researchers

Threats arising from within the four non-TriV domains of the Personal Wellbeing Index have a generally weak link to SWB. This includes the domain of health. The reasons are, first, people generally adapt to deteriorating physical health. For example, people with Multiple Sclerosis experience a gradual loss of motor functioning over many years, and yet some continue to report normal levels of SWB even when they can no longer independently breathe and require mechanical ventilation (Bach et al. 1991).

Second, increasing the health of people with normal levels of SWB will not significantly increase SWB. For example, people with normal body weight and no major medical condition exhibit similar levels of SWB to people who are overweight and have high blood pressure (Cummins 2012). Provided that someone is sufficiently healthy, such that their level of health does not challenge the buffering capacity of the homeostatic system, improved health will not raise SWB further.

Third, if baseline health is causing SWB to be low, due either to persistent pain or gross impairment of self-care, then increasing health may increase SWB. A caveat is that the associated symptoms of pain and self-care are also ameliorated. Even then, however, the increase in SWB will continue only up to the point that health satisfaction lies within its normal range.

Implications for Depression, Anxiety, and Stress

Depression, stress and anxiety scales simply record the level of emotional challenge, not the influence of such conditions on SWB. Because of this, a low level of SWB is a more valid measure of pathology than scores on these scales. Low SWB signals the defeat of homeostasis and is, therefore, the dividing line between an emotional challenge and the distress of psychopathology.

Implications for Intervention Studies

Almost universally within the SWB literature, researchers who study the outcome of interventions assume that all members of their sample are equivalent in terms of their capacity to respond to the intervention. That is, while there will be individual differences in responsiveness, there is no systematic factor operating to bias their result. This is incorrect.

If people are already operating normally within their set-point-range, interventions that attempt to raise SWB are simply wasting resources. Homeostatic control will defeat such attempts. However, this does not apply to people who are operating below their normal range.

The three ranges established earlier (≤50, 51–69, 70≥ points) are predictive of very different responsiveness to any attempt to increase SWB. This has been demonstrated by Tomyn et al. (2015) who studied the influence of an intervention designed to support adolescents disengaged from education, employment and post-secondary training, their families and/or their communities. The 4243 adolescents were assessed before and after the intervention, a period of about 4 months. Consistent with theory, the degree of gain in SWB for each of the three groups was: ≤50 (23.75 points), 51–69 (12.08 points), 70+ (2.1 points).

Implications for Social Policy

The most effective distribution of government resources within a population can be informed by the discrepancy between the level of SWB for the population as a whole and the level within disadvantaged subgroups. For example, there are abundant reports to support the relatively low SWB of informal caregivers (Fadden et al. 1987). Raising the SWB of such disadvantaged subgroups, to a level that is not statistically different from the general population, should be considered nationally aspirational.

Acknowledgements I gratefully acknowledge advice from the following people on an earlier version of this chapter: Christine Baxter, Tanja Capic, Matthew Fuller-Tyszkiewicz, Anna Lau, Mark Stokes, Adrian Tomyn, and Melissa Weinberg.

References

Affleck, G., & Tennen, H. (1996). Construing benefits from adversity: Adaptational significance and dispositional underpinnings. *Journal of Personality, 64*(4), 899–922.

Andrews, F. M., & Withey, S. B. (1976). *Social indicators of well-being: American's perceptions of life quality*. New York: Plenum Press.

Bach, J. R., Campagnolo, D. I., & Hoeman, S. (1991). Life satisfaction of individuals with Duchenne Muscular Dystrophy using long-term mechanical ventilatory support. *American Journal of Physical Medicine & Rehabilitation, 70*, 129–135.

Bernard, C., & Cannon, W. B. (1998). What is Homeostasis?: California State University
Best, C. J., Cummins, R. A., & Lo, S. K. (2000). The quality of rural and metropolitan life. *Australian Journal of Psychology, 52*, 69–74.
Block, J. (1981). Some enduring and consequential structures of personality. In A. I. Rabin, J. Aronoff, A. M. Barclay & R. A. Zucker (Eds.), *Further Explorations in Personality* (pp. 27–43). New York: Wiley.
Blore, J. D., Stokes, M. A., Mellor, D., Firth, L., & Cummins, R. A. (2011). Comparing multiple discrepancies theory to affective models of subjective wellbeing. *Social Indicators Research, 100*(1), 1–16. doi: 10.1007/s11205-010-9599-2.
Campbell, A., Converse, P. E., & Rodgers, W. L. (1976). *The quality of American life: Perceptions, evaluations, and satisfactions*. Russell Sage Foundation: New York.
Cannon, W. B. (1932). *The wisdom of the body*. New York NY: Norton.
Carver, C. S. (1998). Resilience and thriving: Issues, models, and linkages. *Journal of Social Issues, 54*, 245–266.
Clark, A. E., Diener, E., Georgellis, Y., & Lucas, R. E. (2008). Lags and leads in life satisfaction: A test of the baseline hypothesis. *Economic Journal, 118*, F222-F243. doi: 10.1111/j.1468-0297.2008.02150.x.
Conger, R. D., & Conger, K. J. (2002). Resilience in midwestern families: Selected findings from the first decade of a prospective, longitudinal study. *Journal of Marriage and Family, 64*, 361–373.
Costa, P. T., & McCrae, R. (1980). Influence of extraversion and neuroticism on subjective well-being: Happy and unhappy people. *Journal of Personality and Social Psychology, 38*, 668–678.
Cummins, R. A. (1995). On the trail of the gold standard for life satisfaction. *Social Indicators Research, 35*(2), 179–200. doi: 10.1007/BF01079026.
Cummins, R. A. (1998). The second approximation to an international standard of life satisfaction. *Social Indicators Research, 43*(3), 307–334. doi: 10.1023/A:1006831107052.
Cummins, R. A. (2000). Personal income and subjective well-being: A review. *Journal of Happiness Studies, 1*(2), 133–158.
Cummins, R. A. (2010). Subjective wellbeing, homeostatically protected mood and depression: A synthesis. *Journal of Happiness Studies, 11*, 1–17. doi: 10.1007/s10902-009-9167-0.
Cummins, R. A. (2012). The relationship between subjective wellbeing and health. In M. L. Caltabiano & L. A. Ricciardelli (Eds.), *Applied topics in health psychology* (pp. 101–111). West Sussex, UK: John Wiley & Sons.
Cummins, R. A. (2013). Limitations to Positive Psychology Predicted by Subjective Wellbeing Homeostasis. In M. L. Wehmeyer (Ed.), Oxford Handbook of Positive Psychology and Disability. New York: Oxford University Press (in press).
Cummins, R. A. (2014). Can Happiness Change? Theories and Evidence. In K. M. Sheldon & R. E. Lucas (Eds.), *Stability of Happiness: Theories and Evidence on Whether Happiness Can Change* (pp. 75–97). Amsterdam: Elsevier.
Cummins, R. A., Li, L., Wooden, M., & Stokes, M. (2014). A demonstration of set-points for subjective wellbeing. *Journal of Happiness Studies, 15*, 183–206. doi: 10.1007/s10902-013-9444-9.
Cummins, R. A., & Nistico, H. (2002). Maintaining life satisfaction: The role of positive cognitive bias. *Journal of Happiness Studies, 3*(1), 37–69.
Cummins, R. A., Woerner, J., Weinberg, M., Collard, J., Hartley-Clark, L., & Horfiniak, K. (2013). Australian Unity Wellbeing Index: -Report 30.0 - The Wellbeing of Australians: Social media, personal achievement, and work. Melbourne: Australian Centre on Quality of Life, School of Psychology, Deakin University. http://www.deakin.edu.au/research/acqol/reports/auwbi.php.
Davern, M., Cummins, R. A., & Stokes, M. (2007). Subjective wellbeing as an affective/cognitive construct. *Journal of Happiness Studies, 8*(4), 429–449. doi: 10.1007/s10902-007-9066-1.
DeWall, C. N., Twenge, J. M., Koole, S. L., Baumeister, R. F., Marquez, A., & Reid, M. W. (2011). Automatic Emotion Regulation After Social Exclusion: Tuning to Positivity. *Emotion, 11*(3), 623–636.

Diener, E., Emmons, R. A., Larsen, R. J., & Griffin, S. (1985). The satisfaction with life scale. *Journal of Personality Assessment, 49*, 71–75.
Diener, E., Scollon, C. N., & Lucas, R. E. (2004). The evolving concept of subjective well-being. The multifaceted nature of happiness. In P. T. Costa & I. C. Siegler (Eds.), *Recent Advances in Psychology and Aging* (pp. 188–219). Amsterdam, The Netherlands: Elsevier Science BV.
Eiser, J. R., & Stroebe, W. (1972). *Categorization and social judgement.* London: Academic Press.
Emmons, R. A., & Diener, E. (1985). Personality correlates of subjective well-being. *Personality and Social Psychology Bulletin, 11*, 89–97.
Ensel, W. M., & Lin, N. (1991). The life stress paradigm and psychological distress. *Journal of Health and Social Behavior, 32*(4), 321–341.
Fadden, G., Bebbington, P., & Kuipers, L. (1987). The burden of care: The impact of functional psychiatric illness on the patient's family. *British Journal of Psychiatry, 150*, 285–292.
Graham, L., & Oswald, A. J. (2010). Hedonic capital, adaptation and resilience. *Journal of Economic Behavior & Organization, 76*(2), 372–384.
Gutheil, I. (1991). Intimacy in nursing home friendships. *Journal of Gerontological Social Work, 17*(1–2), 59–73.
Hartmann, G. W. (1934). Personality traits associated with variations in happiness. *Journal of Abnormal and Social Psychology, 29*, 202–212.
Headey, B., Muffels, R., & Wagner, G. G. (2010). Long-running German panel survey shows that personal and economic choices, not just genes, matter for happiness. *PNAS, 107*(42), 17922–17926. doi: 10.1073/pnas.1008612107.
Headey, B., & Wearing, A. (1989). Personality, life events, and subjective well-being: Toward a dynamic equilibrium model. *Journal of Personality and Social Psychology, 57*, 731–739. doi: 10.1037/0022-3514.57.4.731.
Heidemeier, H., & Göritz, A. S. (2013). Individual Differences in How Work and Nonwork Life Domains Contribute to Life Satisfaction: Using Factor Mixture Modeling for Classification. *Journal of Happiness Studies, 14*(6), 1765–1788.
Helson, H. (1964). *Adaptation-level theory: An experimental and systematic approach to behavior*. New York: Harper and Row.
International Wellbeing Group. (2013). *Personal Wellbeing Index Manual 5th Edition* Retrieved from http://www.deakin.edu.au/research/acqol/instruments/wellbeing-index/pwi-a-english.pdf
Kennedy, P., Marsh, N., Lowe, R., Grey, N., Short, E., & Rogers, B. (2000). A longitudinal analysis of psychological impact and coping strategies following spinal cord injury. *British Journal of Health Psychology, 5*(2), 157–172.
Lai, L. C. H., & Cummins, R. A. (2013). The contribution of job and partner satisfaction to the homeostatic defense of subjective wellbeing. *Social Indicators Research 111*(1), 203–217. doi: 10.1007/s11205-011-9991-6.
Longo, Y. (2014). The Simple Structure of Positive Affect. *Social Indicators Research*, before publication. doi: 10.1007/s11205-014-0776-6.
Lowenthal, M. F., & Boler, D. (1965). Voluntary vs involuntary social withdrawal. *Journal of gerontology, 20*(3), 363–371.
Lykken, D., & Tellegen, A. (1996). Happiness is a stochastic phenomenon. *Psychological Science, 7*(3), 186–189.
Lyubomirsky, S., King, L., & Diener, E. (2005). The benefits of frequent positive affect: Does happiness lead to success? *Psychological Bulletin, 131*(6), 803–855.
Masten, A. S. (2007). Resilience in developing systems: progress and promise as the fourth wave rises. *Development and Psychopathology, 19*, 921–930.
McEwen, B. S., & Wingfield, J. C. (2003). The concept of allostasis in biology and biomedicine. *Hormones and behavior, 43*(1), 2–15.
McGue, M., Bacon, S., & Lykken, D. T. (1993). Personality stability and change in early adulthood: A behavioral genetic analysis. *Developmental Psychology, 29*, 96–109. doi: 10.1037/0012-1649.29.1.96.

Mendel, R., Hamann, J., Traut-Mattausch, E., Bühner, M., Kissling, W., & Frey, D. (2010). 'What would you do if you were me, doctor?': randomised trial of psychiatrists' personal v. professional perspectives on treatment recommendations. *The British Journal of Psychiatry, 197*(6), 441–447. doi: 10.1192/bjp.bp.110.078006.
Palmore, E., & Kivett, V. (1977). Change in life satisfaction: A longitudinal study of persons aged 46–70. *Journal of Gerontology, 32*, 311–316.
Richardson, B., Fuller-Tyszkiewicz, M. D., Tomyn, A. J., & Cummins, R. A. (2015). The Psychometric equivalence of the Personal Wellbeing Index for normally functioning and homeostatically defeated Australian adults. *Journal of Happiness Studies*. doi: http://link.springer.com/article/10.1007/s10902-015-9613-0
Robins, R. W., & Beer, J. S. (2001). Positive illusions about the self: short-term benefits and long-term costs. *Journal of Personality and Social Psychology, 80*(2), 340–352.
Røysamb, E., Nes, R. B., & Vittersø, J. (2014). Well-Being: Heritable and Changeable. In K. M. Sheldon & R. E. Lucas (Eds.), *Stability of Happiness: Theories and Evidence on Whether Happiness Can Change* (pp. 9–36). USA: Elsevier.
Russell, J. A. (2003). Core affect and the psychological construction of emotion. *Psychological Review, 110*(1), 145–172.
Russell, J. A. (2009). Emotion, core affect, and psychological construction. *Cognition & Emotion, 23*, 1259–1283.
Ruthig, J. C., Perry, R. P., Hall, N. C., & Hladkyj, S. (2004). Optimism and Attributional Retraining: Longitudinal Effects on Academic Achievement, Test Anxiety, and Voluntary Course Withdrawal in College Students. *Journal of Applied Social Psychology, 34*(4), 709–730.
Rutter, M. (1985). Resilience in the face of adversity: Protective factors and resistance to psychiatric disorder. *British Journal of Psychiatry, 147*(1), 598–611.
Sarason, B. R., Sarason, I. G., & Pierce, G. R. (1990). *Social support: An interactional view*. New York: John Wiley & Sons.
Schulz, R., & Heckhausen, J. (1996). A life span model of successful aging. *American Psychologist, 51*(7), 702–714.
Smith, H. C. (1961). *Personality adjustment*. New York: McGraw-Hill.
Taylor, S. E., & Brown, J. D. (1988). Illusion and well-being: A social psychological perspective on mental health. *Psychological Bulletin, 103*, 193–210.
Tellegen, A., Lykken, D. T., Bouchard, T. J. J., Wilcox, K., Segal, N., & Rich, S. (1988). Personality similarity in twins reared apart and together. *Joumal of Personality and Social Psychology, 54*, 1031–1039.
Thompson, R. F. (2009). Habituation: A history. *Neurobiology of Learning and Memory, 92*, 127–134.
Tomyn, A. J., & Cummins, R. A. (2011). Subjective wellbeing and homeostatically protected mood: Theory validation with adolescents. *Journal of Happiness Studies, 12*(5), 897–914. doi: 10.1007/s10902-010-9235-5.
Tomyn, A. J., Weinberg, M. K., & Cummins, R. A. (2015). Intervention efficacy among 'at risk' adolescents: A test of Subjective Wellbeing Homeostasis Theory. *Social Indicators Research*. doi: 10.1007/s11205-014-0619-5.
Vallacher, R. R., & Nowak, A. (1997). The emergence of dynamical social psychology. *Psychological Inquiry, 8*, 73–99.
Werner, E. E. (1995). Resilience in development. *Current Directions in Psychological Science, 3*, 81–85.
Williams, D. E., & Thompson, J. K. (1993). Biology and behavior: A set-point hypothesis of psychological functioning. *Behavior Modification, 17*, 43–57. doi: 10.1177/01454455930171004.
Yap, S. C. Y., Anusic, I., & Lucas, R. E. (2014). Does happiness change? Evidence from longitudinal studies. In K. M. Sheldon & R. E. Lucas (Eds.), *Stability of Happiness: Theories and Evidence on Whether Happiness Can Change* (pp. 127–145). USA: Elsevier.

Chapter 5
Do People Adapt to Poorer Health? Health and Health Satisfaction over the Life Cycle

Richard A. Easterlin

Introduction

As editor and contributor to Social Indicators Research, Alex Michalos did much to advance knowledge of the relation between health and quality of life. The present paper is offered as a modest addition to this literature.

Traditionally, economists have been taught that well-being can be inferred from people's objective circumstances alone. But in the faraway land where psychology borders economics, a serious attack has been launched on this proposition. In 1999, three psychologists edited an encyclopedic tome entitled Well-Being: The Foundations of Hedonic Psychology (Kahneman et al. 1999). Running throughout much of this volume is the view that how happy or satisfied people are with their lives, that is, their *subjective* well-being, depends not only on their objective circumstances, but also on their goals – their subjective norms or aspirations. This, of course, is precisely the idea behind Michalos' "multiple discrepancies theory" (Michalos 1985). One's objective circumstances may improve, but whether subjective well-being also improves depends on whether goals change too, and by how much.

In psychology, however, proponents of the so-called "setpoint theory" have carried this view to an extreme. They see goals as adjusting rapidly and fully to changes in objective conditions, and well-being centering at a setpoint given by genetics and personality (Costa et al. 1987; Cummins 2010, 2012; Lykken and Tellegen 1996; Myers 1992). In this conception, life events such as serious injury or disease, a substantial salary increase, loss of a job, or death of one's child or lifelong partner may deflect a person above or below his or her setpoint, but hedonic

R.A. Easterlin (✉)
Department of Economics, University of Southern California,
Los Angeles, CA 90089-0253, USA
e-mail: easterl@usc.edu

F. Maggino (ed.), *A Life Devoted to Quality of Life*, Social Indicators Research Series 60, DOI 10.1007/978-3-319-20568-7_5

adaptation will fairly quickly return the individual to the initial level given by personality and genes. For example, in the volume just mentioned, Nobel Laureate Daniel Kahneman writes:

> Each individual may be on a personal treadmill that tends to restore well-being to a predetermined setpoint after each change of circumstances (Kahneman et al. 1999, 14).

In a similar vein, two other advocates of set point theory state:

> Chance events like personal tragedies, illness, or sudden strokes of good fortune may drastically affect the level of happiness, but apparently these effects do not last long (Csikszentmihalyi and Hunter 2003, 185–6).

Recently there has been a modest retreat from setpoint theory (Diener et al. 2006; Headey 2010; Headey et al. 2010; Lucas 2007; Yap et al. 2012), but its grip among psychologists seemingly remains strong, especially in regard to health.

The most widely cited article in psychology in the domain of health and well-being is undoubtedly a point-of-time study by Brickman et al. (1978). This article, in the words of Headey and Wearing (1989) "is often cited as showing that adaptation is so rapid and so complete that events have no detectable impact" (as examples Headey and Wearing reference Argyle 1987; Costa and McCrae 1980; Diener 1984). Actually, a careful reading of the Brickman et al. article indicates that in regard to health this study provides no support for the setpoint model. The article asserts only that accident victims (paraplegics and quadriplegics, numbering a mere 29) "did not appear nearly as unhappy as might have been expected" (p. 921). What "might have been expected" is never stated. The statistical analysis itself clearly demonstrates that relative to a group of controls (numbering 22), the accident victims "rated themselves significantly less happy" (p. 924).

There have been a number of studies since, some supporting the conclusion of complete adaptation to adverse health as some claim the 1978 study shows; others, contradicting it. To my knowledge the most comprehensive point-of-time investigation is one that compares the life satisfaction of disabled and nondisabled persons in two large national samples, each numbering over 600 (Mehnert et al. 1990). The principal result of this study is that the life satisfaction of disabled persons is, on average, significantly less than those who report no disabilities, a finding consistent with that of the Brickman et al. statistical analysis. Of even more importance is the finding by Mehnert and his collaborators that when persons with disabilities are classified in several different ways – according to the severity of the disability, whether the respondent suffers from one or multiple conditions, to what extent the respondent is limited in daily activities, and whether close others are thought to perceive the respondent as disabled – life satisfaction is less for those with more serious problems on every single one of these dimensions. Powdthavee (2009) also finds a significant decrease in life satisfaction associated with increased severity of disability. These results reinforce the inference that the state of one's health affects significantly one's life satisfaction.

Both the Mehnert et al. and Brickman et al. studies are based on cross-sectional data and one might argue that not enough time has been allowed for complete adaptation to occur to an adverse health event. In response, one might point to statements in the literature such as those quoted above that "these effects do not last long" or that "adaptation is so rapid and so complete that events have no discernible impact." But clearly what is needed is a study that follows a group of people over time to see whether adverse health change has a long-lasting impact on well-being. My purpose here is to contribute to this end, using the demographic technique of birth cohort analysis – what is sometimes termed, a "synthetic panel."

In what follows, I compare a summary measure of people's actual health over the life cycle with one on how they feel about their health, that is, their health satisfaction. The comparison here of health and health satisfaction is similar to earlier work by Michalos and Zumbo (2002). If people adapt fully to adverse health changes and adjust their standard of good health to conform to their actual circumstances, then satisfaction with health should remain unchanged, despite deterioration in their actual health. If they adapt less than fully (or not at all) to an adverse change in health, then satisfaction with health should decline. I also examine differences within the population by gender, race, birth cohort, and education to see whether differences in health are accompanied by corresponding differences in health satisfaction.

Data and Methods

The data are from the National Opinion Research Center's General Social Survey (GSS), a nationally representative sample of the population, conducted almost annually since 1972 (National Opinion Research Center 2011). For my measure of health I use a summary health measure, self-reported health. The question asked is, "Would you say your own health, in general, is excellent, good, fair or poor?" I have scaled the responses from "excellent" = 4 down to "poor" = 1.

There is ample evidence of the consistency of self-reported health with the presence of chronic diseases and of disabilities (e.g., Golini and Calvani 2001, p. 6; McNeil 1997, p. 14). An indication of the substantive significance of self-reported health is that it is found in longitudinal studies to be a significant predictor of both functional disability and mortality, even after controlling for health conditions identified in medical examinations and health histories (Idler and Kasl 1995; Idler et al. 1997; Smith et al. 2001). It is also found to be a significant predictor of expected retirement age after correcting for possible endogeneity of self-rated health (Dwyer and Mitchell 1999).

For my measure of subjective well-being I use satisfaction with health. This is the response to the following question:

> For each area of life I am going to name, tell me the number that shows how much satisfaction you get from that area: [The fifth item named is] your health and physical condition.

The numerical options for health satisfaction range from 7 (= "a very great deal") down to 1 (= "none"). I use health satisfaction here rather than overall happiness or life satisfaction because one would expect that changing health would directly affect satisfaction with health. For the total population and its components, mean values of health satisfaction, and also of self-rated health, are computed as averages of the individual numerical responses.

Unfortunately, GSS data on health satisfaction were only collected in the period 1973–1994. I have therefore confined the analysis of both self-reported health and health satisfaction to the data for 1973–1994 to ensure maximum comparability between the two measures. The wording of both questions has been constant over time, and their placement in the very lengthy GSS questionnaire has been the same in most years. The question on health satisfaction is typically separated from that on health by queries about people's helpfulness and trustworthiness, and the respondent's satisfaction with his or her place of residence, leisure time, family life, and friendships. It is unlikely, therefore, that a respondent when reporting satisfaction with health has in the forefront of his or her mind the answer about self-reported health given earlier, and to a different scale.

For the present analysis I have re-cast the data in life cycle form so that health and health satisfaction can be followed over the life course as people age from 18 to 89. Although any given birth cohort is observed at most for a period of about two decades, the full life cycle is inferred by piecing together the experience of eight 10-year birth cohorts, from the youngest of 1963–1972 to the oldest of 1893–1902. For example, the cohort of 1953–1962 is observed as it progresses from ages 20 to 32; the cohort of 1943–52 as it ages from 30 to 42; the cohort of 1933–1942 from ages 40 to 52; and so on. I also subdivide the data into gender, race (black and non-black), and education (those with at least 1 year of college and those with no college education). I confine the analysis of each cohort to the age span for which calendar year data are available for the entire 10-year birth cohort. For example, the cohort of 1953–1962 is observed in its entirety at age 25 in the calendar years 1978–1987, but only partially at age 35, because data are not available for those born in 1960–1962 who reach age 35 after 1994. Hence, data for the cohort of 1953–1962 are not included beyond age 32.

The analysis is based on OLS regressions (reported in Appendix A) of both health and health satisfaction on age and age squared, cohort, gender, race, and education using the individual data for 1973–1994. In what follows, the relationship reported of health (or health satisfaction) to any given independent variable is after controlling for the other variables in the regression.

Results

The story is quickly told, because it is so consistent. Over the life cycle health and health satisfaction decline steadily. Differences in health by gender, race, education, and cohort are all positively associated with differences in health satisfaction. I detail briefly the specific patterns in what follows.

Life Cycle Changes The National Health Interview Surveys (NHIS) document the deterioration of physical health with age. Chronic conditions such as cardiovascular disease, diabetes, emphysema, arthritis, musculo-skeletal conditions, and orthopedic impairments all get progressively worse, and the proportion of the population unable to work or limited in major activity increases (Reynolds et al. 1998, Tables 2 and 3).

Consistent with the NHIS health data, self-reported health, as surveyed in the GSS, declines steadily over the life course. Between ages 18 and 89 self-reported health falls from an initial mean value of 3.6 to 2.9, on a scale where 4=excellent and 1=poor (Fig. 5.1, dotted line). This is a substantial decline, equivalent to a downward shift of 70 % of the population by one out of four categories.

It should be emphasized that the association between health and age observed here is not based on point-of-time data. Because I control for cohort, one is observing the relationship of health to age as eight overlapping cohorts progress through the life span from age 18 to 89.

What about the life cycle pattern of satisfaction with health? The answer is that as health gets worse, so too do people's judgments of their health. At age 18, the mean value of health satisfaction, on a scale of 1 to 7, is 6.4; by 89 it has fallen to 5.0 (Fig. 5.1, solid line). Again, the decline is substantial, equivalent to a downward shift of 70 % of the population by two out of seven categories. (Because the numerical range of the response scale for health satisfaction is almost twice that for self-reported health, I have halved the scale in Fig. 5.1 for health satisfaction relative to that for health.)

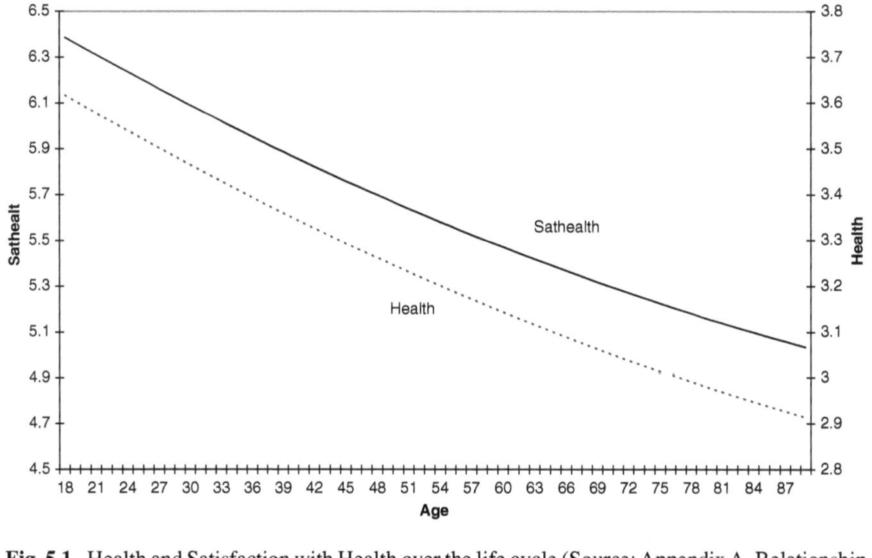

Fig. 5.1 Health and Satisfaction with Health over the life cycle (Source: Appendix A. Relationship is for nonblack males born 1933–1942 with at least some college education)

Population Differentials The health of blacks is substantially worse than that of nonblacks; so too is the health of less compared with more educated persons. Females are less healthy than males (Appendix A, col. 1). Although the gender difference is small compared with the race and education differences, it is statistically significant. The gender, race, and education differences in self-reported health all correspond to reports on presence of disease and limitation of activity found in the entirely independent National Health Interview Survey (Crimmins et al. 2004).

The differentials within the population in satisfaction with health are the same as those for health (Fig. 5.2). Blacks, less-educated persons, and females are all less satisfied with their health than their counterparts in the population. The positive association between health and health satisfaction between groups within the population is consistent with the positive association found in the life cycle trends.

Cohort Differences The four 10-year cohorts born prior to 1933 are significantly less healthy than the birth cohort of 1933–1942 (the reference group in the regression reported in Appendix A). Later born cohorts do not differ significantly from that of 1933–1942, except for the youngest cohort, that born in 1963–1972, which reports significantly poorer health than the birth cohort of 1933–1942. A plot, ranging from the earliest-born cohorts to the most recent, of the cohort deviations in health from that of 1933–1942 takes the form roughly of a hill tilted toward the left (Fig. 5.3, solid line). This cohort pattern for self-rated health corresponds to that for limitation of activity and functional disability found in NHIS data (Reynolds et al. 1998, Table 2).

The cohort pattern for satisfaction with health also takes the shape of a hill, but for health satisfaction the hill is tipped sharply to the right (Fig. 5.3, broken line). There is no significant difference in health satisfaction between the cohort of 1933–1942 and the four 10-year cohorts born earlier. Those born later, however, report progressively less health satisfaction, with the most recent cohort, that of 1963–1972, least satisfied of all.

There is, then, a general similarity in the hill-like pattern of health and health satisfaction, but the hills tilt in different directions. The gap between health satisfaction and health becomes progressively more negative among recent cohorts. One possible explanation is that the GSS question on satisfaction with health asks about "your health *and physical condition*" (emphasis added). It is possible that the recent and much-publicized rise in obesity affects responses adversely, particularly for younger cohorts because of dissatisfaction with their physical condition.

Magnitude Differences by age, cohort, gender, race, and education in health satisfaction are in the same direction as those in self-reported health. How, on average, do the two variables compare with regard to the magnitude of these differences? To answer this, the annual data here for individuals are pooled, and health satisfaction is regressed on health. The results are as follows (t-stat in parentheses):

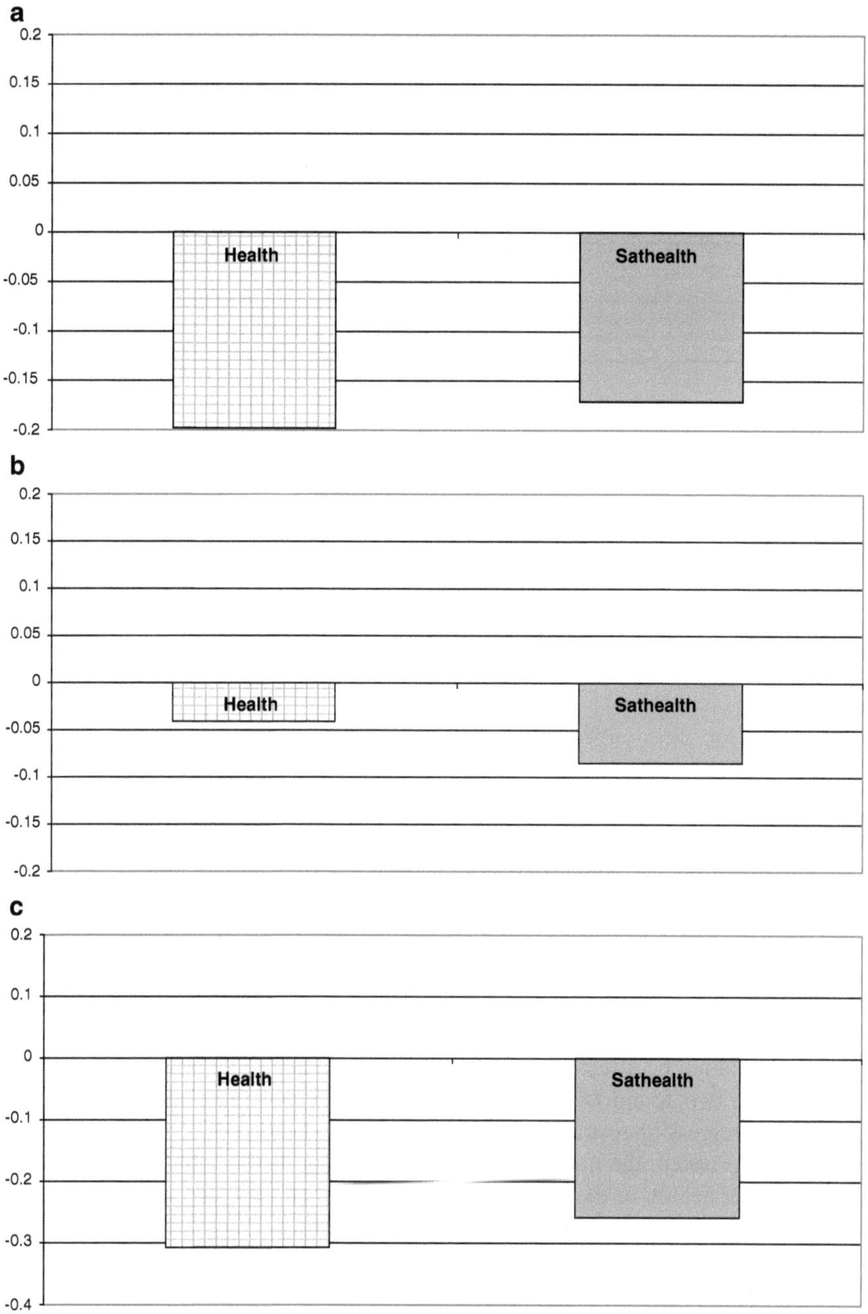

Fig. 5.2 Differences between specified population groups in Health and Satisfaction with Health, 1973–1994. (**a**) Deviation of blacks from nonblacks (**b**) Deviation of females from males (**c**) Deviation of persons with no college education from those with some college education (Source: Appendix A. Differences are after controlling for age, cohort and other population groups)

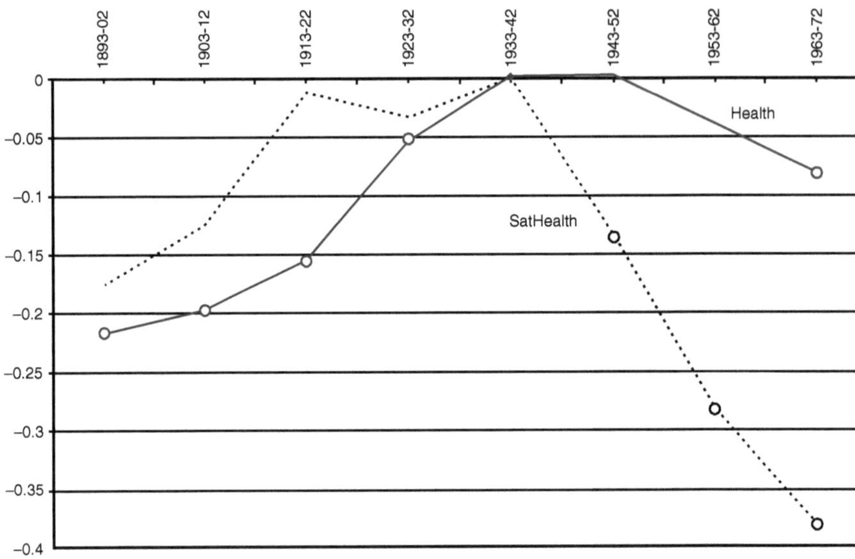

Fig. 5.3 Deviation of specified Cohort from Cohort of 1933–1942 in Health and Satisfaction with Health, 1973–1994 (Source: Appendix A. Circled points are differences from the 1933–1942 cohort with $p<0.1$. Differences are after controlling for age, gender, race and education)

$$\text{Sathealth} = 1.0770\ \text{Health} + 2.2469$$
$$(90.94)\quad(60.87)$$
$$n = 12{,}981\quad \text{Adj.}R^2 = .3892$$

The coefficient of health satisfaction on health is positive and highly significant, indicating that differences among individuals in satisfaction with health typically correspond to differences in their self-reported health status – the better one's health, the better one feels about it.

If people adapted fully to adverse health circumstances, then there would be no significant association between health and health satisfaction, because health satisfaction would not be affected by changes in actual health. The positive association between the two found here implies that people do not fully adapt to changing health. The regression results, however, do give an indication of some adaptation. In the questions asked, the numerical response scale for health satisfaction is almost twice that for health. In the absence of adaptation, therefore, one would expect the regression coefficient, the change in health satisfaction per unit change in health, to be about two. In fact, the regression coefficient only slightly exceeds one. This suggests that while standards of good health do change in the same direction as actual health, they only change by about half as much.

Discussion

If, as the setpoint model implies, people simply change their standards of good health commensurately with changes in their actual health status, so that their well-being is unaffected by such changes, then satisfaction with health should not change as actual health changes. In fact, over the life course, satisfaction with health tends to decline as health itself deteriorates. Moreover, differences in health and health satisfaction by gender are positively associated, as are differences by race, education, and cohort. The results suggest that changes and differences in health do, on average, have a corresponding effect on well-being, contrary to the setpoint model.

It might be argued that the positive association between the responses to health and health satisfaction is because both are influenced in a similar way by personality characteristics. It is well-known, for example, that neuroticism is negatively associated with life satisfaction, and extroversion, positively associated (Diener and Lucas 1999). Thus neurotics with a serious disability might give more negative assessments on both health and health satisfaction than others in the population in the same health circumstances. It is unlikely, however, that the positive association between health and health satisfaction found here in the differences by race, gender, and education are due to personality. For this to be true, one would have to argue that blacks, women, and less educated persons are, on average, more neurotic and/or less extroverted than others in the population. Nor is it likely that the life course trends in health and health satisfaction are due to personality, because it is hard to see how personality might account for the fact that the decline in health satisfaction is about half what one would expect due to the decline in actual health. In general, therefore, it seems unlikely that personality could account for the results reported here.

Although the present results contradict the psychologists' setpoint model, they do lend support to psychologists' emphasis on the relevance to well-being of subjective norms, as well as actual life circumstances. Health satisfaction does change in the same direction as actual health, but it changes by only about half of what one might expect. This implies that health standards do change with actual health, and that the effect on well-being of a deterioration in health is mitigated by this change in standards. Thus, the economists' assumption that objective circumstances alone are sufficient to infer well-being is called into question. The most reasonable model of well-being seems to be one that includes norms along with objective circumstances, a middle ground between the economists' "objective circumstances" approach and the psychologists' setpoint model.

Why does health satisfaction decline with age, but seemingly not as rapidly? A speculative answer can be suggested. Following Michalos's multiple discrepancies theory, one may distinguish between the course of health goals and actual health. The course of health goals is determined by two types of comparison: with others (interpersonal) and with one's past experience (intrapersonal). If comparison with others were the *only* determinant of health goals, then one might expect health goals to decline to the same extent as actual health ("the health of everyone my age is getting worse too"). As a result there would be no change in the gap between health goals and actual health and hence, no change in satisfaction with health. If, in contrast, health goals were fixed at their early adulthood peak, then the gap between health goals and actual health would widen commensurately with the decline in actual health ("I can't do the things I used to do"). The result would be a decline in satisfaction with health equal in magnitude to the decline in actual health.

The finding that health satisfaction declines about half as much as might be expected based on the actual decline in health suggests that both interpersonal and intrapersonal comparisons play about an equal role in determining health goals. In answer to the question posed in the title to this article: people do adapt to poorer health, but only partly.

Acknowledgements I am grateful for the assistance of Donna Hokoda Ebata, Pouyan Mashayekh-Ahangarani, and Shaked Peleg. Financial support was provided by the University of Southern California.

Appendix A

OLS regression of Health and Satisfaction with Health on specified variables, 1973–1994

	(1)	(2)	(3)	(4)	(5)	(6)
Variable	Health			Sathealth		
	Coef.	t	p>|t|	Coef.	t	p>|t|
age	−0.149813	−5.89	0.000	−.0292475	−4.87	0.000
age^2	.0000473	1.83	0.067	.0000954	1.55	0.121
coh.1963–1972	−.0807686	−2.68	0.007	−.3805667	−5.20	0.000
coh.1953–1962	−.0391296	−1.63	0.104	−.2816966	−5.15	0.000
coh.1943–1952	.0031637	0.16	0.873	−.1347602	−3.29	0.001
coh.1923–1932	−.0508889	−2.31	0.021	−.0326354	−0.73	0.466
coh.1913–1922	−.1550985	−5.50	0.000	−.0120409	−0.20	0.844
coh.1903–1912	−.1969902	−4.98	0.000	−.1237737	−1.40	0.162
coh.1893–1902	−.2161338	−3.61	0.000	−.1761639	−1.34	0.181
male (=1)	.0410763	3.90	0.000	.084954	4.08	0.000
black (=1)	−.1981374	−13.27	0.000	−.1708531	−5.77	0.000
ed ≤ 12 (=1)	−.3068997	−27.81	0.000	−.2582432	−11.74	0.000
constant	3.830732	54.42	0.000	6.796419	41.92	0.000
n	23,531			19,992		
Adj R^2	0.1237			0.0497		

Source: National Opinion Research Center (2011)
Note: Reference groups for dummy variables: cohort 1933–1942, female, nonblack, education more than 12 years

References

Argyle, M., 1987. The Psychology of Happiness. London: Methuen.

Brickman, P. D. Coates and R. Janoff-Bulman, 1978. "Lottery Winners and Accident Victims: Is Happiness Relative?" Journal of Personality and Social Psychology, 36, 917–927.

Costa, Paul T. Jr. and Robert R. McCrae, 1980. "Influence of Extraversion and Neuroticism on Subjective Well-Being," Journal of Personality and Social Psychology, 38, 668–678.

Costa, Paul T. Jr., Alan B. Zonderman, Robert R. McCrae, Joan Cornoni-Huntley, Ben Z. Locke, and Helen E. Barbano, 1987. "Longitudinal Analyses of Psychological Well-Being in a National Sample: Stability of Mean Levels," Journal of Gerontology, 42:1, 50–55.

Crimmins, Eileen M., Mark D. Hayward, and Teresa Seeman, 2004. "Race/Ethnicity, Socioeconomic Status, and Health," in N. Anderson, R. Bulatao, and B. Cohen, eds., Critical Perspectives on Race and Ethnic Differences in Health in Later Life, National Academy of Sciences, 310–352.

Csikszentmihalyi M, Hunter J (2003) Happiness in Everyday Life: The Uses of Experience Sampling. Journal of Happiness Studies 4(2): 185–199.

Cummins RA (2010) Subjective Wellbeing, Homeostatically Protected Mood and Depression: A Synthesis. Journal of Happiness Studies 11(1): 1–17.

Cummins RA (2012). The Determinants of Happiness. International Journal of Happiness and Development 1(1): 86–101.

Diener, Ed, 1984. "Subjective Well-Being," Psychological Bulletin, 45, 542–575.

Diener, Ed, and Richard E. Lucas, 1999. "Personality and Subjective Well-Being," in Daniel Kahneman, Ed Diener, and Norbert Schwarz (eds.), Well-Being: The Foundations of Hedonic Psychology, New York: Russell Sage, 213–229.

Diener E, Lucas RE, Scollon CN (2006) Beyond the Hedonic Treadmill: Revising the Adaptation Theory of Well-Being. American Psychologist 61(4): 305–14.

Dwyer, Debra Sabatini and Olivia S. Mitchell, 1999. "Health Problems as Determinants of Retirement: Are Self-Rated Measures Endogenous?" Journal of Health Economics 18, 173–193.

Golini, Antonio and Plautilla Calvani, 2001. Relationships Between Perceptions of Health, Chronic Diseases and Disabilities, Nihon University, Population Research Institute.

Headey, Bruce and Alexander Wearing, 1989. "Personality, Life Events, and Subjective Well-Being: Toward a Dynamic Equilibrium Model," Journal of Personality and Social Psychology, 57:4, 731–739.

Headey B (2010), The set point theory of well-being has serious flaws: On the eve of a scientific revolution? Social Indicators Research (97): 7–21.

Headey B, Muffles R, Wagner GG (2010). Long-running German panel survey shows that personal and economic choices, not just genes, matter for happiness. Proceedings of the National Academy of Sciences 107(42): 17922–17926.

Idler, Ellen L. and Yael Banyamini, 1997. "Self-Rated Health and Mortality: A Review of Twenty-Seven Community Studies," Journal of Health and Social Behavior, 38:1 (March), 21–37.

Idler, Ellen L. and Stanislav V. Kasl, 1995. "Self-Ratings of Health: Do They Also Predict Change in Functional Ability?" Journal of Gerontology: Social Sciences, 50B(6), S344–S353.

Kahneman, Daniel, Ed Diener, and Norbert Schwarz, eds., 1999. Well-Being: The Foundations of Hedonic Psychology. New York: Russell Sage.

Lucas, RE (2007). Adaptation and the Set-Point Model of Subjective Well-Being: Does Happiness Change after Major Life Events? Current Directions in Psychological Science 16(2): 75–79.

Lykken, David and Auke Tellegen, 1996. "Happiness is a Stochastic Phenomenon," Psychological Science, 7:3 (May), 180–189.

McNeil, Jack, 1997. "Americans with Disabilities," U.S. Census Bureau, Current Population Reports, Series P-70-73, Household Economic Studies, 1–17.

Michalos, A. C., 1985. "Multiple Discrepancies Theory (MDT)." Social Indicators Research 16(4), 347–413.

Michalos, A.C. and Bruno Zumbo, 2002. "Healthy Days, Health Satisfaction and Satisfaction with Overall Quality of Life," Social Indicators Research, 59(3), 321–338.
Mehnert, Thomas, Herbert H. Kraus, Rosemary Nadler, and Mary Boyd, 1990. "Correlates of Life Satisfaction in Those with Disabling Conditions", Rehabilitation Psychology, 35(1), 3–17.
Myers, David G., 1992. The Pursuit of Happiness. New York: Avon.
National Opinion Research Center, 2011. General Social Surveys, 1972–2010. Chicago: National Opinion Research Center.
Powdthavee, Nattavudh, 2009. "What Happens to People Before and After Disability? Focusing Effects, Lead Effects and Adaptation in Different Areas of Life," Social Science and Medicine 69, 1834–1844.
Reynolds, Sandra L., Eileen M. Crimmins, and Yasuhiko Saito, 1998. "Cohort Differences in Disability and Disease Presence," The Gerontologist, 38:5, 578–590.
Smith, V. Kerry, Donald H. Taylor, Jr., and Frank A. Sloan, 2001. "Longevity Expectations and Death: Can People Predict their Own Demise?" American Economic Review 91:4 (September), 1126–1134.
Yap SCY, Anusic I, Lucas RE (2012). Does personality moderate reaction and adaptation to major life events? Evidence from the British Household Panel Survey. Journal of Research in Personality 46: 477–488.

Chapter 6
Progress: Concept and Measurement

Heinz-Herbert Noll

Introduction

Progress, or – more specifically – societal progress[1] appears to be a normative concept, which in its essence may be understood as the change or advancement of major conditions of societies and people's lives in a direction considered to be desirable based on prevailing social values and shared political goals of societal development. Seen from the retrospect, progress thus means that present conditions of life and society are considered as an improvement compared to the past, in a prospective view, it means that future conditions are envisaged to be better than those of present times.

Even though the "demise of the idea of progress" (Sztompka 1994: 33) had already been noticed and (prematurely) pronounced by notable scholars quite some decades ago, the concept has seen an unexpected and remarkable renaissance more recently. The renewed interest in and popularity of the concept of progress is closely related to the currently flourishing debate on measuring well-being "beyond GDP" and thus to alternative approaches of defining and measuring betterments of people's living conditions, societal characteristics and life quality in ways, which are not restricted to economic terms. Particularly the "OECD – Global Project on Measuring the *Progress* of Societies", that was first presented at the "World Forum on Key Indicators" in 2004 as well as recommendations of the so-called 'Stiglitz

---

This article is a revised and extended version of a long entry on "Societal Progress" in the "Encyclopedia of Quality of Life and Well-Being Research", edited by Alex Michalos.

[1] I prefer to use the broader term 'societal progress' rather than 'social progress' as the latter has a strong connotation to social issues as they are addressed by welfare state policies.

H.-H. Noll (✉)
Formerly Social Indicators Research Centre of GESIS, 122155, 68072 Mannheim, Germany
e-mail: hh.noll@t-online.de

F. Maggino (ed.), *A Life Devoted to Quality of Life*, Social Indicators Research Series 60, DOI 10.1007/978-3-319-20568-7_6

Commission' on the "Measurement of Economic Performance and *Social Progress*" (Stiglitz et al. 2010) have stimulated a new debate on societal progress and its meaning in our present times.

Conceptual Issues

History

Although it has been shown that the idea of directed change towards better human conditions is ancient and can be traced back to Greek and Roman philosophers (Nisbet 1980), the concept of progress is usually considered to be a child of the age of enlightenment and modern times. Characterized by a strong belief in the power of human reason, the gradual replacement of religious and traditional beliefs by scientific thinking as well as the fights for civil rights and liberties, the age of enlightenment gave birth to optimistic views of being capable to shape and improve human conditions and thus promoted the idea of and hope for progress. As a representative of this age, the French philosopher and politician Marquis de Condorcet saw "the human race, freed from its chains and marching with a firm tread on the road of truth and virtue and happiness" (see Bossard 1931/1932: 8). The notion of progress thus became a characteristic if not 'trademark' of modernity, flourishing particularly during the industrial age, and it was not least closely related to working class movements, unions, and 'progressive' political parties aiming to improve working and living conditions of employees and their families successfully.

In social theory the notions and ideas of progress have always played a crucial role, beginning with the works of Auguste Comte (law of three stages) and Herbert Spencer (evolution as the progressive development of society) until our present times, although in varying intensity. For example, the concept of progress was explicitly addressed in a series of articles published in the Journal "Social Forces" during the 1930s. In one of those articles, James Bossard (1931/32: 14) interestingly characterizes progress as a "term, which is used to indicate a consciousness of movement in a given direction, considered at the time to be desirable. There are involved …not one, but three ideas in the modern concept of progress: the idea of change, …the idea of valuation, and …the idea of control". In his book on "life chances", the eminent German sociologist Ralf Dahrendorf (1979: 11 ff.) emphasizes the normative character of the concept of progress, a concept that in his notion is useful in order to determine and analyze the direction of social change. Referring to Kant, Dahrendorf adopted a regulative rather than a constitutive understanding of progress, which means that progress is not supposed to be constitutive for human history, but only as a possibility. More recently scholars as prominent as Jeffrey Alexander, Piotr Sztompka (1990), Claus Offe (2011) and others have taken up the issue again with major contributions to clarify the concept and to discuss its present day meanings.

Notions of the Idea of Progress

The concept of progress has been used in a variety of different notions, changing over time. There is a common understanding however, that progress indicates a directional valued social or societal change, which is to be distinguished clearly from other sorts of societal developments like neutral change, stagnation, cyclical change, or regress. Beyond this basic notion, the literature exhibits numerous differences in ways of understanding and attributing basic characteristics to the concept of progress.

According to Sztompka (1994: 27ff.), important variations in the understanding and usage of the concept of progress are related to a set of basic components, such as the 'shape of the process', the 'necessity' of progress, the 'manner of operation', and the 'moving forces'. Regarding the shape of the process, approaches understanding progress as continuous, gradual, cumulative or even linear changes towards better states of society may be distinguished from understandings of progress as a stepwise, incremental, uneven or eventually even revolutionary process. While progress may be considered a necessity in the course of history, at least in the long run, as for example suggested by Marxist approaches, but eventually also by modernization theory,[2] it may alternatively also be regarded as a possibility or chance only, which must not necessarily occur. A third variation in the understanding of progress concerns the 'manner of operation': While progress can be understood as an outcome of an harmonious unfolding of inherent potentials and thus a peaceful process, it may also be considered a result of tensions, contradictions, conflict and fights, as for example 'class struggle' proposed in Marxist theory. Another important distinction concerns the forces bringing progress about: Is progress considered as a result of unintended processes, as for example evolution and market activities,[3] or even side effects of certain forces, or is progress deemed to be the result of human agency, which has to be aimed at and to be achieved. Offe (2011: 79), for example, represents the latter view, proposing an understanding of progress as "the outcome of collective intentional efforts driven by reason" and "not the evolutionary outcome of the blind forces of change". Sztompka, after all, arrives at the conclusion of a new conceptualization of progress "(1) as a potential capacity, rather than ultimate achievement, (2) as a dynamic, evolving, relative quality of a concrete process, rather than absolute, universal, external standard, (3) as a historical possibility, opportunity, open option rather than necessary, inevitable, inexorable tendency, (4) as a product – often unintended, and even unrecognized – of human pluralistic and collective actions, rather than a result of divine will, good intensions of exceptional individuals, or operation of automatic social mechanisms" (Sztompka 1990: 251).

---

[2] Modernization theory, which is not undisputed, addresses and analyses the processes of modernization of societies as a sequential and progressive transition from traditional to modern' societies, eventually distinguishing different preconditions – such as value and life style changes – as well as different stages.

[3] E.g. according to Norbert Elias (1969), the progressive evolution of civilization is to be considered as unintended and not rationally achieved progress.

Current Views and Discourses

The period of 'triumphant modernity' (Touraine 1992: 21–108) has been considered by many observers as the 'true' era of societal and social progress. Particularly in the second half of the twentieth century citizens of many nations – primarily in the so-called Western World – enjoyed unprecedented betterments of living conditions and quality of life: substantial reductions of working hours and increase in leisure time, improved working conditions, expanded welfare state regulations and benefits, better education for large parts of the population, rising incomes and living standards, advanced health and extended longevity, to name just a few. All these developments were unequivocally welcomed as improvements of individual and collective quality of life and considered as progress by the large majority of the populations almost everywhere. More recent societal developments in European and other well-off Western nations however seem to undermine the notion of progress: stagnating or even decreasing real incomes, enduring high levels of unemployment, increasing inequalities, growth of poverty and 'the working poor', expansion of precarious jobs and working conditions, as well as the dismantling of welfare state institutions and cutbacks in welfare state benefits are some of the changes observed in various nations raising doubts about the progressive character of current societal developments. These doubts have also been fueled by numerous negative side effects of the raising material level of living in many societies, such as environmental impairments, but also strain and stress or even mental illness (Eckersley 2008) and other diseases of civilization. Even if changes seem to be positive and progressive at first glance, it is not always clear whether or not they are making life ultimately really better, as for example the debate about the quality of the additional life years resulting from extended longevity has demonstrated impressively. Moreover, there are good reasons to assume, that the social consensus about the elements of a 'good life' and the desirable directions of social change has weakened due to a differentiation of needs and a pluralization of value orientations and life styles.

Given this background, it is perhaps not too surprising, that considerable parts or even majorities of the populations in many European societies recently assessed the changes of the social situation in their countries in a way that 'life is getting worse', perceiving a decline of their quality of life rather than improvements and progress. Results from the European Social Survey 2006 suggest, that more than 50 % of the respondents in 11 of the 23 nations covered 'agree' or 'strongly' agree that "for most people in their country life is getting worse" (Fig. 6.1). In some countries this percentage even extends 80 % and thus reaches alarming levels.

The prevailing skepticism and pessimism in contemporary theoretical discourses on progress are to a considerable degree due to postmodernism and related views of history and social change. As Anthony Giddens (1993: 665) put it more than 20 years ago, "modern societies…took their inspiration from the idea that history has a 'shape' – it 'goes somewhere', and leads to 'progress'. … The advocates of the idea of postmodernity suggest today that this notion has collapsed". Also Gordon Marshall notices a significant change in the attitude toward progress in the postmodern age: "For most of the twentieth century, theories of progress followed the pattern

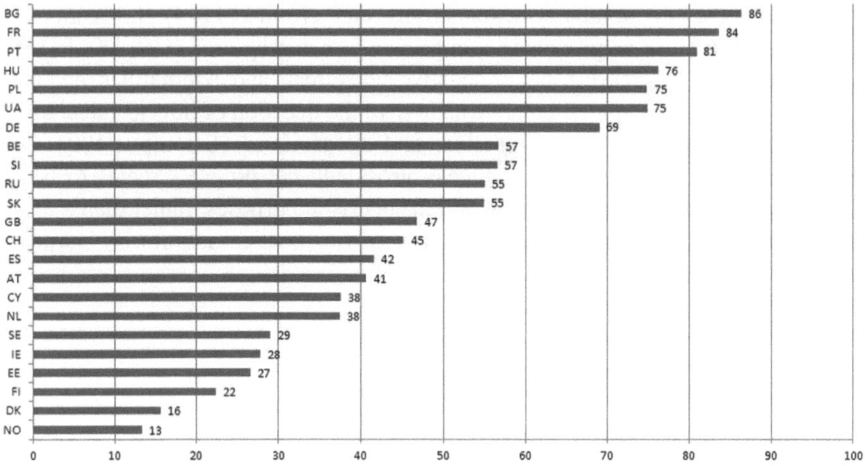

Fig. 6.1 "For most people in country life is getting worse" – % Agree/strongly agree (2006) (Source: Noll and Weick 2011; Database: European Social Survey 2006)

of the nineteenth – optimistic, rationalistic, materialistic. ... At the century's end, however, the idea of progress seems to be in eclipse" (Marshall 1994: 420). The skeptical and pessimistic views grounded in postmodern thinking even seem to have been reinforced by the recent economic crisis and the negative consequences on people's living conditions it had or still has in many societies around the globe.

Even though it was apparently premature to proclaim the "demise of the idea of progress" (Sztompka 1994: 33), it seems to be obvious that there is a need to rethink or eventually even redefine the meaning and notion of progress in the twenty first century. Another important line of skepticism concerning the possibility and meaningfulness of further progress is rooted in the paradigm shift toward sustainable development initiated at the end of the twentieth century and related doubts and concerns about the sustainability of progress in its traditional notion,[4] particularly in its understanding as a further advancement of the material level of living in rich as well as developing societies. According to the German sociologist Claus Offe, these sorts of concerns have turned the notion of progress into a 'logic of preventing regression', shifting the emphasis from 'moving ahead' to sustaining the achieved level of well-being and to prevent decline and regress. Thus, in other words, the metaphor of 'marching forward' is going to be replaced by "establishing effective stop signs" (Offe 2011: 86). As an alternative to such a de facto abandoning of the goal of achieving progress, which seems to be rather unlikely to be accepted by human mankind, it has been proposed to eventually re-conceptualize the idea of progress "in such a way that it captures all those elements which may have been

[4]As a policy goal sustainability or sustainable development was for the first time proposed by the Brundtland Commission in its 1987 report "Our Common Future".

neglected in the past: solidarity, sustainability, etc." (Kohl 2011: 4). Suggestions of this sort come close to proposing a concept of "net progress" (Offe 2011: 88f), which means gross-progress, net of negative side effects and externalities, and may thus also be understood as a tentative answer to the question of how to calculate "a balance of benefits and harms, functions and disfunctions" (Sztompka 1994: 29). However, as yet, the distinction between gross and net progress seems to be an option solely at the conceptual level and for heuristic purposes, rather than a feasible methodological approach, ready to be used for practical monitoring purposes and empirical research.

Measurement and Monitoring of Progress

Countless statistical measures of societal progress have been proposed over many years and decades. First suggestions of how to monitor progress empirically have been presented as early as at the beginning of the twentieth century (see Bossard 1931/1932: 13). With his book "*Les indices numérique de la civilisation et du progress*" (1921) the Italian statistician and criminologist Alfredo Niceforo made an important early effort to systematically "identify quantifiable symptoms of living conditions in a broad sense – indicators in our modern terminology – in order to measure and monitor levels and degrees of civilisation and social progress across time and space" (Noll 2004: 152). Seen from the retrospect, Nicefero thus apparently was an important predecessor of the social indicators movement,[5] which emerged in the 1960s and put the measurement of progress – in terms of improvements of living conditions and quality of life and societies – explicitly at the agenda of research institutes, statistical offices and governments at national and supranational levels. The character of social indicators as measures of progress is pretty well reflected in some of the early definitions. Raymond Bauer – one of the pioneers of the movement – defined social indicators as "statistics …and other forms of evidence that enable us to assess where we stand and are going with respect to our values and goals" (Bauer 1966: 1). Mancur Olson considered a social indicator as "a statistic of direct normative interest which facilitates concise, comprehensive and balanced judgements about the condition of major aspects of a society. …It is a direct measure of welfare and is subject to the interpretation that if it changes in the 'right' direction… things have gotten better, or people are 'better off'" (Department of Health, Education, and Welfare 1969: 97). Both definitions thus emphasize the function of social indicators to measure and monitor societal progress in the sense

[5]Alex Michalos has been an eminent member and protagonist of this movement over a long period of time in many respects. Apart from his countless well-respected scholarly contributions, he was not only the founder and longtime editor of the first and most esteemed specialized international journal on "Social Indicators Research", but also a main driver of a successful institutionalization of social indicators research, e.g. in his role as a 'founding father' of the Working Group (now Research Committee) 'Social Indicators' in the International Sociological Association (see Noll and Michalos 2014).

of improvements in well-being over time, or societal change relative to normative standards, such as values and development goals. In subsequent years, research on social indicators has resulted in different sorts of measurement tools and instruments, indicators and indicator systems, composite indices as well as population surveys, with a view to empirically monitor progress continuously.[6]

The ongoing activities of monitoring societal progress as part of social indicators research and social reporting activities have received new stimuli and momentum by a recently renewed interest in the measurement of well-being and progress "beyond GDP" among economists, official statistics and policy makers. This renewed interest and debate has been triggered off by initiatives like the "OECD – Global Project on Measuring the *Progress* of Societies" (Hall et al. 2010), the report of the so-called 'Stiglitz Commission' on the "Measurement of Economic Performance and *Social Progress*" (Stiglitz et al. 2010), but also the "beyond GDP" initiative of the European Commission (www.beyond-gdp.eu/) and diverse projects on measuring well-being and progress at the national level, e.g. in Australia and Ireland. Apart from few exceptions, theoretical and conceptual issues are however rarely reflected thoroughly within this new debate on the measurement of progress.

Since the concept of progress is multidimensional by nature, as it is the case with underlying concepts like well-being and quality of life, it seems to be obvious first of all, that measurement approaches, like e.g. indicator systems (Noll 2014) or so-called indicator dashboards, suggest a multitude of measures to comprehensively cover the diverse dimensions and sub-dimensions deemed to be relevant. Actually, such an approach based on a multitude of single indicators, seems to be the only way to arrive at a detailed diagnosis, whether or not the various elements have been changing in the desired direction and to which degree goals and objectives have been achieved. Since the different domains and dimensions considered to be relevant, may change in an uneven or asynchronous way, a measurement approach based on a variety of single indicators may however not necessarily lead to a clear cut and unequivocal overall assessment that things have gotten better or worse. Rather it turns out to be quite likely that changes in different domains and dimensions will not only taking place at different rates, but also go in different – more or less desirable – directions, e.g. increasing unemployment may go together with extended longevity, and raising household incomes may be accompanied by increasing crime rates. In other words: because 'uni-dimensional' change must not result in 'syndromatic' change (Novak 1990: 235f), there is a good chance that "progress in certain sectors of society does not add up to a comprehensive progress throughout the whole that earns the name of progress in the singular" (Joas 1990: 188).

Against this background there is thus a demand – first and foremost expressed by policy makers – for measures allowing to balance the various developments in different domains and dimensions of life and to allow unidimensional measurement of a multidimensional concept or phenomenon. This demand is being addressed by constructing so-called 'composite indices' of progress. To our knowledge, Niceforo

[6] For an extensive review of currently existing social monitoring and reporting activities in Europe see Noll and Berger (2014).

(1921) was also among the first scholars aiming to develop a composite index of progress, which he considered as an improvement of the total of living conditions across time. However, his efforts to develop such an index were not successful and apparently he dismissed this idea with some disillusionment:

> …one may measure the most palpable characteristics – mortality, average wealth, tobacco consumption, number of persons able to read and write, severe crimes – by indicators and summarize those indicators by a total index. By doing so, one would eventually arrive at a single synthetic measure, but would it be really useful? Not to mention the countless difficulties to be faced by calculating a summary index, which – to my knowledge – cannot all be solved. (my own translation from the German edition: Niceforo 1930: 136f)

In recent years, research aiming to develop composite indices of wellbeing and progress has been flourishing and currently there are plenty composite index measures available, which have been proposed as measures of progress. Among the most popular are the "Genuine Progress Index", which comprises 26 separate indicators (http://genuineprogress.net/genuine-progress-indicator/), the "Human Development Index" (http://hdr.undp.org/en/content/human-development-index-hdi), the "Happy-Planet-Index" (http://www.happyplanetindex.org/) and not least the "OECD-Better-Life-Index" (www.oecdbetterlifeindex.org/). Also at national level several composite indices of progress have been proposed, such as the Canadian Index of Wellbeing[7] (https://uwaterloo.ca/canadian-index-wellbeing) or the Australian National Development Index (www.andi.org.au/), responding to the requirement to take national particularities into account. Although the composite index approaches mentioned differ in their conceptual foundations, aims, coverage in terms of domains and dimensions, number and sorts of indicators employed, and not least their underlying methodologies, all of them are characterized by the ambitious objective of providing unidimensional quantitative measures for the multidimensional concept of wellbeing and societal progress. All of these measures obviously have their particular strengths and weaknesses, also in methodological terms. However as yet, no general agreement has been achieved of how a composite index of societal progress should look like, neither in terms of which single domains, dimensions, and indicators are to be included, nor methodologically, e.g. concerning weighting, best practices of standardization, aggregation etc.

Rather than relying on a composite-index-approach, it has also been argued, that summary measures of subjective well-being, such as individual life satisfaction and happiness, may actually do better than objective measures on this account and should be used to measure societal progress – exclusively or in addition to other sorts of indicators. Proponents of such an approach argue first of all, that summary measures of subjective well-being as measures of ultimate outcomes were much closer to what "really counts" and what is considered to be important in terms of societal progress. Moreover, compared to composite indices, the superiority of subjective well-being measures, such as life satisfaction, is deduced from the fact, that unidimensionality in this case is not the result of mathematical operations, but rather

[7] Alex Michalos actually is one of the "foundational leaders" of the Canadian Index of Well-Being project and continues to be a member of the "CIW Canadian Research Advisory Group".

the outcome of cognitive and emotional psychological processes within the individual, who takes stock of the various components and elements of his or her life. Under these circumstances the methodological challenges and difficulties of calculating composite indices, such as the normalization and standardization of indicators, selecting and applying weights, choosing a specific aggregation calculus, obviously can be avoided.

However, the usefulness of subjective well-being indicators as measures of progress is all but undisputed, and there are several reasons why indicators of subjective well-being – particularly life satisfaction – do not seem to be well qualified for the measurement of progress. Among those reasons is first of all the observation, that life satisfaction scores are typically rather stable and do not change much across time, even under circumstances of significant improvements of objective living conditions, which are usually considered as progress. The evolution of life satisfaction in West- and East-Germany (Fig. 6.2) seems to be a good example for this observation, but more or less unchanged levels of life satisfaction over extended periods of time have also been observed in numerous other European and non-European societies.[8]

A most impressive case is East-Germany, which underwent a radical economic, political and social change, and faced major improvements of living conditions, while the average life satisfaction score – 6.6 at the 0–10 scale[9] – in 2011 turns out to be at exactly the same level as it was in 1990! The apparently very limited sensitivity of life satisfaction measures to changes in objective circumstances have been explained by the finding that "changes in the environment, although important for short-term well-being, lose salience over time through processes of adaptation, and have small effects on long-term SWB" (Diener and Lucas 1999: 227), an observation, which may be considered as a generalized explanation of the Easterlin-Paradox (Easterlin 1974), which initially was focused on economic growth and its impact on SWB only. Adaptation thus seems to be the key mechanism, which makes life satisfaction and other indicators of subjective well-being particularly insensitive to objective social change and – in consequence – poor measures of societal progress.[10] In a recent paper on "The financial crisis and the well-being of Americans", Angus Deaton (2012) identifies not only strong questionnaire-context-effects on measures of subjective well-being, but also finds that "in a world of bread and circuses, measures like happiness that are sensitive to short-term ephemera, and that are affected more by the arrival of St Valentine's Day than to a doubling of unemployment, are measures that pick up the circuses but miss the bread" (Deaton 2012:

[8] This does not mean, that average life satisfaction levels turn out to be totally invariant across time. Average satisfaction may go up or down in certain periods of time (Noll 2008: 7f), but – according to the available empirical evidence – in the long run there seems to be little change overall.

[9] Doubts that satisfaction or happiness indicators are well qualified to measure progress, result also from the fact that the answering scales used are closed rather than open ended, e.g. 0–10, 1–7, and thus – contrary to household income, GDP, and almost all other objective progress-indicators – do not allow unlimited increase of scale values (Noll 2013: 8).

[10] This is not to say that subjective social indicators in general are necessarily poor measures of progress. There are other sorts of subjective social indicators, which seem to be much less affected by adaptation.

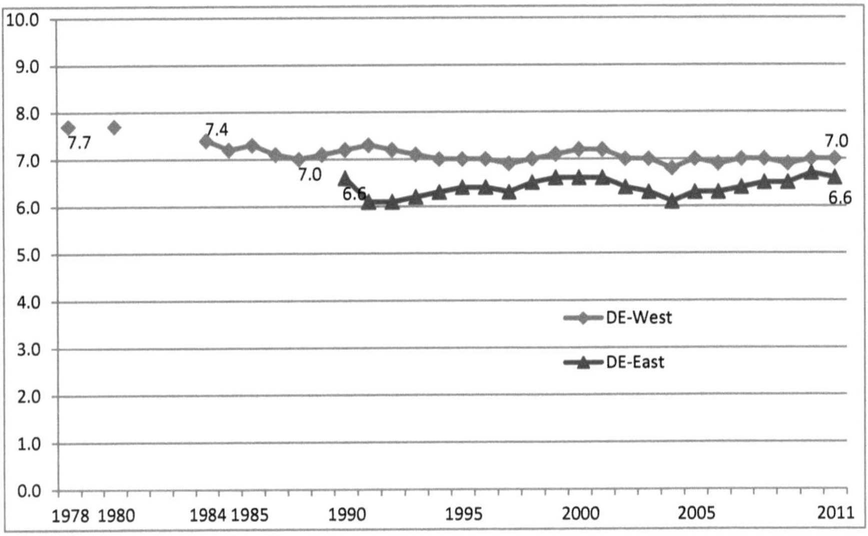

Fig. 6.2 Life satisfaction: West- and East-Germany; 1978–2011. Database: 1978, 1980 German Welfare Survey; 1984–2011 German Socio-Economic Panel Study (Source: Social Indicators Monitor – SIMon (www.gesis.org/simon))

14). His conclusions in terms of the usefulness of SWB measures for measuring progress and temporal changes in general seem to reveal quite some disillusionment: "there are serious problems in using well-being measures for tracking the performance of the economy over time. They cannot be expected to change much in response to even historically large changes in macroeconomic activity – the predicted (and actual) effects are just too small." (Deaton 2012: 13f)

Overall it thus seems as yet to be rather unlikely that there will be an undisputable and broadly accepted single measure – objective or subjective – of progress available in the near future. The current debate about the measurement of progress has nevertheless stimulated numerous promising research activities, which may hopefully lead to scholarly progress in measurement and empirical monitoring of societal progress in years to come.

References

Alexander, J. C., & Sztompka, P. (1990). Rethinking Progress. Movements, Forces, and Ideas at the End of the 20th Century. Boston: Unwin Hyman Inc.

Bauer, R. A. (1966). *Social Indicators*. Cambridge, Mass./London: The M.I.T. Press.

Bossard, J. H. S. (1931/1932). *The Concept of Progress*. Social Forces, 10:1/4, 5–14.

Dahrendorf, R. (1979): Lebenschancen. Anläufe zur sozialen und politischen Theorie. Frankfurt a.M: Suhrkamp.
Deaton, A. (2012). The financial crisis and the well-being of Americans. Oxford Economic Papers; 64(1): 1–26.
Diener, E., & Lucas, R. E. (1999). Personality and subjective well-being. In D. Kahneman, E. Diener, & N. Schwarz (Eds.), Well-being: The foundations of hedonic psychology (pp. 213–229). New York: Russell Sage Foundation.
Department of Health, Education, and Welfare (1969). *Toward a Social Report.* Washington: US Government Printing Office.
Easterlin, R.: 1974, 'Does Economic Growth Improve the Human Lot?', in P. David & M. Reder (Eds.), *Nations and Households in Economic Growth: Essays in Honor of Moses Abramovitz.* New York: Academic Press.
Eckersley, R. (2008). Wretched or contented? The politics of past life. Journal of Futures Studies, Vol. 13, No. 2, 87–92.
Elias, N. (1969). *Über den Prozeß der Zivilisation.* Two Volumes. 2nd Edition. Bern/München: Francke.
Giddens, A. (1993). *Sociology. Second Edition.* Oxford: Polity Press.
Hall, J., Giovannini, E., Morrone, A., & Ranuzzi, G. (2010). A Framework to Measure the Progress of Societies. Statistics Directorate, Working Paper No. 34. Paris: OECD.
Joas, H. (1990). The democratization of differentiation: on the creativity of collective action. In J. C. Alexander, & P. Sztompka (Eds.), *Rethinking Progress. Movements, Forces, and Ideas at the End of the 20th Century* (pp. 182–201). Boston: Unwin Hyman.
Kohl, J. (2011). Comments to Claus Offe: *What, if anything, might we mean by "progressive" politics today?* 6th Conference Social Reporting in Europe: "Measuring and Monitoring Social Progress in European Societies – Is Life Still Getting Better?". Villa Vigoni 2011. (www.gesis.org/en/events/events-archive/social-indicators-research-centre/villa-vigoni-2011/).
Marshall, G. (1994). *The Concise Oxford Dictionary of Sociology.* Oxford, New York: Oxford University Press.
Niceforo, A. (1921). Les Indices numériques de la civilisation et du progrés. Paris: Flammarion.
Niceforo, A. (1930). *Kultur und Fortschritt im Spiegel der Zahlen.* Wien/Prag/Leipzig: Strache.
Nisbet, R. (1980). *History of the Idea of Progress.* New Brunswick: Basic Books.
Noll, H.-H. (2004). Social Indicators and Quality of Life Research: Background, Achievements and Current Trends. In: N. Genov (Ed.), *Advances in Sociological Knowledge Over Half a Century.* Wiesbaden: VS Verlag für Sozialwissenschaften.
Noll, H.-H. (2008). European Survey Data: Rich Sources for Quality of Life Research. In: V. Møller, D. Huschka, A. Michalos (eds.): *Barometers of Quality of Life Around the Globe.* Social Indicators Research Series, Vol. 33. Dordrecht: Springer, pp. 1–21.
Noll, H.-H. (2013). Subjective Social Indicators: Benefits and Limitations for Policy Making—An Introduction to this Special Issue. Social Indicators Research, Volume 114, Issue 1, pp. 1–11.
Noll, H.-H. (2014). Systems of Social Indicators. In: Michalos, Alex C. (ed.), *Encyclopedia of Quality of Life and Well-Being Research*, Heidelberg: Springer, pp. 6579–6582.
Noll, H.-H., & Berger, C. (2014). *Stocktaking Report on Social Monitoring and Reporting in Europe.* E-Frame Project. Mannheim. Published online: http://www.eframeproject.eu/fileadmin/Deliverables/Deliverable5.2.pdf
Noll, H.-H., & Michalos, A. C. (2014). International Sociological Association Working Group / Research Committee on Social Indicators. In: Michalos, Alex C. (ed.), *Encyclopedia of Quality of Life and Well-Being Research*, Heidelberg: Springer, pp. 3331–3336.
Noll, H.-H., & Weick, S. (2011). *Progress, Regress, Stagnancy? Changes in Living Conditions and Subjective Well-Being in Germany.* Conference "Social Reporting in Europe 2011: Measuring and Monitoring Social Progress in European Societies – Is Life Still Getting Better?" (http://www.gesis.org/en/events/events-archive/social-indicators-research-centre/villa-vigoni-2011/).

Novak, S. (1990). Models of directional change and human values: the theory of progress as an applied science. In: J. C. Alexander, & P. Sztompka (Eds.), *Rethinking Progress. Movements, Forces, and Ideas at the End of the 20th Century* (pp. 229–246). Boston: Unwin Hyman.
Offe, C. (2011). What, if anything, may we mean by "progressive" politics today? In: The Council of Europe (Ed.), *Rethinking progress and ensuring a secure future for all: what we can learn from the crisis. Trends in social cohesion, no. 22* (pp. 79–92). Strasbourg: Council of Europe Publishing.
Stiglitz, J. E., Sen, A., & Fitoussi, J.-P. (2010*). Mismeasuring Our Lives: Why GDP Doesn't Add Up*. New York: The New Press.
Sztompka, P. (1990). Agency and progress: the idea of progress and changing theories of change. In: J. C. Alexander, & P. Sztompka (Eds.), *Rethinking Progress. Movements, Forces, and Ideas at the End of the 20th Century* (pp. 247–263). Boston: Unwin Hyman.
Sztompka, P. (1994). *The Sociology of Social Change.* Oxford and Cambridge: Blackwell Publishers.
Touraine, A. (1992). *Critique de la Modernité*. Paris. Les Éditions Fayard.

Chapter 7
A Hierarchy of Unsatisfied Needs: A Subjective Well-Being Study

Mariano Rojas and Jorge Guardiola

Introduction

This chapter studies the role that unsatisfied needs have in depressing people's well-being. The chapter studies how the discrepancy between what people have and what they would like to have influences their life satisfaction. Even though it is less ambitious, the research project gets inspiration from Alex Michalos' Multiple Discrepancy Theory (MDT). Michalos proposes that life satisfaction depends on people's perceived discrepancies in several dimensions and areas of life. In our case we are dealing with a person's selection of that unsatisfied need which is considered of the greatest relevance by the person, suggesting that it is in this need where the most important discrepancy takes place.

There is an association between people's well-being and the satisfaction of their needs. This association is the reason for needs occupying a central place in the study of well-being, as well as in the design of economic and social policies. The fundamental claim is that people do attain greater well-being by satisfying their needs, and that the role of the economic and social organization is to provide the conditions for this satisfaction of needs taking place.

Needs do also play a central role in explaining human behavior: By pursuing greater well-being people are motivated to undertake those actions that contribute to the satisfaction of their needs.

M. Rojas (✉)
FLACSO- Mexico & UPAEP, Carretera al Ajusco 377, Colonia Héroes de Padierna, Delegación Tlalpan, México D.F. C.P. 14200, Mexico
e-mail: mariano.rojas.h@gmail.com

J. Guardiola
Department of Applied Economics, Universidad de Granada, Campus de Cartuja sn, 18012 Granada, Spain

F. Maggino (ed.), *A Life Devoted to Quality of Life*, Social Indicators Research Series 60, DOI 10.1007/978-3-319-20568-7_7

Needs are usually understood as 'sense or feeling of lacking' which calls for immediate action. In fact, both satisfied and unsatisfied needs are associated to essential experiences of being well such as: physical pain and pleasure, negative and positive affects, and a sense of failure and achievement (Rojas 2014). Unsatisfied needs create discomfort and induce people to act because they are associated to experiences of failure, negative affects, and physical pain which people want to avoid, as well as to the potential attaining of experiences of achievement, positive affects, and physical pleasure which people would like to reach. Thus, by satisfying their needs people aspire to greater life satisfaction. However, for most people the list of unsatisfied needs may be very large, and the possibilities of satisfying some of them are limited. In consequence, people – as well as policy makers- do face the challenge of identifying those needs that should have priority in any strategy to raise well-being.

It has been widely accepted that not all needs are equally important and that a hierarchy of needs exists. It is stated that satisfying some needs is more important than satisfying others; in other words, leaving some needs unsatisfied is more harmful than leaving others. There seems to be agreement on the postulate that not all needs are equally important; however, there is substantial disagreement and confusion on the appropriate methodology to delineate the hierarchy of needs. In fact, the definition of a hierarchy of needs has been dominated by normative approaches which leave the issue in the hands of scholars and thoughtful people. Other approaches use people's behavior (their so-called revealed preference) to infer a hierarchy of needs. The subjective well-being approach provides an alternative methodology using the impact of needs satisfaction on people's satisfaction with life to find out what the hierarchy of needs is.

This chapter uses the first official subjective well-being survey in Mexico (applied by Mexico's National Statistical Office in 2012) to study the role some unsatisfied needs have in depressing people's well-being. The survey is representative at the country level, with about 10,600 observations, and it contains many subjective well-being questions. The survey also asked people about the most important unsatisfied need they had – from a large list of about 40 needs-. It is then possible to apply econometric techniques to study these needs as well as to find out which unsatisfied need has a larger impact on people's well-being. The estimates allow us to elaborate a hierarchy of unsatisfied needs on the basis of their impact on people's satisfaction with life. The paper finds out that relational and psychological needs are of greater importance in reducing people's well-being.

The chapter is structured as follows: Section "Human needs and their hierarchy" presents a review of the relevant literature on needs; the focus of this section is on methodological approaches dealing with the ranking of needs. Section "Database" explains the database and presents some descriptive statistics on the relevant variables. Section "Subjective well-being estimation of a hierarchy of unsatisfied needs" estimates a hierarchy of unsatisfied needs on the basis of the subjective well-being approach, while section "Explaining relevant needs" goes deeper in an explanation of those unsatisfied needs which resulted of greater relevance. Section "Final considerations" presents the main conclusions from the analyses.

Human Needs and Their Hierarchy

On Human Needs

Human needs are part of people's condition, and there are many approaches and understandings of human needs (Alkire 2002; Gasper 2007; Guillén-royo 2007). In some occasions the term makes reference to those requirements human beings have for their survival, in other cases a broader conception incorporates all those requirements people need to lead a decent life – either according to her own standards or according to somebody else' standards-. The relevant literature incorporates terms as needs, basic needs, wants, desires, cravings, human and social rights which are presented as needs (Gasper 2007), and even the needs of the nature (Galtung 2012). Some authors use these terms indistinctly – as in economics textbooks-, but other authors try to make a distinction between needs and wants, as well as between human needs and basic needs (Guillén-Royo 2007).

The understanding of needs has occupied the attention of many scholars; however, most of them have worked from a normative perspective. The using of normative approaches to rank needs is a common practice in psychology (human psychology), as well as in sociology (human rights) and in economics (flourishing, basic-needs). The famous Maslow (1943) pyramid constitutes a good example in psychology; Alkire (2002) presents a review of many of normative approaches.

Needs make reference to a sense of lacking. Most scholars assume that people are aware of their needs because, under their perspective, needs play an informational role. If needs motivate people to undertake those actions which are required either to survive or to enhance their well-being, it is necessary, then, for people to be aware of their needs. Within this view there is a close relationship between the concept of needs and that of well-being. Well-being is enhanced when people satisfy their needs, and unsatisfied needs constitute a source of ill-being (Fuentes and Rojas 2001; Guillén-Royo et al. 2009, 2013; Guillén-Royo and Velazco 2006; Guardiola and Guillen-Royo 2014; Lelkes 2006). The satisfaction of needs requires resources that are not always within people's control; and in many cases the satisfaction of needs is subject to contingencies nobody can easily foresee and plan about. There are some approaches that do not require from people to be aware of their needs; in these cases it is a third party who states what needs are important to people and how important they are. This is, for example, the case of the human and social-rights literature as well as of the human-flourishing literature. It is also the case of the basic-needs approach, as Gasper (2007) states: "The World Bank of the 1970s had espoused and to some degree pursued a policy priority to basic needs, largely interpreted as basic material needs that were to be conceptualized and specified by government planners, especially economists.".

Needs, in their material form, received great attention starting in the late 1970s, particularly by institutions aiming to eradicate poverty, such as the World Bank, whose strategy was to increase and redistribute production to provide basic goods and services to the most disadvantaged. Criticism to this view arose within the academy; scholars questioned the arbitrary hierarchical classification of needs, as well as the arbitrary setting of threshold levels (Stern 1989; Streeten 1984).

There are some important works proposing taxonomies of needs; for example, Doyal and Gough (1991) propose a theory of needs with an emancipatory purpose in mind; they claim that needs are universal and elaborate a sophisticated taxonomy of needs. Their approach is basically normative and, as such, it is beyond empirical corroboration because its role is to provide a conceptual framework to study needs. An empirical application of this theory is implemented by Camfield and Guillen-Royo (2010) and Guillén-Royo et al. (2013). Max-Neef (1991) also proposes taxonomy on the basis of a matrix that identifies four different categories for existential needs and nine categories for axiological needs. One common feature these approaches have is that the needs are assumed to be universal, but the ways of satisfying needs (the list of satisfiers) are culturally -and even personally- dependent. Therefore, there is a distinction between the need – which is assumed to be universal- and the culturally-dependent "satisfier" (see Guillén- Royo 2007 for discussion). Some researchers have used Max-Neef's approach in order to assess environmental concerns and social-cohesion issues (Guillen-Royo 2010, 2012). Nussbaum (2000) formulates ten different capacities which she claims to be universal and which can be considered as human needs. The human and social-rights movement is also inspired by these normative approaches when proposing and justifying new rights.

The economics discipline has not given much attention to the study of needs; economists are more concerned about people's preferences and about the process of producing those satisfiers people express a preference to. Microeconomic theory supports the view that the price of satisfiers provides some guidance about how people rank their needs. However, this view would marginalize all those needs that are satisfied through non-market processes. In addition, a ranking based on people's willingness to pay may end up confusing the importance people give to some needs with the purchasing capacity people do have.

Even though the term 'theory' is frequently used, most of these approaches are essentially normative; the approaches do not provide a methodological framework to testing the main hypotheses derived from the theory. Thus, the fundamental issue is not whether needs are universal or not or whether there is a specific hierarchy of needs, but the relevant issue is how these propositions can be empirically tested.

Normative Approaches in the Hierarchy of Needs

Hierarchies of needs have proliferated in the literature. Some of these hierarchies are intrinsically normative in their definition and ranking of needs; this is: they assume either that people are not necessarily aware of their needs or that their experience of being well is irrelevant. In consequence, it is the role of a third-agent (the expert) to define their needs as well as to rank them.

Other approaches rely on normative methodologies to rank needs because they are skeptical about measuring people's well-being. These approaches recognize that needs are related to people's well-being and that people are aware of both their well-being and their needs. However, they are forced to rely on a third-party (the expert) defining the ranking of needs because of reluctance to the directly measure well-being.

Humanist psychologists, such as Abraham Maslow, have proposed normative hierarchies of needs as part of a theory on human motivation. The theory leads to the well-known Maslow's pyramid of needs, which suggests a hierarchy of needs. The theory defines five -or even six, in Maslow's late-years version- steps in the pyramid which end up defining a hierarchy of needs: Physiological needs are at the basis, which means that these needs call for immediate attention. Safety needs do follow up; implying that their satisfaction takes precedence to other needs placed in the upper layers. The need of love and belonging is positioned in the middle of the pyramid; followed up by the need of esteem. Self-actualization is placed at the top of the pyramid; with some versions incorporating a sixth layer associated to self-transcendence (Maslow 1943, 1954).

It is important to state that this hierarchy can be read either bottom-up (according to the calling for immediate attention) as well as top-down (in terms of significance of the pursued goal). What needs are more important? In explaining human motivation and behavior the bottom-up reading is, according to the theory, useful because the theory points toward the sequence in which human beings address the satisfaction of their needs. However, if human fulfillment is in mind and the purpose is to define human goals then a top-down reading defines the hierarchy of needs. Following its psychological development inspiration, it is presumed that self-actualized people constitute the final goal in human development. It is in this sense that the theory becomes normative, proposing a common path all human beings are expected to transit through and a common goal all human beings are expected to have.

There is an old debate both on the hierarchy of needs proposed by Maslow's Theory and on its universality (Wahba and Bridwell 1976; Hofstede 1984; Doyal and Gough 1991; Cianci and Gambrel 2003). However, this chapter is not interested in pursuing normative debates but on proposing and exploring empirical tests to study the hierarchy of needs. Following a subjective well-being approach it is possible to study whether Maslow's theory can be contrasted on the basis of people's experience of being well. It is widely accepted that people's well-being increases with the satisfaction of needs as they move upwards from the basis of the pyramid; however, it is not clear whether well-being increases at a decreasing or at an increasing rate. Does the satisfaction of physiological needs provide more or less well-being than the satisfaction of the self-actualization needs?

During the 1960s and 1970s some economists developed a basic-needs approach which aimed to classify human needs on the basis of their importance from a policy-making perspective. This approach proposed a -somehow ambiguous- hierarchy of needs. As a matter of fact, a rudimentary classification divided needs into two broad categories: basic needs and everything else. The main purpose of this theory was to call the attention of policy makers to the satisfaction of a subset of human needs which was considered – by scholars- to be of the greatest importance (JavedBurki and UlHaq 1981; Streeten and JavedBurki 1978). Some needs which are frequently considered as basic are food, shelter, clothes, healthcare and education; however, the list is not well-delimited and it is arbitrarily expanded or contracted by scholars and policy makers.

The basic-needs approach was used to define poverty lines and to classify people as poor on the basis of their purchasing-power capacity to satisfy needs. Some economists criticized the basic-needs approach because it provided no welfare foundation to classify human needs. For example, Nicholas Stern stated: "*the basic needs ideas have real problems. What needs are basic and more worryingly what levels are held to be essential minima? What if these levels are infeasible…? Who decides which needs are basic and the appropriate level? In what sense are they basic if people who can afford to attain them do not choose to do so?*" (Stern 1989: 645)

In fact, the basic-needs approach was widely criticized in the 1980s. However, the idea of establishing a hierarchy of needs re-emerged at the dawn of the new millennium (Gasper 2007). The Millennium Development Goals initiative established a list of needs which scholars and politicians considered of greatest relevance, such as hunger alleviation, achieving primary education enrolment, and improving child and maternal health, among others. The establishment of a list of goals also fostered the idea of defining a multiplicity of needs as relevant for addressing the conceptualization of poverty (Rojas 2015; Alkire 2002). Thus, during the past years the United Nations Development Program has promoted a multidimensional understanding of poverty on the basis of a list of deprivations considered as relevant (Alkire and Foster 2011). The definition of the list of deprivations has been inspired by ethical considerations as well as by consensus reached among scholars and policy makers. The academic discussion on basic needs and their relationship with well-being is now at the peak of interest with the design of the post-2015 Development Agenda, which will reshape the Millennium Development Goals after 2015.

Well-Being and Human Needs

The emergence of the subjective well-being (SWB) approach has provided a methodology to test the hypotheses derived from the many theories of needs. Research has also assessed the impact of needs on SWB. The SWB approach empowers people by avoiding the patronizing role that policy makers and researches play within the presumption and imputation approaches (Rojas 2014). Some researchers have studied how SWB relates to needs and how this relationship is explained by variables such as employment condition and income (Camfield and Guillen-Royo 2010; Guardiola and García- Muñoz 2011; Guardiola and Guillen-Royo 2014).

Traditional studies in happiness economics aim to determine a basic-needs income threshold by finding out at what level the contribution of income to happiness vanishes, understanding income as a source to satisfy human needs. This income is estimated to be around $10,000–$15,000 per year (Frey and Stutzer 2002; Layard 2005). The assumption of wealth and basic needs being strongly associated is challenged by Guillen-Royo et al. (2013), who find out that basic needs and wealth are weakly associated in a sample from Thailand. The authors also found out that wealth might contribute to happiness for personal or symbolic reasons, which go beyond its normal role of allowing accessing more basic-needs satisfiers. They elaborate an approach to needs valuation related to the intermediate needs from Doyal and Gough (1991), finding that needs are only related to happiness in several regions of their sample.

The SWB approach has also been used to empirically study the importance of needs. Tay and Diener (2011) use a sample of 123 countries to test the importance of several needs in different SWB measures: life evaluation, positive feelings, and negative feelings. They find that need fulfillment is closely associated with SWB, and basic material needs such as food and shelter were mostly associated with life evaluation and negative feelings. They also find that Maslow pyramid theory holds to the extent that people tend to achieve basic material needs before others.

Similarly to Tay and Diener (2011), Rojas and Guardiola (2012) estimate the influence in life evaluation, positive feelings, and negative feelings of different material satisfiers, that can be found in many societies, such as having electricity or phone. They find that a person's subjective well-being is not only influenced by her access to needs-satisfiers but also by others' access to satisfiers; this is an empirical finding that points towards the existence of comparative effects. Michalos' Multiple Discrepancies Theory (MDT) gives support to this statement from an empirical and theoretical view (Michalos 1985, 1986).

Database

The Survey and Information Gathered

This investigation takes advantage of a recent survey enquiring about self-reported well-being which was applied by the National Statistical Office in Mexico in 2012. This is, in fact, the first official survey on self-reported well-being which is carried out in Latin America. With more than 10,600 observations the survey is representative at national level. As expected, there is a large list of questions regarding people's well-being; this research works with the life satisfaction question, which constitutes an overall assessment of how life is going on. The survey also contains information on socio-economic and demographic conditions. In addition, one question in the survey gathers information about which is (from a given list) the most important need the person has.

Life satisfaction is measured on the basis of the following question: "In a scale of 0–10, in general, how satisfied are you with your life?" The response scale also states that 0 is associated to 'not satisfied at all' and 10 to 'completely satisfied'. In principle, this is a categorical scale which can also be treated as cardinal. For simplicity of analyses the variable is treated as cardinal; some exploratory analyses show that there are not substantial differences in the main conclusions when treating the life-satisfaction variable as categorical or as cardinal; this is a common finding in happiness research (Ferrer-i-Carbonell and Frijters 2004). Life satisfaction has a mean value of 8.04 in Mexico, which can be considered as relatively high according to international levels.

The needs question states: "Please, within this list (options are shown or read) which need is, at this moment, more important for you?"; the list of needs contains 40 options. These needs are classified into the following broader categories on the basis of the needs literature: Economical, Psychological, Relational, Health, Personal Development, Occupational, Environmental, Affective, Care, Others. This classification does not aspire to be precise; as a matter of fact, specific needs could involve many aspects which make it difficult to generate a strict classification. In consequence, this broader classification must be considered as illustrative and simplified.

It is important to state that each person in the survey was asked to select only one need from the list: that need which was the most important for him or her at the moment. This is a need that is not being satisfied at the moment of the interview; the Spanish phrasing is clear on this regard. Thus, people are not being asked about providing a ranking of all needs -satisfied or unsatisfied-, but about telling the interviewer which unsatisfied need they considered to be the most important one; that which they would like to be satisfied first in case they were granted the option of satisfying one of the needs in the list. There may be many reasons explaining why the interviewed person focuses on one particular need rather than on other: It could be that more important needs in the list are already satisfied, but it could also be that other unsatisfied needs in the survey are considered by the person to be less important. Hence, the information basically tells us which unsatisfied need from the list is considered to be the most important; this information points towards that aspect where the person has the greatest sense of lacking.

Table 7.1 shows the needs under study, it also presents a general classification of these needs into some global categories. The Table also shows the frequency for each need being selected as most important, and the average life satisfaction of those persons selecting each need.

It is observed that the most frequently mentioned needs are: 'See that the country gets better' (7.72 %), finding 'a job' (6.65 %), having a 'better house' (6.53 %), having 'better working conditions' (6.24 %), 'changing job, a better job' (5.57 %), 'companionship, not been alone' (5.10 %), and having 'harmony in the family' (5.08 %).

The following needs have a frequency of less than 1 %: 'Being forgiven', 'A loan, access to credit', 'Receiving comfort and hope', 'Looking better', 'Living in a cleaner and well-organized city', being 'Accepted by others', 'Being asked for forgiveness', 'Access to medical care', 'Better public transportation', 'Living in a better community', 'A lawyer, legal advice', and 'Attending a better school'.

Table 7.1 List of needs in the study and life satisfaction

Needs	Frequency %	Life satisfaction mean
See that the country gets better	7.72	8.57
Having a job	6.65	7.69
Better house	6.53	7.73
Better working conditions	6.24	8.33
Changing job, a better job	5.57	7.79
Companionship, not been alone	5.10	7.42
Harmony in the family	5.08	7.89
More public security in the community	4.37	8.62
More help and collaboration at home	4.25	8.07
More education, having a diploma	4.01	8.34
Pay and cancel out debts	3.79	7.74
Better health	3.14	7.74
More achievements and success	3.04	8.19
Less anxiety and fear	2.63	8.13
Being more free and more autonomous	2.33	7.99
More time to take care of myself	2.32	8.45
Better care of nature and environment	2.21	8.64
Being heard and taken into account	2.12	7.67
Being able of saving more	2.06	8.42
Less stress	2.04	8.31
Feeling respected by others	1.94	7.58
Having an exciting life, out of boring routine	1.94	8.01
Better medical care	1.82	8.28
Having affection/love in life	1.8	7.71
Obtaining justice	1.44	7.5
Meeting more people, more social life	1.38	8.33
More culture and refinement	1.06	8.62
Receiving recognition and/or gratitude	1.02	7.86
Being forgiven	0.98	8.19
A loan, access to credit	0.85	7.81
Receiving comfort and hope	0.71	7.17
Looking better	0.61	7.97
Living in a cleaner and well-organized city	0.57	8.52
Accepted by others	0.54	7.59
Being asked for forgiveness	0.53	7.86
Access to medical care	0.52	7.89
Better public transportation	0.47	8.70
Living in a better community	0.34	8.33
A lawyer, legal advice	0.20	8.48
Attending a better school	0.09	8.60
	N = 10,654	

Source: BIARE 2012, INEGI. Self-reporting well-being Survey, National Statistical Office of Mexico

The needs that are associated to lower mean life satisfaction are: 'Receiving comfort and hope' (7.17), 'Companionship, not been alone' (7.42), 'Obtaining justice' (7.50), 'Feeling respected by others' (7.58), being 'accepted by others' (7.59), and 'Being heard and taken into consideration' (7.67). While the needs associated to higher mean life satisfaction are: 'Better public transportation' (8.70), 'Better care of nature and environment' (8.64), 'More public security in the community' (8.62), 'More culture and refinement' (8.60), 'Attending a better school' (8.57), 'Seeing that the country gets better' (8.52), and 'Living in a cleaner and well-organized city' (8.48).

The survey also gathered information regarding some socio-demographic and economic characteristics. In specific, we have information about marital status, schooling, gender, age, total household expenditure, and number of persons in the household.

Subjective Well-Being Estimation of a Hierarchy of Unsatisfied Needs

It is important to state that the association – shown in Table 7.1- between some needs and mean life satisfaction may result from other variables that are correlated to both life satisfaction and the propensity to have such a need. For example, it may be that both the propensity for having need Z and life satisfaction depend on people's income; in this case, the association between life satisfaction and need Z could be, in part, spurious. In consequence, it is necessary to control for other variables in order to estimate the correct association between life satisfaction and having a specific need Z. The following regression is run to study this relationship:

$$LS_i = \propto_0 + \sum_{n}^{j=1} \beta_j N_{ji} + \alpha_1 Gender_i + \alpha_2 Age_i + \alpha_3 Age_i^2 + \propto_4 \log(Y_i) \\ + \propto_5 \log(S_i) + \propto_6 Edu_i + \sum_{6}^{k=1} \gamma_k MS_{ki} + \mu_i \quad (7.1)$$

Where:

LS_i: life satisfaction of person *i*. This variable is measured in a 0 to 10 scale.

N_{ji}: Need *j* of person *i*. This is a dichotomous variable, with a value of 1 when person *i* selects this need *j* as 'most important' and 0 otherwise. 'Better public transportation' is the reference category.

$Gender_i$: gender of person *i*, with a value of 1 for women and 0 for men.

Age_i: age in years.

Y_i: Household total expenditure, in Mexican pesos.

S_i: Number of household members.

Edu_i: schooling of person *i*, in education levels.

MS_i: marital status of person *i*; six categories are used: stable partner, separated, divorced, widowed, single, and married (reference category).
μ_i: error term, assumed *i.i.d.*

Table 7.2 presents the results from the econometric analysis.

Table 7.2 Life satisfaction and needs ordinary least squares regression

Variable	Coef.	Std. err.	P>t
Women	0.005	0.04	0.90
Age	−0.042	0.01	0.00
Age_squared	0.000	0.00	0.00
Edu	0.025	0.01	0.00
Log(S)	−0.278	0.04	0.00
Log(Y)	0.281	0.03	0.00
Stable partner	−0.113	0.05	0.04
Separated	−0.498	0.08	0.00
Divorced	−0.574	0.11	0.00
Widowed	−0.269	0.10	0.01
Single	−0.228	0.05	0.00
Companionship, not been alone	−1.199	0.28	0.00
Accepted by others	−1.091	0.36	0.00
Having affection/love in life	−0.964	0.30	0.00
Being forgiven	−0.574	0.32	0.08
Being asked for forgiveness	−0.897	0.37	0.01
Feeling respected by others	−1.104	0.30	0.00
Receiving recognition and/or gratitude	−0.987	0.32	0.00
Being heard and taken into account	−0.971	0.29	0.00
Obtaining justice	−1.221	0.31	0.00
More help and collaboration at home	−0.618	0.28	0.03
Being more free and more autonomous	−0.792	0.29	0.01
Harmony in the family	−0.827	0.28	0.00
Receiving comfort and hope	−1.432	0.34	0.00
Meeting more people, more social life	−0.455	0.31	0.14
Having an exciting life, out of boring routine	−0.721	0.30	0.02
More achievements and success	−0.612	0.29	0.03
Less anxiety and fear	−0.626	0.29	0.03
Less stress	−0.463	0.30	0.12
More time to take care of myself	−0.364	0.29	0.21
Looking better	−0.800	0.35	0.02
More culture and refinement	−0.175	0.32	0.58
More education, having a diploma	−0.482	0.28	0.09
Attending a better school	−0.146	0.65	0.82
Having a job	−0.925	0.28	0.00
Changing job, a better job	−0.832	0.28	0.00

(continued)

Table 7.2 (continued)

Variable	Coef.	Std. err.	P>t
Better working conditions	–0.411	0.28	0.14
Better care of nature and environment	–0.130	0.29	0.66
See that the country gets better	–0.228	0.27	0.41
A lawyer, legal advice	–0.213	0.49	0.66
Being able of saving more	–0.415	0.30	0.16
A loan, access to credit	–0.793	0.33	0.02
Pay and cancel out debts	–1.004	0.28	0.00
Better house	–0.839	0.28	0.00
Living in a better community	–0.363	0.41	0.38
Living in a cleaner and well-organized city	–0.305	0.36	0.40
More public security in the community	–-0.170	0.28	0.55
Better health	–0.866	0.29	0.00
Access to medical care	–0.658	0.37	0.07
Better medical care	–0.356	0.30	0.23
Intercept	7.108	0.40	0.00
R-squared	0.065		
R-squared without needs variables	0.039		

Source: Regression analyses using data from BIARE 2012, INEGI (Self-reporting well-being Survey, National Statistical Office of Mexico)

Our interest is not to study the relationship between socio-economic and demographic variables and life satisfaction. Most results regarding these variables are consistent with previous findings in the subjective well-being literature: There is no gender difference; life satisfaction increases with household purchasing power and declines with the number of members in the household; education raises life satisfaction; there is a U-shaped relationship between life satisfaction and age, with a minimum about 47 years old; married people are happiest than other marital statuses, while divorced and separated people are unhappiest.

The goodness of fit in the regression analyses is absolutely low, with an R-squared of about 0.065; however, low R-squared coefficients are normal when dealing with subjective well-being variables. It is also observed that the introduction of the needs variables does contribute to the goodness of fit; the R-squared coefficient passes from 0.039 to 0.065 when these variables are introduced.

Table 7.3 presents a hierarchy of needs that uses the estimated coefficients presented in Table 7.2; needs are ranked on the basis of their negative impact on life satisfaction.

The top ten needs on the basis of their impact on life satisfaction are: 'Receiving comfort and hope' (−1.43), 'Obtaining justice' (−1.22), 'Companionship, not been alone' (−1.20), 'Feeling respected by others' (−1.10), 'Accepted by others' (−1.09), 'Pay and cancel out debts' (−1.00), 'Receiving recognition and/or gratitude' (–0.99), 'Being heard and taken into account' (–0.97), 'Having affection/love in life' (–0.96), and 'Having a job' (–0.93). The coefficients in parentheses make

Table 7.3 Hierarchy of (unsatisfied) needs on the basis of their impact on life satisfaction

General needs classification	Rank	Need	Coefficient	Frequency percentages
Psychological	1	Receiving comfort and hope	–1.432	0.71
Psychological	2	Obtaining justice	–1.221	1.44
Relational	3	Companionship, not been alone	–1.199	5.10
Relational	4	Feeling respected by others	–1.104	1.94
Relational	5	Accepted by others	–1.091	0.54
Economical	6	Pay and cancel out debts	–1.004	3.79
Psychological	7	Receiving recognition and/or gratitude	–0.987	1.02
Psychological	8	Being heard and taken into account	–0.971	2.12
Affective	9	Having affection/love in life	–0.964	1.80
Occupational	10	Having a job	–0.925	6.65
Relational	11	Being asked for forgiveness	–0.897	0.53
Health	12	Better health	–0.866	3.14
Economical	13	Better house	–0.839	6.53
Occupational	14	Changing job, a better job	–0.832	5.57
Relational	15	Harmony in the family	–0.827	5.08
Other	16	Looking better	–0.800	0.61
Economic	17	A loan, access to credit	–0.793	0.85
Psychological	18	Being more free and more autonomous	–0.792	2.33
Psychological	19	Having an exciting life, out of boring routine	–0.721	1.94
Health	20	Access to medical care	–0.658	0.52
Affective	21	Less anxiety and fear	–0.626	2.63
Relational	22	More help and collaboration at home	–0.618	4.25
Psychological	23	More achievements and success	–0.612	3.04
Relational	24	Being forgiven	–0.574	0.98
Development	25	More education, having a diploma	–0.482	4.01
Affective	26	Less stress	–0.463	2.04
Relational	27	Meeting more people, more social life	–0.455	1.38
Economical	28	Being able of saving more	–0.415	2.06
Occupational	29	Better working conditions	–0.411	6.24
Care	30	More time to take care of myself	–0.364	2.32
Environmental	31	Living in a better community	–0.363	0.34
Health	32	Better medical care	–0.356	1.82
Environmental	33	Living in a cleaner and well-organized city	–0.305	0.57
Environmental	34	See that the country gets better	–0.228	7.72
Other	35	A lawyer, legal advice	–0.213	0.20

(continued)

Table 7.3 (continued)

General needs classification	Rank	Need	Coefficient	Frequency percentages
Development	36	More culture and refinement	–0.175	1.06
Environmental	37	More public security in the community	–0.170	4.37
Development	38	Attending a better school	–0.146	0.09
Environmental	39	Better care of nature and environment	–0.130	2.21
Environmental	40	Better public transportation	Ref.cat.	0.47

Source: Regression analyses using data from BIARE 2012, INEGI (Self-reporting well-being Survey, National Statistical Office of Mexico)

reference to the impact of this need in comparison to that of the reference category: 'Better public transportation'.

It is important to remark that psychological and relations needs dominate the top-five list of needs. This results points towards the importance that psychological and relational needs have in explaining human well-being. From a policy-making perspective the importance of needs depends on a combination of their life-satisfaction impact and their incidence. Three of the top ten needs have a large incidence: 'Having a job' (with a frequency of 6.65 %), 'Companionship, not being alone' (5.10 %), and 'Pay and cancel out debts' (3.8 %). These are (unsatisfied) needs that should be at the center of policies because they are widely spread and they substantially depress happiness.

Explaining Relevant Needs

What factors influence the probability of people selecting a specific (unsatisfied) need as 'most important'? This section further explores the role played by the socio-economic and demographic condition. Some probit-regression analyses are carried out to study the probability of selecting need j (N_j) as most important on the basis of a group of explanatory variables. It is important to recall that N_{ij} is a dichotomous variable with a value of 1 when person i selects it as most important (unsatisfied) need and a value of 0 otherwise. The following specification is used:

$$N_{ij} \underset{Probit}{=} \varnothing_0 + \varnothing_1 Gender_i + \varnothing_2 Age_i + \varnothing_3 Age_i^2 + \varnothing_4 \log(Y_i) + \varnothing_5 \log(S_i) + \varnothing_6 Edu_i + \sum_{6}^{k=1} \vartheta_k MS_{ki} + \tau_i \tag{7.2}$$

Table 7.4 presents the results from the probit analyses. It is observed that the global capability of the socio-economic and demographic variables in explaining the selection of a specific need is very low (low pseudo R squared). In other words, these variables may influence the probability, but they do not determine it.

Table 7.4 Probability of selection an (unsatisfied) need as most important probit regressions

	Receiving comfort and hope	Obtaining justice	Companionship, not being alone	Feeling respected by others	Accepted by others	Pay and cancel out debts	Receiving recognition and/or gratitude	Being heard and taken into account	Having affection/ love in life	Having a job
Women	0.088	–0.133[b]	0.009	0.112[c]	–0.074	0.032	–0.040	0.044	0.141[b]	0.009
Age	–0.014	0.044[a]	0.019[c]	–0.005	–0.029	0.044[a]	–0.023	–0.006	0.009	0.006
Age 2	0.000	0.000[b]	0.000	0.000	0.000	–0.001[a]	0.000	0.000	0.000	0.000
Edu	–0.010	0.006	–0.031[a]	0.002	–0.033	0.011	0.043[a]	–0.023[c]	–0.028[b]	0.013[c]
Log(Y)	–0.098	0.062	0.013	–0.026	0.007	0.036	0.035	–0.059	0.010	–0.276[a]
log(S)	0.072	–0.046	–0.421[a]	0.009	–0.005	0.006	–0.111	0.165[a]	–0.092	0.265[a]
Stable partner	–0.144	0.074	0.147[b]	0.012	0.058	–0.041	–0.037	0.152[b]	0.059	0.111[b]
Separated	0.063	0.211[c]	0.593[a]	0.020	0.068	–0.166	–0.533[b]	–0.007	–0.028	0.090
Divorced	0.296	0.251	0.778[a]	–0.122	–0.148	–0.170	–0.183	–0.076	0.246	0.103
Widowed	0.330[b]	–0.232	0.609[a]	0.045	–0.421	0.108	–0.145	–0.068	–0.065	–0.047
Single	0.080	–0.082	0.596[a]	–0.166[c]	–0.024	–0.251[a]	–0.130	0.036	0.075	0.271[a]
_cons	–1.371[b]	–3.644[a]	–1.977[a]	–1.811[a]	–1.935[a]	–2.931[a]	–2.274[a]	–1.568[a]	–2.220[a]	0.733[a]
Pseudo R^2	0.02	0.02	0.11	0.01	0.01	0.02	0.03	0.01	0.01	0.04

Source: Regression analyses using data from BIARE 2012, INEGI (Self-reporting well-being Survey, National Statistical Office of Mexico)

Note: Coefficient is statistically significant at: [a](0.01 %), [b](0.05 %), [c](0.10 %)

Some variables show statistical significance in the selection of specific needs. For example, being a woman reduces in 13 % the probability of selection 'obtaining justice', but it increases in 11 % the probability of selection 'feeling respected by others' and in 14 % the probability of selection 'having affect/love in life'.

The probability of selecting 'obtaining justice', and 'companionship, not being alone', tends to increase with age, while the probability of selection 'pay and cancel out debts' shows an inverted-U relationship with age.

Household income is inversely related to the probability of selecting 'having a job'; which is not surprising at all. However, what is really surprising is for the other nine needs under study to show no significant relationship with income.

The probability of selecting 'companionship, not being alone' declines with household size; however, as the size of the household increases there is also a rise in the probability of selecting 'being heard and taken into account' and 'having a job'.

Marital status plays an important role in selecting some needs. For example, the probability of selection 'Companionship, not being alone' is significantly lower for people who are married in comparison to any other marital status. Widows have a larger probability of selecting 'Receiving comfort and hope' in comparison to married people.

Final Considerations

The subjective well-being (SWB) approach constitutes an alternative to normative approaches to rank the importance of needs. While normative approaches rely on the arbitrariness of scholars and policy makers, the SWB approach is based on the experience of well-being people do report. When people's well-being is the main concern it is clear that people is in a privileged position to judge their experience. Thus, SWB constitutes a superior approach to study the hierarchy of needs.

It is not difficult to delineate a hierarchy of needs on the basis of reported well-being and information about satisfactors people do have access to. This study has relied on a modified methodology which takes advantage of information on the unsatisfied need which people consider as the most important one.

It has been found that not satisfying some psychological and relational needs may have a large depressing impact on people's satisfaction with life. Of particular importance are needs such as: 'Receiving comfort and hope', 'Obtaining justice', 'Companionship, not been alone', 'Feeling respected by others', 'Accepted by others', 'Receiving recognition and/or gratitude', 'Being heard and taken into account', and 'Having affection/love in life'. The only top-ten needs which are not relational or psychological are: 'Pay and cancel out debts' and 'Having a job'.

That income has little impact in the satisfaction of the most important relational and psychological needs is a noteworthy finding. Thus, policies which aim to increase people's well-being by raising income face the obstacle of income being a very inefficient instrument to ensure the satisfaction of some relevant needs. It is necessary to have a broader perspective when designing public policies which aim to raise well-being; increasing income is neither effective nor efficient because some important needs are relational and psychological rather than economic. With a broader perspective it is possible to bring new instruments into the public-policy sphere; as well as to think about better ways of using income.

Hierarchies of needs are important to guide policy making as well as to inform people. Policy makers do need some guidance in order to efficiently allocate scarce resources; the resources must go to the satisfaction of those needs that have the larger impact on people's well-being. In addition, people know their experience of being well; however, they may err in assessing the well-being impact of satisfying some needs. Thus, subjective well-being estimated hierarchies of needs may inform people about what unsatisfied needs they should attend first.

It is important to acknowledge the limitations this study faces regarding the lack of information on satisfied needs. Complete information regarding the availability of satisfactors would allow for estimating a comprehensive hierarchy of needs.

References

Alkire, S., and J. Foster (2011). Counting and Multidimensional Poverty Measurement. *Journal of Public Economics*, 95, 476–487.

Alkire, S. (2002). Dimensions of Human Development. *World Development*, 30(2), 181–205.

Camfield, L., and M. Guillen-Royo (2010). Wants, Needs, Satisfactions: A Comparative Study in Thailand and Bangladesh. *Social Indicators Research*, 96(2), 183–203.

Cianci, R., and P.A. Gambrel (2003). Maslow's Hierarchy of Needs: Does it Apply in a Collectivist Culture?. *Journal of Applied Management and Entrepreneurship* 8(2), 143–161.

Doyal, L., and I. Gough (1991). *A Theory of Human Need*, Macmillan.

Ferrer-i-Carbonell, A., and P. Frijters (2004). How Important is Methodology for the Estimates of the Determinants of Happiness? *The Economic Journal*, 114, 641–659.

Frey, B., and A. Stutzer (2002). *Happiness and Economics*. Princeton: Princeton University Press.

Fuentes, N., and M. Rojas (2001). Economic Theory and Subjective Well-Being: Mexico. *Social Indicators Research*, 53, 289–314.

Galtung, J. (2012). *Peace Economics: From a Killing to a Living Economy*. Transcend University Press.

Gasper, D. (2007). Conceptualizing Human Needs and Human Well-Being. In I. Gough and A McGregor, eds., *Wellbeing in Developing Countries: From Theory to Research*, 139–165. Cambridge, Cambridge University Press.

Guardiola, J., and T. García-Muñoz (2011). Fulfillment of Basic Needs from a Subjective Point of View in Rural Guatemala. *International Journal of Social Welfare*, 20(4), 393–403.

Guardiola, J., and M. Guillén-Royo (2014). Income, Unemployment, Higher Education and Wellbeing in Times of Economic Crisis: Evidence from Granada (Spain). *Social Indicators Research*, in press.

Guillén-Royo, M. (2007). Well-being and Consumption: Towards a Theoretical Approach based on Human Need Satisfaction. In L. Bruni (ed.) *Handbook on Happiness in Economics*. Cheltenham: Edward Elgar.

Guillen-Royo, M.(2010). Realising the 'Wellbeing Dividend'. An Exploratory Study using the Human Scale Development Approach. *Ecological Economics*, 70(2), 384–393.

Guillen-Royo, M. (2012). The Challenge of Transforming Consumption Patterns: A Proposal using the Human Scale Development Approach. In K. Bjørkdahl and B. Nielsen, eds., *Development and the Environment*, 99–118. Oslo: Akademika.

Guillen Royo, M., and J. Velazco (2006). Exploring the Relationship between Happiness, Objective and Subjective Well-Being: Evidence from Rural Thailand. WeD Working Paper 16. Bath: Wellbeing in developing countries WeD Research Group, University of Bath.
Guillen-Royo, M., J. Velazco, and L. Camfield (2009). Basic Needs and Happiness in Thailand: Exploring the Linkages between Objective and Subjective Wellbeing. In C. Brassard and T. Kusago, eds., *Development Paths and Happiness: Alternative Frameworks*. Asia.
Guillen-Royo, M., J. Velazco, and L. Camfield (2013). Basic Needs and Wealth as Independent Determinants of Happiness: An Illustration from Thailand. *Social Indicators Research*, 110(2), 517–536.
Hofstede, G. (1984). The Cultural Relativity of the Quality of Life Concept. *Academy of Management Review*, 9 (3): 389–398.
JavedBurki, S. and M. UlHaq (1981). Meeting Basic Needs: An Overview. *World Development*, 9, 167–182.
Layard. R. (2005). *Happiness, Lessons from a New Science*. The Penguin Press, New York.
Lelkes, O. (2006). Knowing What is Good for You: Empirical Analysis of Personal Preferences and the "Objective Good". *Journal of Socio-Economics*, 352, 285–307.
Maslow, A. (1943). A Theory of Human Motivation. *Psychological Review*, 50(July), 370–396.
Maslow, A. (1954). *Motivation and Personality*. New York: Harper and Row.
Max-Neef, M. (1991). *Human-Scale Development. Conception, Application and Further Reflection*. New York: The Apex Press.
Michalos, A. (1985). Multiple Discrepancies Theory (MDT). *Social Indicators Research*, 16 (4), 347–413.
Michalos, A. (1986). An Application of Multiple Discrepancies Theory (MDT) to Seniors. *Social Indicators Research*, 18 (4), 349–373.
Nussbaum, M. (2000). *Women and Human Development: The Capabilities Approach*. Cambridge: Cambridge University Press.
Rojas, M. (2014), *El Estudio Científico de la Felicidad*. Mexico City: Fondo de Cultura Economica.
Rojas, M. (2015). Poverty and Well-being Deprivation. In W. Glatzer, V. Moller, L. Camfield, and M. Rojas (eds.), *Global Handbook of Quality of Life*, Springer.
Rojas, M., and J. Guardiola (2012). Satisfaction of Basic Needs and Subjective Well-Being. Paper presented at the XI ISQOLS conference. Venice, 1st of November, 2012.
Stern, N. (1989). The Economics of Development: A Survey. *Economic Journal*, 99, 597–685.
Streeten, P. (1984). Basic Needs: Some Unsettled Questions. *World Development*, 12(9), 973–997.
Streeten, P. and S. JavedBurki (1978) Basic Needs: Some Issues. *World Development*, 6(3), 411–421.
Tay, L., and E. Diener (2011). Needs and Subjective Well-Being around the World. *Journal of Personality and Social Psychology*, 101(2), 354–365.
Wahba, M., and L. Bridwell (1976). Maslow Reconsidered: A Review of Research on the Need Hierarchy Theory. *Organizational Behavior and Human Performance*, 15(2), 212–240.

Chapter 8
An Essay in Honors of Alex Michalos: Finding Community in Quality of Life

Rhonda Phillips

It is not often enough that we encounter others who have a profoundly positive impact on our well-being. Yes, we meet many in the course of living, but how many can one truly single out as having a major influence and helping shape the direction of our working and professional lives for the better? I think it is no small coincidence that Alex is a scholar of quality of life and has this kind of profound influence on others – many of whom are contributing to this volume. I like to think of this influence as adding to our community of scholars, and improving our quality of life as researchers, academics, colleagues, and practitioners. In other words – creating "community" by his leadership, direction, care, and concern for pushing forward research in quality of life. I write this essay to honor, in a small way, this ability of Alex to create and foster a sense of community and collaboration. It begins with a bit of history, followed by an exploration of connecting and finding community in quality of life.

My background is in community development, focusing on places and people in those places across a range of considerations – economic, social, physical, cultural and so on. I came at this notion of quality of life from a somewhat different angle than many of our colleagues. My first readings and study into quality of life were works by Alex. (Indeed, it is hard to search the terminology without his name quickly emerging!). Essays, articles, and books abounded with his careful consideration of the topic, and its relation to other disciplines and theoretical bases. My reaction to this body of work was first to feel stunned by the magnitude of it and also felt the excitement of finding a connection to community development via a new pathway, one that expanded the construct and framework from which I had operated for over two decades. This was, and continues to be, an exciting vista opening up to expand and change the way community development researchers and practitioners

R. Phillips (✉)
Purdue Honors College, Purdue University, 205 N. Russell Street, West Lafayette, IN, USA

Agricultural Economics Department, Purdue University, 205 N. Russell Street, West Lafayette, IN, USA
e-mail: rphillips@purdue.edu; http://www.purdue.edu/honorscollege

F. Maggino (ed.), *A Life Devoted to Quality of Life*, Social Indicators Research Series 60, DOI 10.1007/978-3-319-20568-7_8

think and operate. (I realize of course that this is not the only sphere of influence of Alex's work as other disciplines and inquiries benefit from his contributions and shaping of quality of life research.)

And then I met him! All of this tremendous influence on perceptions and approaches to a long standing discipline in which I was working was occurring before I had the opportunity to cross paths with Alex. It was at a Community Indicators Consortium meeting, several years ago, when the idea of indicators was beginning to take off at a rapid pace with more communities designing and implementing systems to gauge conditions. I had just written a planning guide to community indicators and quality of life dimensions were included as one of my first forays into this arena. And here was a luminary figure in this still a bit mystifying area of research talking to me and other colleagues and sharing his knowledge, wisdom, and wit about applying quality of life to community concerns. Sharing readily and providing considerate answers to a range of diverse questions, his participation was invaluable. It was, luckily, one of the first encounters that has led to other discussions and opportunities for engaging in this arena of research that crosses boundaries easily since it resonates deeply with many, regardless of disciplinary specialty.

One of the most striking characteristics Alex possesses is his ability to bring others into the excitement of his work, and generate a sense of belonging to the greater goal of fostering an important and beneficial area of inquiry and research. This could indeed be considered "community." For example, he compiled *The Encyclopedia of Quality of Life and Well-Being Research*! Literally, he made this monumental contribution of over 7000 pages happen, bringing together writers from across the world to contribute on thousands of topics (Michalos 2014). So I think of Alex as a community builder, not in the physical sense of designing a plan for a city, but rather in building a community of quality-of-life scholars as well as influencing me and others in the realm of community development and community well-being. And I suspect many others have found him to serve this role as well, and his work will continue to inspire others to follow.

Defining Community

As with many elements in life that are not concrete and fundamentally tangible, defining community can be challenging. Perhaps the reason for this is the underlying notion that community depends on who is attempting the definition. Similar to quality of life, there are several nebulous characteristics surrounding the concept. These are the "soft" elements, often more qualitative than quantitative in nature and described in nontangible terms. We can recognize community when we encounter it, and can feel a part of one or several different types – that of interest, special concern, or of place. Most of us can state which community we live in, or name some we enjoy visiting, and even recognize other communities for their unique attributes, but how many can really describe what a community is? I like to think of community (in the context of place) as somewhere we have connection, whether by interests, history, culture, physical dimensions, emotions, political aspects, or any range of combinations that people identify with and feel a part of that area. Neighborhoods are the level where many of us feel the strongest connection, while communities may be thought of as a larger place enveloping the neighborhoods and other features of the place (this is not too far afield as housing – where we live – takes up the majority of land use in a typical town or city). And to be sure, quality of life is impacted by where we live, interact, work, play, and conduct the business of life, so communities in this sense have a profound and direct influence on perceived well-being whether we give credit to it or not.

Let us reverse course for a moment and digress to exploring this word. Numerous definitions exist, although we will center on those that are more place-based in nature for purposes of this chapter. Definitions of community include the following: (1) People who live within a geographically defined area and who have social and psychological ties with each other and with the place where they live (Mattessich and Monsey 2004: 56). Community can also be thought of as, "a general term to describe what occurs outside systems and institutions. It also refers to an aggregation of people or neighborhoods that have something in common. It is both a place and an experience of connectedness" (McKnight and Block 2010: 5). There is something different, or special, about community, and this has been recognized as long as people have gathered to share in the tasks and pleasures of life. Etymological roots date back to the late fourteenth century, with the word translated as roughly meaning "everyone," from the Old French comunité. Earlier still, the Latin noun, communitas, has the definition of "fellowship, friendly intercourse; courtesy, condescension, affability" (OED 2014). Further, these definitions convey a sense of community spiritedness with a united feeling of being together.

Community development in many ways can be thought of as both a process (developing and enhancing the ability to act collectively) and an outcome (taking collective action to improve a community in any or all realms – physical, environmental, social, cultural, political, economic, etc.) (Phillips and Pittman 2015). As an interdisciplinary topic of research, study, and practice, it is defined in myriad manners including local economic development, urban or regional planning, civic engagement, and political empowerment (Green and Haines 2002; Phillips and Pittman 2015). The underlying idea of building or creating something is inherent as well, with the processes and outcomes of it helping solve community problems and improving overall quality of life (Green and Haines 2002; Haines 2009; Phillips and Pittman 2015). There is an explicit link to quality of life, with Green and Haines (2002, 5) positing "community development as a planned effort to build assets that increase the capacity of residents to improve their quality of life."

The assets of community here are called "community capital" in terms of social, human, physical, financial and environmental community level resources. An important capital in community development is that of social capital – this includes social relationships and networks in communities and the strength of those relationships for facilitating collective action for solving problems (Green and Haines 2002; Phillips and Pittman 2015). This concept of mutuality is further explored by Wilkinson (1991) who presents community as a contingent phenomenon, dependent on a number of conditions to realize social interactions for the benefit of mutual interests. Putnam (2000) presents social capital as impacting individual well-being via impacts on safe neighborhoods, health and happiness, education, and children's welfare, for example. Seung et al. (2015, 8) describe other dimensions of community capitals as:

- Human capital is the abilities and skills including labor market skills, leadership skills, education background, health, and others related to human abilities.
- Physical capital, in the context of community development, refers to buildings (houses, factories and stores) and infrastructures (roads, rail tracks, and sewer).
- Environmental capital refers to natural resources and other resources related to community environment.
- Financial capital indicates economic infrastructures such as financial institutions, and community businesses to enhance community development.

It is clear that all five types of community capital are essential to achieve desirable community development outcomes, along with improved quality of life (Haines 2009; Phillips and Pittman 2015; Vincent 2009).

Community development, both as a practice and a discipline, can be considered a complementary concept to quality of life and community well-being (more on this later in the essay). The overriding focus and value inherent in community development is to help make people's lives better – improving quality of life. Community development is practiced at the local, regional and national levels in the public sector along with nonprofit and private as well. Around the world, most governments embed community development within their policies and practices. In the US, the Community Development Society represents both researchers and practitioners. It has a long history of striving to foster improved quality of life, and was established right after the social turmoil of the 1960s as a way to promote effective scholarship and practice. I mention it here because their Principles of Good Practice reflect the underlying values of community development and have relevance for quality of life and well-being. These principles are:

- Promote active and representative participation toward enabling all community members to meaningfully influence the decisions that affect their lives.
- Engage community members in learning about and understanding community issues, and the economic, social, environmental, political, psychological, and other impacts associated with alternative courses of action.
- Incorporate the diverse interests and cultures of the community in the community development process; and disengage from support of any effort that is likely to adversely affect the disadvantaged members of a community.
- Work actively to enhance the leadership capacity of community members, leaders, and groups within the community.
- Be open to using the full range of action strategies to work toward the long-term sustainability and well-being of the community (Community Development Society 2014).

It seems clear that many of these values or guiding principles have similarity to community well-being and quality of life. This society is not the only group to base their actions on principles such as these. The International Association for Community Development is a nonprofit/nongovernmental association representing members across the globe. Take a look at their principles or priorities, most of which center on their mission of sustainable community development for social justice:

- Promote community development as a key method for addressing challenges, opportunities and priority issues in rural and urban areas locally, regionally and internationally.
- Facilitate quality practice exchange, education, training, research and publications in support of practitioners, educators, researchers, policy analysts, activists and other community workers and organizers.
- Engage practitioners, educators, researchers, policy analysts, activists and other community workers and organisers at country and regional levels and thereby promote their community-based planning and development work.
- Ensure the short, medium and longer term sustainability of IACD (2014).

At this point, another definition would likely help confirm the relationships between community development, community well-being and quality of life. Here is one that reflects the collectivity, action, and capitals:

> Community development is "a process of developing and enhancing the ability to act collectively and an outcome: (1) taking collective action and (2) the result of that action for improvement in a community in any or all realms: physical, environmental, cultural, social, political, economic, etc." (Phillips and Pittman 2009: 6)

Seung et al. (2015: 9) describe community development as the following:

> It centers on capacity building and taking action. As seen, a vital part of the term community development is that of community. Connecting this special feeling of the common or togetherness with action to impart improvements is community development. There is a related area, that of community economic development, which is highly interrelated with community development itself although focused more on economic dimensions. Schaffer et al. (2006: 61) provide a description of this relationship: Community economic development occurs when people in a community analyze the economic conditions of our community, determining its economic needs and unfilled opportunities, deciding what can be done to improve economic conditions that community and then moving to achieve agreed upon economic goals and objectives. Newer definitions incorporate vital concepts of sustainability and equity, reflecting the triology eluded to earlier. These include discussion of opening opportunities for the poor (Anglin 2011). A slightly different view on community economic development is provided by Phillips and Besser (2013: 6) as a "merging of aspects of the fields of community development and economic development, implying practice aimed at community betterment and economic improvement at the local level, preferably encompassing sustainable development approaches."

Community Well-Being

As discussed, there is much overlap with conceptions of community well-being and community development. Let's look a little deeper at community well-being, exploring its dimensions. This very topic was recently addressed in a work by Sung and Phillips (2015). The following excerpt is provided from that work to help explain these ideas.

Community well-being encompasses comprehensive and integrated concepts developed by synthesizing research constructs related to residents' perceptions of the community, residents' needs fulfillment, observable community conditions, and the social and cultural context of the community. Community well-being is a relatively new idea in social science, it still lacks the theoretical structure for explanatory purposes. From hedonic and positive psychology perspectives, well-being indicates how well a person's life is going. Prilleltensky and Prilleltensky (2012) emphasize that relational and collective dynamics of well-being consist of five components: site, signs, sources, strategies and synergy. On the other hand, Seligman (2012) constructs well-being theory into five elements: positive emotion, engagement, relationships, meaning and achievement. He argues that, "the way we choose our course in life is to maximize all five of these elements" (p. 25) and that these elements contribute to well-being as a whole. Diener (2000) focuses on subjective well-being, which refers to peoples' cognitive and affective evaluations of their lives. Defining a good life requires evaluating subjective well-being, and it is connected to a subjective quality of life. He also suggests that well-being results from components of subjective well-being such as life satisfaction, satisfaction with important domains, positive affect, and low levels of negative affect. However, even though he posits a subjective viewpoint of well-being, he agrees that cultural and social factors influence subjective well-being as well (Diener 2000). It might be hard for individuals to change their level of well-being without environmental changes, and vice versa. Well-being has to embrace not only an individual's pleasure, enjoyment, and satisfaction but also the environmental conditions under which people live; it can be seen as germane to community well-being.

The term *quality of life* (QOL) is generally deemed the overall well-being of individuals and societies. The World Health Organization Quality of Life Group (1993) defines QOL as:

> An individual' perception of their position in life in the context of the culture and value systems in which they live … incorporating in a complex way the person's physical health, psychological state, level of independence, social relationships, personal beliefs and their relationship to salient features of the environment. (as cited in Rapley 2003, p. 50)

There are several common views of QOL studies. QOL embraces "the totality of human life" (Cummins 2000); QOL has multidimensional factors measured by different life domains regardless of an emphasis on either subjective or objective aspects of life; and QOL encompasses various units of society from individual to community, to national, and to global level (Sirgy et al. 2011). Additionally, as a reflection of values that exist in a community (Phillips and Pittman 2009), assessment of QOL is not only germane to residents' well-being, happiness, and satisfaction status quo, but also conducive to building and improving a healthy community which embodied community well-being. Quality of life then accounts for a significant component within a construction of community well-being.[1]

Is the Whole Greater Than the Sum of Its Parts?

Aristotle may have been thinking about a variety of applications when he looked at the idea of synergy of the "whole," but one can certainly see the relevance in his words for gauging quality of life in the *whole of a community*. The idea that one can achieve a view of a community's overall quality of life and well-being by adding up individual's subjective measures does not necessarily reflect the idea of synergy. It can certainly help gauge the trends and majority views, but does it really fully gauge the range of considerations that influence a community's situation, issues and outlook? It does not, for a variety of reasons (Sirgy 2011). From a community development perspective, it most definitely does not convey the overall picture of community well-being. There are numerous other considerations that influence a community, as discussed previously, and it is unlikely that we can fully gauge the situation based on subjective measures reported from individuals. These valuable data can however be integrated with objective measures to provide more of a complete picture, along with tools such as community indicator systems. Community indicators essentially paint a picture of the current situation, and whether a community is making progress towards goals and desired outcomes (Phillips 2003). It is discussed here because it relates to measuring, gauging and guiding progress in societies as opposed to indicators such as the Gross Domestic Product, commonly used to assess economic development outcomes. Efforts such as the Genuine Progress Indicator from Canada are more comprehensive although still include economic dimensions as a vital component in the now well-known trilogy of economics, equity and environmental domains (See Alex's 2003 work for more insights). This more closely aligns with the concepts of community well-being, which can be viewed as encapsulating both community development and community economic development, as components fostering overall community well-being. The future of research is rich in this area, and the foundation of quality of life research can serve as a strong basis on which to develop further understanding.

Now, back to the original question – can we find community in quality of life? I hope you will agree that we have and can continue to find more connections, especially given the contributions of Alex Michalos and others who are interested in the application and range of considerations within quality-of-life research.

[1] Excerpted with permission from Sung, H. & Phillips, R. (2015) Conceptualizing a Community Well-Being and Theory Construct. In Kee, Y., Lee, S. & Phillips, R. *Social Factors and Community Well-Being*, Springer, forthcoming.

References

Anglin, R. (2011). Promoting sustainable local and community economic development. London: CRC Press.

Community Development Society. (2014). Principles of good practice. http://www.comm-dev.org/. Accessed 1 December 2014.

Cummins, R. A. (2000). Objective and subjective quality of life: An interactive model. *Social Indicators Research, 52*, 55–72.

Diener, E. (2000). Subjective well-being: The science of happiness, and a proposal for national index. *American Psychologist* 55: 34–43.

Green, G. P., & Haines, A. (2002). *Asset building & community development*. Thousand Oaks, CA: Sage Publications, Inc.

Haines, A. (2009). Asset-based community development. In R. Phillips & R. H. Pittman (Eds.), *An introduction to community development* (pp. 38–48). New York, NY: Routledge.

International Association for Community Development (IACD). (2014). http://www.iacdglobal.org/about. Accessed 1 December 2014.

Mattessich, P., & Monsey, M. (2004). Community building: What makes it work. St. Paul, MN: Wilder Foundation.

McKnight, J., & Block, P. (2010). The abundant community. San Francisco: Berrett-Koehler.

Michalos, A. (2003). Combining Community, Social, Economic, and Environmental Indicators to Measure Sustainable Human Well-Being. In Michalos, A., *Essays on the Quality of Life*. Dordrecht, The Netherlands: Springer.

Michalos, A. (2014). (Ed). *Encyclopedia of Quality of Life and Well-Being*. Dordrecht, The Netherlands: Springer.

Online Etymology Dictionary (OED). (2014). Community. http://www.etymonline.com/index.php?term=community. Accessed 13 Jan 2015.

Phillips, R. (2003). *Community indicators measuring systems*. Aldershot: Ashgate Publishing.

Phillips, R., & Besser, T. (2013). Community economic development. London: Routledge.

Phillips, R. & Pittman R. (eds). (2009) Introduction to community Development, London: Routledge.

Phillips, R. & Pittman, R. (2015) *Introduction to Community Development* 2nd edition. London: Routledge

Prilleltensky, I., & Prilleltensky, O. (2012). Webs of well-being: The interdependence of personal, relational, organizational and community well-being. In J. Haworth & G. Hart (Eds.), *Well-being: individual, community and social perspectives*. New York, NY: Palgrave Macmillan.

Putnam, R. D. (2000). *Bowling alone: The collapse and revival of America community*. New York: Simon & Schuster.

Rapley, M. (2003). Quality of life research. Los Angeles: Sage.

Shaffer, R., Deller, S., & Marcouiller, D. (2006). Rethinking community economic development. *Economic Development Quarterly* 20(1): 59–74.

Seligman, M. E. P. (2012). Flourish: A visionary new understanding of happiness and well-being. New York, NY: Free Press.

Seung, J.L., Kim, Y. & Phillips, R. (2015). Exploring the Intersection of Community Well-Being and Community Development. In Seung, J.L., Kim, Y, & Phillips, R. *Community Well-Being and Community Development*. Dordrecht, The Netherlands: Springer.

Sirgy, M. J. (2011). Societal QOL is more than the sum of QOL of individuals: The whole is greater than the sum of the parts. *Applied Research Quality Life, 6*, 329–334.

Sirgy, J., Phillips, R. & Rahtz, D. (2011). *Community Quality-of-Life Indicators: Best Cases V*. Dordrecht, The Netherlands: Springer.

Sung, H. & Phillips, R. (2015). Conceptualizing a Community Well-Being and Theory Construct. In Seung, J.L., Kee, Y. & Phillips, R. *Social Factors and Community Well-Being*.(Forthcoming).

Vincent, J, (2009), Community Development assessments. In R. Phillips & R. Pittman (eds.) Introduction to Community Development. London: Routledge.

Chapter 9
Towards a New Concept of Residential Well-Being Based on Bottom-Up Spillover and Need Hierarchy Theories

M. Joseph Sirgy

Introduction

Many real estate developers and community public official have become increasingly interested in the concept of residential well-being. These practitioners use social indicators to assess quality of life of housing developments, neighborhoods, and communities at large (e.g., Galster 1987; Galster and Hesser 1981; Morris and Winter 1975, 1978). As such, interest has grown to attempts at better understanding and measuring the effects of housing and neighborhood/community amenities on home owners' or home dwellers' overall sense of well-being or quality of life (e.g., Dittman and Goebel 2010). In that vein, quality-of-life researchers usually address issues related to residential well-being (e.g., Grzeskowiak et al. 2003). This chapter briefly describes past conceptualizations of residential well-being and introduces a new concept guided by two well-established theories of human development and quality of life, namely bottom-up theory of subjective well-being and need hierarchy theory.

Past Conceptualizations of Residential Well-Being

Residential well-being has been conceptualized and measured in different ways by quality-of-life researchers (Sirgy 2011). I will first organize these conceptualizations (and the resulting metrics) in terms of objective versus subjective construals. I will then focus on the subjective construals, which are categorized as a direct function of their focal content, namely housing, neighborhood, community, and

M.J. Sirgy, Ph.D. (✉)
Department of Marketing, Pamplin College of Business, Virginia Polytechnic Institute & State University, 880 West Campus Dr, Blacksburg, VA 24061-0236, USA
e-mail: sirgy@vt.edu

F. Maggino (ed.), *A Life Devoted to Quality of Life*, Social Indicators Research Series 60, DOI 10.1007/978-3-319-20568-7_9

integrated construals. I will then focus on the integrated construals and further identify several approaches. Within the integrated category I will then introduce a new concept of residential well-being based on theoretical concepts borrowed from bottom-up spillover theory and need hierarchy theory—theoretical concepts well-established in quality-of-life studies.

Objective Versus Subjective Conceptualizations of Residential Well-Being

Much of the research in residential well-being can be classified in terms of objective versus subjective indicators. Objective indicators of residential well-being may include expert's judgments of housing quality in terms of well-established construction standards and building codes. For example, real estate developers and building and construction professionals typically abide by well-established quality standards (Bubshait and Al-Atiq 1999). The layout of a typical home is decomposed into space for living, sleeping, and utility. Quality standards in residential construction are typically decomposed into housing design, residential site, energy conservation, and neighborhood features. With respect to the housing design, quality judgments are made by focusing on the floor plan. The floor plan adapts the house to three main functions: the living space (i.e., living room, dining room, family room, den, recreation room, and enclosed porches), the sleeping space (i.e., bedrooms, bathrooms, dressing rooms), and service space (i.e., kitchen, utility room, other specialized work areas). The quality of the sleeping space is judged by criteria such as minimum space requirements, storage space, bathrooms, and noise. The quality of living area is judged based on criteria such as space requirements, layout, arrangement within, and location within the house. The quality of the service area is judged by kitchen space requirements, kitchen location, kitchen layout, and laundry facilities. The quality of the floor plan is judged by criteria such as proportionality and balance, storage space, and traffic pattern. With respect to the residential site, quality of the housing unit is judged based on criteria such as topography, site orientation, and landscaping. With respect to energy conservation, quality criteria are quite varied and they tend to differ as a direct function of whether the house is new or old. Finally, we have quality standards related to the neighborhood (or subdivision). These quality standards reflect physical features of the neighborhood, economic features, as well as social features.

At the neighborhood and community levels, planners have their own quality standards that color their judgment of residential well-being. Here is an example. Hovik (1992) conducted a study using a Delphi survey to elicit the judgment of regional planners as to what indicators are significant that reflect quality of life (QOL) of a community. The results of the Delphi survey narrowed the initial list of 113 social indicators into a smaller set involving three groups of indicators:

demographic, sociocultural, and socioeconomic. Indicators judged most useful as a measure of QOL were ranked as follows:

- Air and water quality
- Quality of education
- Percent of population in poverty
- Number of crimes of violence
- Unemployment rate
- Number of crimes of property
- Absence of racial and ethnic bias
- Crime victimization rates
- Distribution of income and wealth
- Employee compensation and earnings
- Number of parks
- Per capita expenditures for social welfare
- Per capita income
- Availability of goods and services
- Percent of income spent on taxes

Now let us turn to the subjective conceptualizations of residential well-being.

Subjective Conceptualizations of Residential Well-Being: Housing, Neighborhood, Community, and Integrated Approaches

Subjective conceptualizations of residential well-being are essentially grounded in *residential satisfaction* (e.g., Walton et al. 2008). Residential satisfaction, in this context, refers to the "experience of pleasure or gratification derived from living in a specific place" (Bonaiuto et al. 2006, p. 24).

Much of the research on residential well-being that use residential satisfaction as a focal concept can be categorized in terms of level of analysis: housing, neighborhood, community, and integrated. At the housing level, residential well-being has also been conceptualized in terms of *satisfaction with dwelling features*. That is, residential well-being involves feelings of the resident in relation to many features that concern his or her immediate dwelling. Operationally-speaking, this translates into a composite of satisfaction with dwelling features such as, plumbing, kitchen facilities, heating equipment, interior condition, exterior condition, modernity, floor space/size, yard space, number of bathrooms, and privacy (e.g., Galster 1987). Also at the housing level, residential well-being was conceptualized in terms of *satisfaction with the various stages of the home consumption life cycle* (Grzeskowiak et al. 2006). That is residential well-being is achieved when the individual is satisfied with the purchase (or rent/lease) of the home (i.e., when the home is purchased or rented with the least amount of effort), with the home preparation (i.e., when the home is prepared for use to meet the needs of the occupant), with home ownership (i.e., home ownership signaling status and enhancing the home owner's financial portfolio), with home use (i.e., the home serves the housing needs of the residents), with home repairs and maintenance (i.e., the maintenance, renovation, and repair in the home are minimal), and with home disposal (i.e., the sale of the home is transacted with the least amount of effort and most financial gain).

At the neighborhood level, researchers have treated residential well-being to mean *residents' attitude toward their immediate living space*. Specifically, residential satisfaction is viewed as an evaluation or attitude toward the neighborhood in question in an expectancy-value sense (Fishbein and Ajzen 1975). Satisfaction with one's residential place is captured as a composite of satisfaction toward the physical and social features of the neighborhood—features such as perceived attractiveness of the neighborhood, evaluations of upkeep of dwellings, similarity to neighbors, and noise level of the block (e.g., Li and Tsai 2014; Miller et al. 1980; Sirgy and Cornwell 2002).

There is also much research on residential well-being that focused on capturing this construct at the community level alone. In this context, residential well-being was conceptualized as involving *residents' feelings of satisfaction with the community at large*. Here, community well-being is captured as residents' satisfaction with the community at large as well as its various conditions and amenities (e.g., Auh and Cook 2009; Jeffres and Dobos 1990, 1992, 1995; Mthembu 1997; Norman et al. 1997; Shin 1980; Sirgy 2011; Sirgy et al. 2000). For example, my colleagues and I (Sirgy et al. 2000) measured community well-being in terms of residents' satisfaction with the community overall. We were able to demonstrate that our measure is nomologically valid by relating it to measures of global satisfaction with life. Another concept of residential well-being that focuses on the community level involves *residents' evaluations of community amenities, services, and conditions*. My colleagues and I (Sirgy et al. 2010) developed a new measure of community well-being based on the notion that community residents perceive the quality-of-life impact of community services and conditions in various life domains (e.g., family, social, leisure, health, financial, cultural, consumer, work, spiritual, and environmental domains). These perceptions influence residents' overall perception of community well-being, their commitment to the community, and their overall life satisfaction. Survey data were collected in the Flint area (Michigan, USA) in four waves (1978, 1990, 2001, and 2006). The data supported the nomological validity of the measure. Other researchers have employed similar composite satisfaction indices. For example, Jeffres and Dobos (1990, 1992) have measured this construct using a series of questions in which respondents rated the quality of housing, public schools, justice/law enforcement, government services, public transportation, cultural events, employment opportunities, and outdoor recreation. Similarly, Santos et al. (2007) conceptualized community well-being as perception and evaluation of a variety of community services and conditions.[1]

[1]There are other conceptualizations of residential well-being at the community level. Here is another example, namely *community pride* (e.g., Baker and Palmer 2006). Community pride in this

Now let's turn our attention to the integrated concepts of residential satisfaction—treating residential well-being in terms of residential satisfaction with aspects of the home, neighborhood, and community.

Integrated Approaches of Residential Well-Being

What do I mean by the integrated approach using the concept of residential satisfaction? There are many studies in residential satisfaction that focused on capturing respondents' satisfaction with aspects of the home itself, the neighborhood, and the community. In other words, the attempt to capture satisfaction in relation to all residential aspects of well-being. For example, Varady and Carrozza (2000) conceptualized residential well-being in terms of residential satisfaction with four residential elements: satisfaction with the dwelling unit, satisfaction with the services provided, satisfaction with the whole housing package (dwelling and service elements), and satisfaction with the neighborhood or surrounding community. Lee and Park (2010) treated residential well-being in terms of two satisfaction elements, namely satisfaction with the home and satisfaction with the neighborhood. Mohit and Nazyddah (2011) treated residential well-being as residential satisfaction of two housing elements (dwelling unit features and housing unit support services) and three non-housing elements (public facilities, social environment, and neighborhood facilities).

The most popular integrated approach to residential satisfaction is the *gap concept*—the gap between actual and desired housing and neighborhood/community conditions (e.g., Erdogan et al. 2007; Galster 1987; Galster and Hesser 1981; Mohit et al. 2010; Wu 2008). This definition focuses on the difference between actual and desired housing and neighborhood/community conditions. In other words, residential well-being is the difference between a resident's actual and desired (or aspired-to) housing and neighborhood/community conditions. Residents make judgments about residential conditions based on their needs and aspirations. Satisfaction with one's residential situation indicates the absence of complaints and a high degree of congruence between actual and desired. Conversely, a discrepancy between their actual housing or neighborhood and desired conditions may lead to dissatisfaction. Consider the following study. Handal et al. (1981) used a congruence measure of housing and neighborhood/community satisfaction involving two dimensions, namely physical and social characteristics. Their measure involved two discrepancy scores: difference between ideal and perceived *physical* characteristics and difference between ideal and perceived social characteristics.

Another conceptualization of residential satisfaction involves the concept of *perceived adequacy*. For example, Ibem and Amole (2013) viewed residential

---

sense refers to the positive feelings of attachment residents feel about their community and their feelings of satisfaction with the community at large. Other research has focused on the *sense of community* (e.g., Yetim and Yetim 2014).

well-being as perceived adequacy of housing unit characteristics (e.g., adequacy of privacy in the residence, the size of the bedrooms, natural lighting), perceived adequacy of neighborhood facilities and environment (e.g., distance to place of work, neighborhood crime, distance to children's school, distance to market), and adequacy of management of housing estate (rules and regulations regarding residency, security services, janitorial/maid services, water supply, electrical services, street lighting).

Yet another concept involves the *goal approach*. The goal concept asserts that residential well-being can be viewed as the extent to which housing facilitates or hinder the attainment of life goals and aspirations (e.g., Amole 2009). For example, how does one's home affect work-related goals? The home is located too far from one's place of employment. The home is not conducive to bringing work at home and completing job-related projects. The home lacks basic information-technology infrastructure (e.g., PC, printer, and Internet access). If so, the home is viewed as a hindrance to one's attainment of job-related goals. As such this situation is viewed as low in residential well-being.

The reader should keep in mind this last conceptualization of residential well-being, namely the goal approach. This concept has a certain degree of affinity to the new concept of residential well-being that I introduce in the next section. Here it is.

Towards a New Conceptualization of Residential Well-Being

The new concept of residential well-being is defined as:

> Residential well-being is satisfaction with one's living arrangement captured by one's home and its immediate surrounding (i.e., community) to the extent that this satisfaction contributes to the sense of well-being in seven major life domains, namely health/safety, financial, family, social, work, leisure/arts/culture, and education/personal development, which in turn all contribute to the overall sense of well-being.

The sense of well-being in three of the seven aforementioned life domains, namely health/safety, financial, and family life, serves to meet basic needs *a la* Maslow. These are essentially low-order needs related to survival such as biological and safety needs (Maslow 1943). In contrast, satisfaction in other life domains such social, work, arts/culture, and education/personal development serves to meet growth needs. Growth needs, *a la* Maslow (1943), are high-order needs related to human flourishing.

I have long argued that satisfaction of the full spectrum of human needs (i.e., both survival and growth needs) is a major predictor of life satisfaction and overall happiness (e.g., Sirgy and Wu 2009). Consider the following. Martin Seligman, the founding father of positive psychology, has long argued that authentic happiness comes about as a function of meeting three major needs: the need to have a pleasant life, the need to have an engaged life, and the need to have a meaningful life (Seligman 2002). The pleasant life is about happiness in a hedonic sense. The engaged life is about happiness through engagement, and the meaningful life is about happiness by achieving virtue. The needs related to the pleasant life, the engaged life, and the meaningful life seem highly akin to Maslow hierarchy of needs. Seligman and his colleagues (Peterson et al. 2005) conducted two studies demonstrating that people who score highly on the three dimensions of authentic happiness (life of pleasure, life of engagement, and life of meaning) score high on traditional measures of subjective well-being.

Also consider the ideas of Raphael et al. (1996). These quality-of-life researchers developed a model of subjective well-being by postulating that satisfaction with three sets of needs related to being, belonging, and becoming contribute significantly to subjective well-being. With respect to the needs related to the *being* dimension, an individual is likely to have a greater sense of subjective well-being if he or she meets his or her needs of physical health (physically healthy, engages in exercise, eats in moderation and nutritiously, etc.) and mental health (good adjustment, positive feelings, positive cognitions, etc.). With respect to needs related to the *belonging* dimension, an individual is likely to have a high level of subjective well-being if he or she experiences a positive immediate environment (home, workplace, neighborhood, school, and community), a positive social environment (family, friends, neighbors, etc.), and a positive community (a community having good job opportunities, healthcare system, educational system, and parks and recreation services). With respect to the *becoming* dimension, the needs here are related to engagement of daily activities (day-to-day activities, domestic work, paid work, schooling, etc.), engagement in leisure activities (activities promoting relaxation and stress reduction), and engagement in growth activities (maintenance and improvement of knowledge and skills and adapting to changed circumstances).

My colleagues and I have also conducted much research using the concept of need hierarchy (e.g., Sirgy et al. 1995). We developed a measure of quality of life based on satisfaction of the totality of human needs. Four need categories were used, namely survival needs, social needs, ego needs, and self-actualization needs. The composite score of human need satisfaction was shown to correlate highly with traditional measures of subjective well-being.

So the argument I am making here is that *subjective well-being is determined mostly by satisfaction of the full spectrum of human developmental needs* (basic and growth needs or low-order and high-order needs *a la* Maslow). Hence, this is the first postulate that I am working with to build my overall model of residential well-being.

The second postulate involves linking satisfaction of the full spectrum of human developmental needs with satisfaction with major life domains. I am doing this because my goal is to link satisfaction with a specific set of housing and neighborhood/community amenities and conditions with domain satisfaction. So my second postulate is as follows: *The sense of well-being in seven major life domains contribute to the overall sense of subjective well-being, namely health/safety, financial, family, social, work, leisure/arts/culture, and education/personal development.* This is clearly represented in Table 9.1.

Table 9.1 The new concept of residential well-being

Subjective well-being (or life satisfaction, happiness, overall positive and negative affect)	Sense of well-being in relation to education and personal development	Housing: personal library, digital educational programming
		Neighborhood/community: community library, educational programs offered nearby
	Sense of well-being in relation to leisure, arts, and culture	Housing: hobby room, nice décor, art pieces and pictures
		Neighborhood/community: theaters, festivals, sports events
	Sense of work well-being	Housing: study room, den, tool room, wiring and other infrastructure in the house to accommodate internet, telephone, mobile phone, etc. to allow the home dweller to engage in job-related activities from home
		Neighborhood/community: workplace within an easy commute, no traffic congestion on the way to work, good road conditions on the way to work, availability of public transportation
	Sense of social well-being	Housing: adequate and quality space for social functions
		Neighborhood/community: restaurants, cafes, shopping malls/centers, park and rec places
	Sense of family well-being	Housing: quality family-related rooms (e.g., kitchen, utility room, family room, porch/deck)
		Neighborhood/community: grocery store(s) close by, department store(s), hardware store(s), childcare centers, eldercare centers
	Sense of financial well-being	Housing: affordable rent or mortgage, investment opportunity, affordable utilities, affordable maintenance and repairs
		Neighborhood/community: affordable cost of living in the community, banks and financial services
	Sense of well-being in relation to health and safety	Housing: safe electrical, safe water, safe heat/air conditioning, safe air
		Neighborhood/community: fitness and sports facilities, hospitals and clinics, crime-free neighborhoods, law enforcement, rescue squad, fire department

The second theoretical postulate is supported by much research on *bottom-up spillover theory* (e.g., Andrews and Withey 1976; Campbell et al. 1976). Here is how I described bottom-up spillover in my book on the *Psychology of Quality of Life* (Sirgy 2012). Bottom-up spillover is the influence of affect from subordinate life domains to superordinate ones, specifically from life domains such as leisure, family, job, and health to overall life. That is, feelings within a given life space within the overall hierarchy of life experiences (captured subjectively as cognitions) spill vertically from bottom (most concrete cognitions) to top (most abstract cognitions). One can view life satisfaction as a satisfaction judgment on top of the cognition hierarchy, domain satisfaction (i.e., satisfaction with health and safety, satisfaction in financial life, satisfaction in family life, satisfaction in social life, satisfaction in work life, satisfaction in relation to arts and culture, and satisfaction in relation to education and personal development) as mid-level cognition (not too abstract and not very concrete). Satisfaction judgments that are concrete are satisfaction related to life events. In relation to residential well-being, satisfaction with certain housing amenities and communities conditions can be considered to be at the bottom of this satisfaction hierarchy.

There is much evidence that suggests that concrete residential life events related to the home and neighborhood/community do indeed influence domain satisfaction and overall life satisfaction (Adams 1984). The home is the place in which people experience intimate experiences and thus tend to affect the quality of their lives (e.g., Andrews and Withey 1976; Campbell et al. 1976; Headey 1981; Morris and Winter 1978; Stoeckler 1977; Stoeckler and Larntz 1986). Major national surveys in the European Union countries (Ireland, Italy, Germany, France, the Netherlands, Belgium, Denmark, and the U.K.) have shown that satisfaction with housing and neighborhood is a significant predictor of life satisfaction (Davis and Fine-Davis 1991). The neighborhood plays an important role in social interactions and relationships with others. The neighborhood affects well-being through health, friendship, work, financial status, and marital relationships (Wagner 1995).

My colleagues and I (Sirgy et al. 2000) developed a method and measures for assessing residents' satisfaction with community-based services, demonstrating that satisfaction with these services determine global satisfaction with the community at large, which in turn plays a significant role in global satisfaction with life. The method is based on the theoretical notion that *consumer satisfaction with individual government services* (e.g., police, fire/rescue, and library), *business services* (e.g., banking/savings, insurance, and department stores), and *non-profit services* (e.g., alcohol/drug abuse services, crisis intervention, and religious services) affect satisfaction with the community at large (global community satisfaction). Ultimately, this global community satisfaction, together with satisfaction with other relevant life domains (work, family, leisure, etc.), affect global life satisfaction. This satisfaction hierarchy was explained using bottom-up spillover theory. That is, residents' overall satisfaction with a community can be decomposed into a variety of subdomains, each of which contributes to their overall feelings about the community. Survey data from four different communities were collected to test the validity of the method. The results provided support to the model and the assessment method and measures used.

We are now at a juncture where the reader is in a position to better understand the next theoretical postulate that I would like to propose—the theoretical link between satisfaction with specific housing amenities and neighborhood/community conditions on domain satisfaction. I will make this case by breaking down and organizing the argument in terms of the seven life domains.

Housing and Neighborhood/Community Amenities Affecting the Sense of Well-Being in Health and Safety

I like to argue that housing and neighborhood/community amenities play a significant role in each of the aforementioned life domains contributing to domain satisfaction, which in turn contribute to overall life satisfaction (Dolan et al. 2008; see Table 9.1). For example, within the health and safety domain, satisfaction with housing basic amenities and infrastructure such as safety of electrical wiring, water and plumbing, heat and air conditioning appliances, and air safety within the home, all contribute to increased positive (or decreased negative affect) within the health and safety domain. Consider the home environment of the elderly and the extent to which these home amenities play a role in the quality of life (e.g., Carp 1976; James 2008). A home can be specifically designed to meet the health and safety needs of the elderly. One-story house is most suitable for the elderly because such a structure does not have stairs to climb. Even with two- or three-story homes, the home may be equipped with a stair lift. Bathrooms are specially designed to make it easier for the elderly to use bathroom facilities with relative ease and safety. Homes are modified with ramps for motorized scooters. And so on. However, most importantly are basic infrastructure that can influence the health and safety of the residents—whether the home has access to clean water, toilets, bath, adequate heating and cooling, electricity, etc. (Royuela et al. 2003).

Similarly, satisfaction with neighborhood/community amenities such as satisfaction with fitness and sports facilities in the community, satisfaction with hospitals and clinics in the area, satisfaction with law enforcement's response to neighborhood crime, satisfaction with community services provided by the rescue squad and fire department, satisfaction with the community healthcare system (e.g., Li and Tsai 2014; Rahtz and Sirgy 2000; Rahtz et al. 2004; Yetim and Yetim 2014), all contribute to sense of well-being in the health and safety domain, which in turn contribute to the individual's overall sense of well-being or life satisfaction (e.g., Sirgy and Cornwell 2001, 2002; Sirgy et al. 2000, 2008, 2010). Furthermore, there are many community conditions that influence the sense of safety and health among community residents. Examples include pollution (e.g., Jacobs et al. 1984; Westaway 2006), airport noise (e.g., Hygge et al. 2002; Van Praag and Baarsma 2005), and neighborhood crime (e.g., Davies and Hinks 2010; Hartnagel 1979). Allow me to formalize this discussion through a formal theoretical postulate (the third postulate). Here it is: *The sense of well-being in the health and safety life domain increases with increased satisfaction with housing amenities related to health and safety* (e.g., *satisfaction with safety of electrical wiring, water and plumbing, heat and air conditioning appliances, and air safety within the home*) *and with increased satisfaction of neighborhood/community services and conditions related to health and safety* (e.g., *satisfaction with fitness and sports facilities, hospitals and clinics, law enforcement, rescue squad, fire department, environmental pollution, congestion, crime*).

Housing and Neighborhood/Community Amenities Affecting the Sense of Well-Being in Financial Life

Satisfaction with housing and community amenities plays a significant role in financial life, which in turn contributes to overall life satisfaction (Dolan et al. 2008; see Table 9.1). Specifically, satisfaction with the financial aspects related to the home such as whether the rent or mortgage is affordable, whether the home is a good investment, whether the utilities are affordable, whether costs related to home maintenance and repairs are low and affordable, etc. For most people, housing is the largest consumption and investment item and an important component of their quality of life (Vera-Toscano and Ateca-Amestoy 2008).

With respect to the neighborhood/community, satisfaction with cost of living in the community is likely to influence the individual's overall sense of financial well-being. There may be other aspects of community amenities that can also influence the individual's overall satisfaction in financial life such as the availability and quality of financial services in the community such as banks and investment services (e.g., Li and Tsai 2014; Sirgy and Cornwell 2001, 2002; Sirgy et al. 2000, 2008, 2010). We can formalize this discussion through a fourth theoretical postulate: *The sense of well-being in the financial life domain increases with increased satisfaction with housing amenities related to one's finances* (e.g., *satisfaction with the rent or mortgage, the market value of the home as investment, the utilities, home maintenance and repairs costs*) *and with increased satisfaction of neighborhood/community services and conditions related to financial life* (e.g., *satisfaction with availability and quality of financial services in the community such as banks and investment services*).

Housing and Neighborhood/Community Amenities Affecting the Sense of Well-Being in Family Life

In the same vein, satisfaction with housing and community amenities plays a significant role in family life, which in turn contributes to overall life satisfaction (e.g., Dolan et al. 2008; see Table 9.1). In other words, housing is critical to family well-being (e.g., Noor et al. 2014). It is the foundation of family life. Most of family activities are carried out within the home. Specifically, satisfaction with many housing amenities related to family life and family functioning may contribute to overall sense of family well-being (e.g., Bratt 2002). Examples of such housing amenities may include availability and quality of rooms conducive to family functioning such as a family room where most of the family members congregate and spend leisure time, the dinning room where the family eat their meals together as a family unit, the kitchen where many family members come together to prepare meals, eat, and socialize. Other places within the home where most family members come together to engage in family-related tasks include the utility room. Hence, satisfaction with this space can influence satisfaction in family life too. Other places around the home such as porches, balconies, and decks are customarily used for socializing purposes; hence, they may influence satisfaction in family life.

With respect to the community, there are many aspects of the community that may impact an individual's sense of family well-being (e.g., Li and Tsai 2014; Sirgy and Cornwell 2001, 2002; Sirgy et al. 2000, 2008, 2010). These include the availability and quality of nearby grocery stores, department stores, hardware stores, and other types of shopping establishments that cater to family needs. There are many community services that also cater to family needs. Examples include restaurants, fast food places, childcare centers, eldercare centers, schools for the children, after school activities, theaters and other entertainment establishments for children, etc. Such community amenities may play a significant role in the individual's sense of family well-being.

Consider the study conducted by Noor et al. (2014). This study developed an index of family well-being in Malaysia. Part of this index involved housing and community-related constructs such as satisfaction with number of bedrooms at home, satisfaction with child care, and satisfaction with community relationships. The other dimensions of family well-being were: resilience, safety, savings, healthy lifestyle, time with family, work-life balance, and importance of religion. The study sample involved 5,616 respondents. The residential satisfaction constructs were found to be highly associated with the other dimensions of the family well-being construct.

Here is the fifth theoretical postulate: *The sense of well-being in the family life domain increases with increased satisfaction with housing amenities related to family life* (e.g., *satisfaction with availability and quality of rooms conducive to family functioning such as a family room, the dinning room, the kitchen, the utility room, porche,balcony,anddeck)andwithincreasedsatisfactionofneighborhood/community services and conditions related to family life* (e.g., *satisfaction with availability and quality of availability and quality of nearby grocery stores, department stores, hardware stores, restaurants, fast food places, childcare centers, eldercare centers, schools for the children, after school activities, theaters and other entertainment establishments for children*, etc.).

Housing and Neighborhood/Community Amenities Affecting the Sense of Well-Being in Social Life

One can also argue that satisfaction with housing and neighborhood/community amenities plays a significant role in social life (e.g., Vera-Toscano and Ateca-Amestoy 2008), which in turn contributes to overall life satisfaction (Bjornskov 2003; Dolan et al. 2008; see Table 9.1). Home dwellers use certain housing amenities to host and entertain associates, friends, neighbors, relatives, and family members. In many homes specific rooms are designed for social functions such as the living room (which is different from the family room). Many of the modern homes have kitchens designed not only to prepare and serve meals but also to serve a social function—guests congregate in the kitchen area to socialize. Hence, the availability and quality of such space in the home is likely to influence the home dweller's sense of social well-being.

With respect to the community, there are many aspects of the community that may impact an individual's sense of social well-being (e.g., Li and Tsai 2014; Sirgy and Cornwell 2001, 2002; Sirgy et al. 2000, 2008, 2010). People get together and socialize with friends, associates, and others at a variety of places in the community. These include restaurants, cafes, shopping malls, park and recreation places, social clubs, among others. Satisfaction with these community facilities may play a significant role in people's sense of social well-being.

Consider the research regarding walkable communities (i.e., neighborhoods designed to allow residents to walk to work, shopping facilities, eating establishments, etc.). There is some evidence suggesting that walkable communities contribute to residents' social well-being (e.g., Leyden 2003; Rogers et al. 2011). Another study conducted by Yetim and Yetim (2014) established the relationship between fulfillment of social needs, social capital, sense of community, and individual well-being. The study involved 677 sample adults from Mersin, Turkey. The construct of satisfaction with social needs was measured using survey items such as "There are places where I can have fun with my friends in my city, and I can utilize them easily." Social capital (measured through two subconstructs, namely civicness and trust) was also found to be an important predictor of subjective well-being in a residential context.

The sixth theoretical postulate can be stated as follows: *The sense of well-being in the social life domain increases with increased satisfaction with housing amenities related to social life* (e.g., *satisfaction with availability and quality of rooms used to host and entertain associates, friends, neighbors, relatives, and family members) and with increased satisfaction of neighborhood/community services and conditions related to social life* (e.g., *satisfaction with availability and quality of places in the community that are used mostly for socializing with friends, associates, and family members such as restaurants, cafes, shopping malls, park and recreation places, social clubs, among others*).

Housing and Neighborhood/Community Amenities Affecting the Sense of Well-Being in Work Life

Housing and community amenities also play a significant role in work life, which in turn impacts one's sense of quality of life or subjective well-being (Dolan et al. 2008; see Table 9.1). There are rooms dedicated to work in many homes. In other words, most people engage in job-related activities not only in traditional work places such as a company office or a manufacturing facility but also at their home place. Also, there is a significant segment of the labor force that work from home (i.e., telecommute). Homes are usually designed with a den, typically used as a home office. Other homes are designed with a study room with built-in book shelves. Still other homes have a tool room. The availability and quality of these work spaces in the home do play a significant role in the home dweller's sense of work well-being.

Similarly, community amenities do play an important role in one's sense of work well-being (e.g., Li and Tsai 2014; Sirgy and Cornwell 2001, 2002; Sirgy et al. 2000, 2008, 2010). Is the home geographically located allowing an easy commute to work? Communting a long distance to work every work day does take an emotional toll on the individual's overall sense of work well-being. How about the experience of constant traffic congestion during the daily work commute? This can also take an emotional toll on satisfaction in work life. How about driving daily to work on roads that are full of pot holes? Roads that have poor street lighting or no lights at all? How about street stop signs and traffic lights related to the daily work commute? Too many stop lights? Too many stop signs? Etc. Again, these community conditions may affect one's sense of work well-being (e.g., Novaco 1992; Novaco and Collier 1994; Novaco et al. 1990, 1991). Is there public transportation to go to work? What is the quality of the public transportation? Again, such experiences are likely to play a role in work life satisfaction.

The seventh theoretical postulate can be stated as follows: *The sense of well-being in the work life domain increases with increased satisfaction with housing amenities related to work life* (e.g., *satisfaction with availability and quality of rooms dedicated to one's job such as a home office, study room with built-in book shelves, and tool room*) *and with increased satisfaction of neighborhood/community services and conditions related to work life* (e.g., *satisfaction with the daily commute to work, the traffic congestion on the way to work, the roads conditions on the way to work, traffic lights and stop signs, availability and quality of public transportation, employment opportunities, among others*).

Housing and Neighborhood/Community Amenities Affecting the Sense of Well-Being in Leisure, Arts, and Culture

The sense of well-being in leisure, arts, and culture contribute to one's overall sense of well-being and housing and community amenities related to arts and culture do contribute to one's sense of well-being in leisure, arts, and culture as well as overall life satisfaction (e.g., Dolan et al. 2008; Lee and Weber 1984; Norman et al. 1997; Stoeckler 1977; Stoeckler and Larntz 1986). See Table 9.1. In regards to housing amenities, some homes are dedicated for leisure and hobbies. For example, some may have a room for exercise and fitness. Some may use space for doing yoga or other forms of meditation. Some may have an theatre entertainment room with other forms of recreation (e.g., pool table). Some may have a library with leisure, arts, and culture books. Some may have have a "cave room" to display special momentos and other nostalgic artifacts of special significance. Having that kind of home space dedicated for leisure, arts, and culture should play a significant role in one's sense of leisure well-being (and one's sense of well-being in relation to arts and culture). Alternatively, instead of specific rooms dedicated for arts and culture, there may be specially designed mantels in the family room (or perhaps the sun room) that can allow the home dweller to post the momentos. The same can be said for placement of paintings and other objects of art and culture (Hafstrom and Chung 1990).

In a community context, there are many communities amenities directly related to leisure, arts, and culture that contribute to people's overall sense of well-being in this life domain (e.g., Baker and Palmer 2006; Li and Tsai 2014; Sirgy and Cornwell 2001, 2002; Sirgy et al. 2000, 2008, 2010). Consider movie theaters, play theaters, sports stadiums hosting sports events, skating rings, swim clubs, golf courses, country club establishments, museums, zoological parks, music concert halls, hiking trails, etc. Again, these community amenities play a significant role in people's sense of well-being in the leisure, arts, and culture domain.

The eight theoretical postulate can be stated as follows: *The sense of well-being in the leisure/arts/culture life domain increases with increased satisfaction with housing amenities related to leisure/arts/culture life* (e.g., *satisfaction with availability and quality of rooms dedicated to leisure/arts/culture such as a room for exercise and fitness, space for doing yoga or other forms of meditation, theatre entertainment center, recreation room, library, cave room, mantels, wall space to hang paintings and other pictures, among others) and with increased satisfaction of neighborhood/community services and conditions related to leisure/arts/culture life* (e.g., *satisfaction with movie theaters, play theaters, sports stadiums hosting sports events, skating rings, swim clubs, golf courses, country club establishments, museums, zoological parks, music concert halls, hiking trails*, etc.).

Housing and Neighborhood/Community Amenities Affecting the Sense of Well-Being in Education and Personal Development

Finally we have the education and personal development domain. There are housing amenities directly and indirectly related to the overall sense of well-being in that domain (Dolan et al. 2008; see Table 9.1). Examples include a library dedicated to collecting educational material related to one's own personal growth. Consider a person who has a passion for photography. Having a studio room dedicated to photography and photographic equipment goes a long way to meet his or her self-actualization needs. Perhaps a space within the family room that allows the person with a photography passion to store his works of art.

In a community context, there may be communities amenities directly related to education and personal development (e.g., Li and Tsai 2014; Sirgy and Cornwell 2001, 2002; Sirgy et al. 2000, 2008, 2010; Yetim and Yetim 2014). Consider the municipal library—a place that a person may seek out educational materials of all kind. How about community services related to adult course offerings (seminars and workshops in dance, pottery, ceramics, yoga, meditation, wine tasting, history, fine arts, foreign languages, religion, etc.). Many of these educational programs are designed to foster personal growth and development, and hence serve to enhance positive affect in the educational/personal development life domain.

The ninth theoretical postulate can be stated as follows: *The sense of well-being in the education/personal development life domain increases with increased satisfaction with housing amenities related to education/personal development life* (e.g., *satisfaction with availability and quality of rooms dedicated to education/personal development such as a room a studio room for those who have a passion for photography*) *and with increased satisfaction of neighborhood/community services and conditions related to education/personal development life* (e.g., *satisfaction with availability and quality of the municipal library and adult course offerings* etc.).

Summary and Conclusion

In this chapter I made an attempt to briefly describe popular conceptualizations of residential well-being and introduce a new conceptualization of my own. With regards to popular conceptualizations of residential well-being, I argued that the concept of residential well-being has been conceptualized and measured very differently by residential researchers. There are those who conceptualize and measure residential well-being using a set of objective indicators (standards of building codes and land use). In contrast, the vast majority of quality-of-life researchers have captured and measured residential well-being using subjective indicators involving satisfaction with housing, neighborhood, and community. I then focused on how quality-of-life researchers captured the concept of residential satisfaction using theoretical concepts such as gap, perceived adequacy, and goal. I then introduced my new concept of residential satisfaction guided by the theoretical concepts of bottom-up spillover and need hierarchy.

In regards to my new concept of residential well-being, I defined the concept as satisfaction with one's living arrangement captured by one's home and its immediate surrounding (i.e., community) to the extent that this satisfaction contributes to the sense of well-being in seven major life domains, namely health/safety, financial, family, social, work, leisure/arts/culture, and education/personal development, which in turn all contribute to subjective well-being. I argued that the sense of well-being in major life domains such as health/safety, financial, and family life serves to meet basic needs *a la* Maslow (low-order needs related to survival such as biological and safety needs). In contrast, satisfaction in other life domains such social, work, leisure/arts/culture, and education/personal development serves to meet growth needs (again *a la* Maslow; high-order needs related to human flourishing). Using the logic of bottom-sup spillover theory, I further argued that housing and community amenities play a significant role in each of the aforementioned life domains contributing to domain satisfaction, which in turn contribute to overall life satisfaction. Within a given life domain, satisfaction with housing and community amenities contribute to positive/negative affect within that domain. Based on this conceptualization of residential well-being, survey measures can be developed and tested to establish the reliability and validity of this construct.

References

Adams, J. S. (1984). The meaning of housing in America. *Annals of the Association of American Geographers, 74*, 515–526.

Amole, D. (2009). Residential satisfaction in students' housing. *Journal of Environmental Psychology, 29*, 76–85.

Andrews, F. M., & Withey, S. B. (1976). *Social indicators of well-being*. New York: Plenum Press.

Auh, S., & Cook, C. C. (2009). Quality of community life among rural residents: An integrated model. *Social Indicators Research, 94*, 377–389.

Baker, D. A., & Palmer, R. J. (2006). Examining the effects of perceptions of community and recreation participation on quality of life. *Social Indicators Research, 75*, 395–418.

Bjornskov, C. (2003). The happy few: Cross-country evidence on social capital and life satisfaction. *Kylos, 56*, 3–16.

Bonaiuto, M., Fornara, F., & Bonnes, M. (2006). Perceived residential environment quality in middle- and low-extension Italian cities. *European Review of Applied Psychology, 56*, 23–34.

Bratt, R. G. (2002). Housing and family well-being. *Housing Studies, 17*, 13–26.

Bubshait, A. A., & Al-Atiq, T. H. (1999). ISO 9000 quality standards in construction. *Journal of Management in Engineering, 15*, 41–46.

Campbell, A., Converse, P. E., & Rodgers, W. L. (1976). *The quality of American life: Perceptions, evaluations, and satisfactions*. New York: Russell Sage.

Carp, F. M. (1976). Housing and living environments of older people. In R. H. Binstock & E. Shanas (Eds.), *Handbook of aging and the social science* (pp. 244–271). New York: Van Nostrand Reinhold.

Davies, S., & Hinks, T. (2010). Crime and happiness amongst heads of households in Malawi. *Journal of Happiness Studies, 11*, 457–476.

Davis, E. E., & Fine-Davis, M. (1991). Social indicators of living conditions in Ireland with European comparisons. *Social Indicators Research, 25*, 103–364.

Dittmann, J., & Goebel, J. (2010). Your house, your car, your education: The socioeconomic situation of the neighborhood and its impact on life satisfaction in Germany. *Social Indicators Research, 96*, 497–513.

Dolan, P., Peasgood, T., & White, M. (2008). Do we really know what makes us happy? A review of the economic literature on the factors associated with subjective well-being. *Journal of Economical Psychology, 29*, 94–122.

Erdogan, N., Akyol, A., Ataman, B., & Dokmeci, V. (2007). Comparison of urban housing satisfaction in modern and traditional neighbourhoods in Edirne, Turkey. *Social Indicators Research, 81*, 127–148.

Fishbein, M., & Ajzen, I. (1975). *Belief, attitude, intention, and behavior.* Reading, MA: Addison-Wesley.

Galster, G. (1987). Identifying the correlates of dwelling satisfaction: An empirical critique. *Environment and Behavior, 19*, 539–568.

Galster, G. C., & Hesser, G. W. (1981). Residential satisfaction: Compositional and contextual correlates. *Environment and Behavior, 13*, 735–758.

Grzeskowiak, S., Sirgy, M. J., Lee, D-J., & Claiborne, C. B. (2006). Housing well-being: Developing and validating a measure. *Social Indicators Research, 79*, 503–541.

Grzeskowiak, S., Sirgy, M. J., & Widgery, R. N. (2003). Residents' satisfaction with community services: Predictors and outcomes. *Journal of Regional Analysis and Policy, 33*, 1–36.

Hafstrom, J. L., & Chung, Y. S. (1990). Housing domain of quality of life: Housing tenure, aesthetic aspects, and environmental attributes. In H. L. Meadow & M. J. Sirgy (Eds.), Quality-of-

life studies in marketing and management (pp. 386–396). Blacksburg, VA: Virginia Tech, Center for Strategy and Marketing Studies.
Hartnagel, T. F. (1979). The perception and fear of crime: Implications for neighborhood cohesion, social activity, and community affect. *Social Forces, 58*, 176–193.
Handal, P. J., Barling, P. W., & Morrissy, E. (1981). Development of perceived and preferred measures of physical and social characteristics of the residential environment and their relation to satisfaction. *Journal of Community Psychology, 9*, 118–124.
Headey, B. W. (1981). The quality of life in Australia. *Social Indicators Research, 9*, 155–182.
Hovik, N. (1992). Using socioeconomic indicators and perceived quality of life in the marketing of a community. In M. J. Sirgy, H. L. Meadow, D. Rahtz, & A. C. Samli (Eds.), *Developments in quality-of-life studies in marketing* (Vol. 4, pp. 128–132). Blacksburg, VA: Academy of Marketing Science.
Hygge, S., Evans, G. W., & Bullinger, M. (2002). A prospective study of some effects of airport noise on cognitive performance in school children. *Psychological Science, 13*, 469–474.
Ibem. E. O., & Amole, D. (2013). Residential satisfaction in public core housing in Abeokuta, Ogun State, Nigeria. *Social Indicators Research, 113*, 563–581.
Jacobs, S. V., Evans, G. W., Catalano, R., & Dooley, D. (1984). Air pollution and depressive symptomatology: Exploratory analyses of intervening psychosocial factors. *Population and Environment, 7*, 260–272.
James, R. N., III. (2008). Residential satisfaction of elderly tenants in apartment housing. *Social Indicators Research, 89*, 421–437.
Jeffres, L. W., & Dobos, J. (1990). Communication and public perceptions of quality of life. In H. L. Meadow & M. J. Sirgy (Eds.), *Quality-of-life studies in marketing and management* (pp. 633–644). Blacksburg, VA: Virginia Tech, Center for Strategy and Marketing Studies.
Jeffres, L. W., & Dobos, J. (1992). Communication and public perceptions of the quality of life: Testing the model. In M. J. Sirgy, H. L. Meadow, D. Rahtz, & A. C. Samli (Eds.), *Developments in quality-of-life studies in marketing* (Vol. 4, pp. 43–49). Blacksburg, VA: Academy of Marketing Science.
Jeffres, L. W., & Dobos, J. (1995). Communication and public perceptions of quality of life. In M. J. Sirgy & A. C. Samli (Eds.), *New dimensions of marketing/quality-of-life research* (pp. 227–252). Westport, CT: Quorum Books.
Lee, E., & Park, N. (2010). Housing satisfaction and quality of life among temporary residents in the United States. *Housing and Society, 37*, 43–67.
Lee, Y., & Weber, M. (1984). Development of an instrument to measure the aesthetic quality of housing environment. *Social Indicators Research, 15*, 255–280.
Leyden, K. (2003). Social capital and the built environment: The importance of Walkable neighbourhoods. *American Journal of Public Health, 93*, 1546–1551.
Li, C-H., & Tsai, M-C. (2014). Is the easy life always the happiest? Examining the association of convenience and well-being in Taiwan. *Social Indicators Research, 117*, 673–688.
Maslow, A. H. (1943). A theory of human motivation. *Psychological review*, *50*(4), 370–385.
Miller, F. D., Tsemberis, S., Malia, G. P., & Grega, D. (1980). Neighborhood satisfaction among urban dwellers. *Journal of Social Issues, 36*, 101–117.
Mohit, M. A., Ibrahim, M., & Rashid, Y. R. (2010). Assessment of residential satisfaction in newly designed public low-cost housing in Kuala Lumpur, Malaysia. *Habitat International, 34*, 18–27.
Mohit, M. A., & Nazyddah, N. (2011). Social housing programme of Selangor zakat board of Malaysia and housing satisfaction. *Journal of Housing and the Built Environment, 26*, 143–164.
Morris, E. W., & Winter, M. (1978). *Housing, family, and society*. New York: Wiley.
Morris, E. W., & Winter, M. (1975). A theory of family housing adjustment. *Journal of Marriage and the Family, 37*, 79–88.
Mthembu, C. Z. (1997). Crime, a continuing national crisis: Its consequences on quality of community life. In H. L. Meadow (Ed.), *Developments in quality-of-life studies* (Vol. 1, p. 60). Blacksburg, VA: International Society for Quality-of-Life Studies.

Noor, N. M., Gandhi, A. D., Ishak, & Wok, S. (2014). Development of indicators for family well-being in Malaysia. *Social Indicators Research, 115*, 279–318.
Norman, W. C., Harwell, R., & Allen, L. R. (1997). The role of recreation on the quality of life of residents in rural communities in South Carolina. In H. L. Meadow (Ed.), *Developments in quality-of-life studies* (Vol. 1, p. 65). Blacksburg, VA: International Society for Quality-of-Life Studies.
Novaco, R. W. (1992). Automobile driving and aggressive behaviour. In M. Wachs & M. Crawford (Eds.), *The car and the city: The automobile, the built environment, and daily urban life* (pp. 234–247). Ann Arbor, MI: University of Michigan Press.
Novaco, R. W., & Collier, C. (1994). Commuting stress, ridesharing, and gender: Analyses from the 1993 state of the commute study in Southern California. *Transportation Board Research, 1433*, 170–176.
Novaco, R. W., Kliewer, W., & Broquet, A. (1991). Home environmental consequences of commute travel impedance. *American Journal of Community Psychology, 19*, 881–909.
Novaco, R. W., Stokols, D., & Milanesi, L. (1990). Objective and subjective dimensions of travel impedance as determinants of commuting stress. *American Journal of Community Psychology, 18*, 231–257.
Peterson, C., Park, N., & Seligman, M. E. P. (2005). Orientations to happiness and life satisfaction: The full life versus the empty life. *Journal of Happiness Studies, 6*, 24–41.
Rahtz, D. R., & Sirgy, M. J. (2000). Marketing of health care within a community: A quality-of-life needs assessment model and method. *Journal of Business Research, 49*, 165–176.
Rahtz, D. R., Sirgy, M. J., & Lee, D.-J. (2004). Further validation and extension and the quality-of-life/community-healthcare model and measures. *Social Indicators Research, 69*, 167–198.
Raphael, D., Renwick, R., Brown, I., & Rootman, I. (1996). Quality of life indicators and health: Current status and emerging conceptions. *Social Indicators Research, 39*, 65–88.
Rogers, S. H., Halstead, J. M., Gardner, K. H., & Carlson, C. H. (2011). Examining walkability and social capital as indicators of quality of life at the municipal and neighbourhood scales. *Applied Research in Quality of Life, 6*, 201–213.
Royuela, V., Surinach, J., & Reyes, M. (2003). Measuring quality of lofe in small areas over different periods of time: Analysis of the province of Barcelona. *Social Indicators Research, 64*, 51–74.
Santos, L. D., Martins, I., & Brito, P. (2007). Measuring subjective quality of life: A survey to Porto's residents. *Applied Research in Quality of Life, 2*, 51–64.
Seligman, M. E. P. (2002). *Authentic happiness: Using the new positive psychology to realize your potential for lasting fulfillment*. New York: The Free Press.
Shin, D. C. (1980). Subjective indicators and the comparative evaluation of the quality of community life. *American Journal of Community Psychology, 8*, 523–535.
Sirgy, M. J. (2011). Theoretical perspectives guiding QOL indicator projects. *Social Indicators Research, 103*, 1–22.
Sirgy, M. J. (2012). *The psychology of quality of life: Hedonic well-being, life satisfaction, and eudomania*. New York: Springer.
Sirgy, M. J., Cole, D. Kosenko, R., Meadow, H. L., Rahtz, D., Cicic, M., et al. (1995). Developing a life satisfaction measure based on need hierarchy theory. In M. J. Sirgy & A. C. Samli (Eds.), *New dimensions of marketing and quality of life* (pp. 3–26). Westport, CT: Greenwood Press.
Sirgy, M. J., & Cornwell, T. (2001). Further validation of the Sirgy et al.'s measure of community quality of life. *Social Indicators Research, 56*, 125–143.
Sirgy, M. J., & Cornwell, T. (2002). How neighborhood features affect quality of life. *Social Indicators Research, 59*, 79–114.
Sirgy, M. J., Gao, T., & Young, R. F. (2008). How does residents' satisfaction with community services influence quality of life (QOL) outcomes? *Applied Research in Quality of Life, 3*, 81–105.
Sirgy, M. J., Rahtz, D. R., Cicic, M., & Underwood, R. (2000). A method for assessing residents' satisfaction with community-based services: A quality-of-life perspective. *Social Indicators Research, 49*, 279–316.

Sirgy, M. J., Widgery, R. N., Lee, D.-J., & Yu, G. B. (2010). Developing a measure of community well-being based on perceptions of impact in various life domains. *Social Indicators Research, 96*, 295–311.
Sirgy, M. J., & Wu, J. (2009). The pleasant life, the engaged life, and the meaningful life: What about the balanced life? *Journal of Happiness Studies, 10*, 183–196.
Stoeckler, H. S. (1977). Aesthetic quality of home interior—a useful indicator of housing satisfaction and other quality of life measures. *Journal of Interior Design Education and Research, 3*, 53–73.
Stoeckler, H. S., & Larntz, K. (1986). Cross-cultural differences in relationships among satisfaction with aesthetic quality of dwelling interior, overall housing, and quality of life. In J. L. Hafstrom (Ed.), *Compendium of quality of life research* (pp. 122–135). Urbana, IL: Illinois Agricultural Experiment Station.
Van Praag, B. M. S., & Baarsma, B. E. (2005). Using happiness surveys to value intangibles: The case of airport noise. *The Economic Journal, 115*, 224–246.
Varady, D. P., & Carrozza, M. A. (2000). Toward a better way to measure customer satisfaction levels in public housing: A report from Cincinnati. Unpublished manuscrpt.
Vera-Toscano, E., & Ateca-Amestoy, V. (2008). The relevance of social interactions on housing. *Social Indicators Research, 86*, 257–274.
Wagner, S. (1995, September). Cities that satisfy. *American Demographics, 17*, 18–20.
Walton, D., Murray, S. J., & Thomas, J. A. (2008). Relationships between population density and the perceived quality of neighbourhood. *Social Indicators Research, 89*, 405–420.
Westaway, M. S. (2006). A longitudinal investigation of satisfaction with personal and environmental quality of life in an informal South African housing settlement, Doornkop, Soweto. *Habitat International, 30*, 175–189.
Wu, C-H. (2008). The role of perceived discrepancy in satisfaction evaluation. *Social Indicators Research, 88*, 423–436.
Yetim, N., & Yetim, U. (2014). Sense of community and individual well-being: A research on fulfillment of needs and social capital in the Turkish community. *Social Indicators Research, 115*, 93–115.

Chapter 10
What We Have Learnt About Happiness

Classic Qualms in the Light of Recent Research

Ruut Veenhoven

Introduction

Over the ages philosophers have reflected on the good life, often denoted by the term 'happiness'. Though most philosophers thought of happiness as a morally good life, some focused on happiness in the sense of a pleasant life e.g. among the ancient Greek philosophers Democritus and among eighteenth century Enlightened thinkers Bentham (1789).

Several questions arose around this kind of happiness. A first question was whether a happy life is possible in the human condition. Are we not doomed to suffer? Isn't a happy life a mere dream? If not, a second question is whether we can become happier than we are. Isn't happiness too relative or too much bound to a set-point from which we can at best temporarily deviate? And, isn't happiness too idiosyncratic to be furthered by social policy? Philosophers addressed these questions in their armchairs, from which they could not provide definitive answers.

Developments in the social sciences with, in particular, the emergence of the social indicator movement in the 1960, opened the way to empirical answers to the questions. Happiness became a common topic in survey research and this resulted in a growing stream of research findings, see Scheme 10.1. The results of this research strand are gathered in the World Database of Happiness (Veenhoven 2015),

This text draws on several of my earlier publications, most of which are mentioned on the list of references.

R. Veenhoven (✉)
Erasmus Happiness Economics Research Organization, EHERO, Erasmus University Rotterdam, 1738, NL3000DR Rotterdam, The Netherlands

Optentia Research Program, North-West University, Vanderbijlpark, South Africa
e-mail: Veenhoven@ese.eur.nl

F. Maggino (ed.), *A Life Devoted to Quality of Life*, Social Indicators Research Series 60, DOI 10.1007/978-3-319-20568-7_10

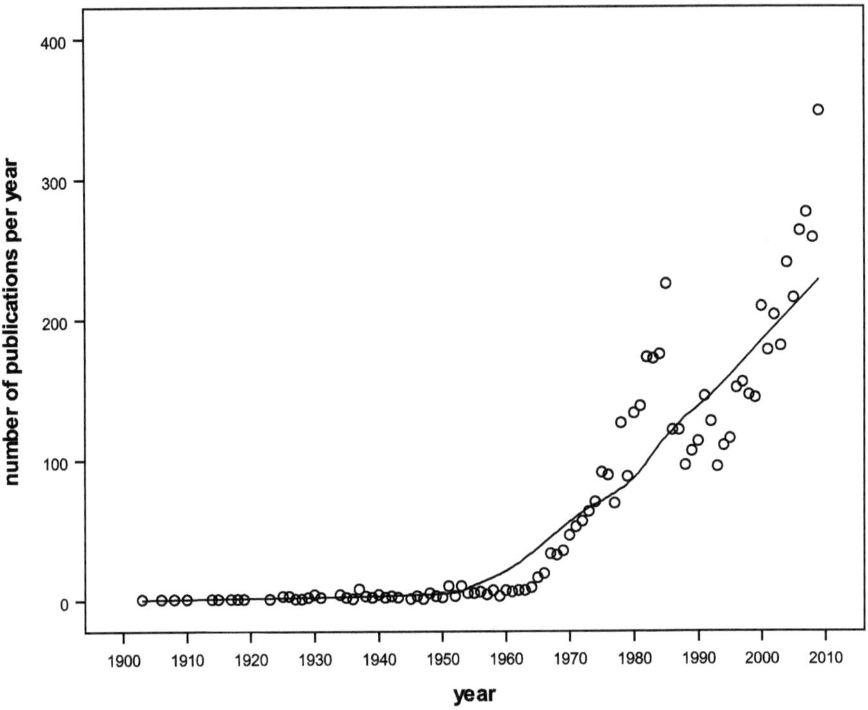

Scheme 10.1 Source: Veenhoven (Source: Bibliography of Happiness Veenhoven 2015a)

the bibliography of which lists currently some 10.000 scientific publications (Veenhoven 2015a). On the basis of this knowledge we can now settle several classic debates, among which the question of whether happiness is too elusive to be pursued.

Qualm 1: Can Happiness Be Defined?

The word 'happiness' has long been used by philosophers to denote a 'good life' and was has commonly been used when giving moral advice on how one should live. Philosophers never agreed on what happiness is precisely and often mixed up happiness-as-such with conditions that promote happiness. As a result, happiness came to be considered an elusive concept, and scientific interest in the subject declined (Buijs 2007). The social indicator movement brought the subject back on the scientific agenda. The practice of measuring quality of life asked for conceptual specificity and required input and output to be distinguished. As a result different notions of the good life crystallized in the literature, one of which is the subject of this chapter.

	Outer qualities	*Inner qualities*
Life chances	Livability of environment	Life-ability of the person
Life results	Usefulness of life	**Satisfaction with life**

Scheme 10.2 Four qualities of life (Source: Veenhoven 2000)

Four Qualities of Life

The different notions of a good life can be ordered in a two by two classification as shown in Scheme 10.2. The top-left quadrant of Scheme 10.2 represents the presence of good external living conditions; with the least livable conditions found in 'hell' and most livable conditions in 'paradise'. This notion is central in 'objective' conceptions of the good life, that is, a notion of conditions in which humans will thrive. This notion is the favorite of policy makers.

The top-right quadrant denotes the inner qualities required to deal with environmental conditions. This notion is central to the 'capability approach' and to the related notion of 'eudemonic happiness'. This meaning is favored by educators and therapists.

The bottom-left quadrant denotes the effects of one's life on the environment, for instance how supportive one is to one's fellow humans and what one contributes to human culture. This rather intangible meaning is favored by moralists.

All three the above notions of quality of life concern objective conditions, that is, conditions that are observable by outsiders of which individual persons are not necessarily aware. In contrast the fourth notion is essentially subjective. The bottom-right quadrant in Scheme 10.2 denotes one's quality of life in the eye of the beholder. This meaning surfaced in social indicators research, among other things because the, in this field, much used technique of survey research involves a focus on subjective experience.

Four Kinds of Satisfaction

There are different kinds of satisfaction, which can also be charted in a fourfold classification, see Scheme 10.3.

The top-left quadrant represents passing enjoyment of aspects of life. Examples are delight in a cup of tea at breakfast, one's fleeting satisfaction with a chore done

	Passing	Enduring
Life domains	Pleasure	Domain-satisfaction
Life as a whole	Peak experience	**Life-satisfaction**

Scheme 10.3 Four kinds of satisfaction with life

or enjoyment of a piece of art. I refer to this category as *pleasures*, Kahneman et al. (1997) call it 'instant-utilities'.

The top right quadrant denotes enduring satisfaction with life-aspects, such as with ones marriage or job. This is currently referred to as *domain-satisfaction*. Although domain-satisfactions depend typically on a continuous flow of pleasures, they also have some continuity. For instance, one can remain satisfied with one's marriage even if one has not enjoyed the company of one's spouse for some time.

The bottom right quadrant in Scheme 10.3 denotes the combination of passing experience and satisfaction with life-as-a-whole. This combination occurs typically in *peak-experiences*, which involve short-lived but quite intense feelings and the perception of wholeness.

Lastly, the bottom-right quadrant represents the combination of enduring satisfaction with life-as-a-whole, that is, how much we like the life we live. The word 'happiness' is increasingly used in this sense. I have defined it as *the degree to which someone evaluates the overall quality of his or her present life-as-a-whole positively* (Veenhoven 1984). This definition is close to what the enlightened philosopher Jeremy Bentham had in mind when he described happiness as 'the sum of pleasures and pains'.

Components of Happiness

When appraising how much we like the life we live, we draw on two sources of information: (1) how well we feel generally, and (2) how well our life-as-it-is compares to standards of how-life-should-be. These sub-appraisals are seen as 'components' of happiness, respectively the *affective component* called 'hedonic level of affect' and the *cognitive component* called 'contentment'. This distinction is discussed in more detail in Veenhoven (2009), in which I propose a theory about difference in the determinants of these components. This distinction is depicted in Scheme 10.4.

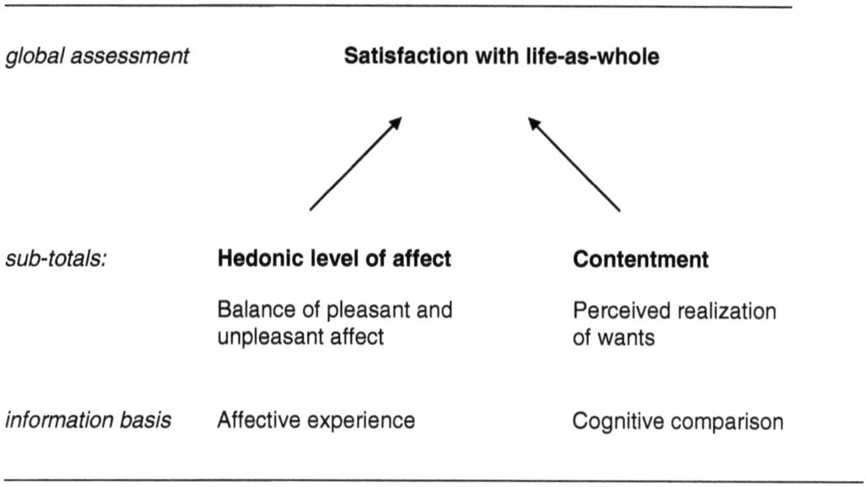

Scheme 10.4 Components of happiness (Source: Veenhoven 1984: section 2/3)

Hedonic Level of Affect
Like other animals, humans can feel good or bad, but unlike other animals, we can reflect on that experience, assess how well we feel most of the time and communicate this to others. This is the feeling-based part of happiness.

Contentment
Unlike other animals, humans can also appraise their life cognitively and compare their life as it is with how they want it to be. Wants are typically guided by common standards of the good life and in this sense contentment is likely to be more culturally variable than affect level. This cognitive appraisal of life assumes intellectual capacity and for this reason this concept does not apply to people who lack this capacity, such as young children who cannot yet oversee their life-as-a-whole and thus can have no clear standards in mind.

In short*: *Happiness can be defined as a specific kind of subjective wellbeing

Qualm 2: Can Happiness Be Measured?

Happiness was long reputed to be immeasurable and many things called 'happines' are indeed difficult to quantify. Yet happiness as defined above is measurable. When defined as the subjective appreciations of one's life, happiness is something we have in mind and what is on our mind can be assessed using questioning.

An overview of acceptable questions is available in the collection 'Measures of Happiness' of the World Database of Happiness (Veenhoven 2015b). To date (March 2015) the collection involves some 1000 slightly different questions. These questions are sorted using the conceptual distinction described above between overall life-satisfaction and its 'components'. Questions that tap overall life-satisfaction are coded 'O' (Overall), questions that address the affective component are coded 'A' (Affect) and questions about the cognitive component are coded 'C' (Contentment). Questions are also sorted by time-frame and rating scale. The collection contains links to studies in which particular questions have been used.

Measures of Overall Happiness

Questions on happiness can be framed in many ways, directly or indirectly, using single or multiple items. Some common questions are presented below.

Single Questions

- "Taking all together, how happy would you say you are: very happy, quite happy, not very happy, not at all happy?" (A standard question in the World Values Surveys)
- "How satisfied are you with the life you lead? Very satisfied, fairly satisfied, not very satisfied, not at all satisfied?" (A standard question in Eurobarometer surveys)

Multiple Questions (Summed)

- Same questions are asked twice: at the beginning and at the end of an interview "How do you feel about your life-as-a-whole? Delighted, pleased, mostly satisfying, mixed, mostly dissatisfying, unhappy, terrible?" (Andrews and Withey's (1976) Life 3)
- Five questions can be used, rated on a 1–7 scale ranging from "strongly agree" to "strongly disagree".
  - In most ways my life is close to ideal
  - The conditions of my life are excellent
  - I am satisfied with my life
  - So far I have gotten the important things I want in life
  - If I could live my life over, I would change almost nothing.[1]
  - (Diener's 1985 Satisfaction With Life Scale SWLS)

[1] I my view this last item is not appropriate. One can be quite satisfied with life, but still be open to the opportunity to try something else.

Measures of Hedonic Level of Affect

There are several ways to ask people how well they feel generally. One way is to invite a person to make a general estimate, for instance using the question: "How often have you felt happy during the past 6 weeks?" Questions of this kind are coded A-TH (Affect: Time Happy), in the above mentioned collection 'Measures of Happiness'.

A second method that can be used to assess hedonic level of affect is a multi-moment assessment. This involves a series of repeated questions such as: "How happy do you feel right now?" Measures of this kind are coded A-ARE, (Affect: Average Repeated Estimates), in the collection 'Measures of Happiness'.

A third approach to assessing an individual's hedonic level is to ask first about various specific affects experienced by that individual in the recent past, both positive affects such as 'joy' and negative affects such as 'anger'. Next an 'affect balance score' is computed by subtracting reported negative affects from reported positive affects. Measures of this kind are coded A-AB (Affect: Affect Balance) in the collection 'Measures of Happiness'.

Measures of Contentment

Contentment can be measured using a general question, such as: "How successful are you in getting what you want from life?" (code C-RW, Contentment: Realize Wants).

A more sophisticated method for measuring contentment requires three steps: First respondents are asked to list the things they want from life. Next they rate how successful they are in reaching each of these things. Finally the investigator computes the respondent's average success in meeting their wants, eventually weighed by importance. Measures of this kind are coded C-ASG (Contentment: Average Success in Goals) in the collection 'Measures of Happiness'.

A variant of the above approach does not ask respondents for personal 'wants', but rather refers to notions of the good life. The first step is to ask people what they think of as the 'best possible life' and next what constitutes the 'worst possible life'. After priming the respondents with these open questions, they are presented with a ladder and asked to imagine that the top of the ladder represents the best possible life as they have just described, and that the bottom of the ladder represents what they imagined as the worst possible life. As a last step respondents are asked to rate their present life on this ladder, in some variants of this approach this is done after the respondents have been asked to rate their life 5 years ago and how they envisage their life 5 years from now. This method is known as Cantril's (1965) 'ladder of life scale' and is coded C-BW (Contentment: Best Worst) in the collection 'Measures of Happiness'.

Validity Doubts

Critics have suggested that responses to questions on life-satisfaction actually measure other phenomena. Rather than indicating how much the respondent enjoys life, the answers to such questions reflect his normative notions and desires. These qualms have been the subject of a lot of research and have been proven to be false (Veenhoven 1993, chapter 5). The main indications for which are summarized below.

No Notion
One of the misgivings about questions on happiness is that most people have no opinion at all of how satisfied they are, they will be more aware of how satisfied they are supposed to be, and report this instead. Though this may happen incidentally, it does not appear to be the rule. Most people know quite well whether or not they enjoy life. Eight out of ten Americans think about it every week. Responses to questions about happiness tend to be prompt. Non-response on these items is low; both absolutely (±1 %) and relative to other attitudinal questions. 'Don't know' responses are also infrequent.

Reflected Appraisal
A related assertion is that respondents mix up how happy they actually are, with how happy other people think they are, given their situation. If so, people considered to be well off would typically report they are very happy, and people regarded as disadvantaged should characterize themselves as unhappy. That pattern is sometimes observed, but it is not general. For instance, in The Netherlands a good education is seen as a pre-requisite for a good life, but the highly educated appear to be slightly less happy with their lives compared to their less educated counterparts.

Colored Answers
Another objection concerns the presence of systematic bias in responses. It is assumed that questions on happiness are interpreted correctly, but that the responses to such questions are often false. People who are actually dissatisfied with their life would tend to answer that they are satisfied, both ego-defense and social-desirability will cause such distortions. This bias is seen to manifest itself in over-report of happiness; most people claim to be happy, at least in modern nations, and most perceive themselves to be more happy than average. Another indication of bias is seen in the finding that psycho-somatic complaints are not uncommon among those that say they are happy.

Yet the above findings allow for other interpretations Firstly, the fact that most people say they are satisfied with their life does not have to imply over-report. It is quite possible that most people are truly happy. Secondly, there are also good reasons why most people think that they are happier than average. One such reason is that most people think like critical scientists and think that unhappiness is the rule. Thirdly, the occurrence of head-aches and worries among happy people does not prove response distortion, life can be a sore trial some times, but can still be satisfying on balance.

The proof of the pudding is in demonstrating response distortion. This has been attempted in a number of clinical studies where responses to single direct questions have been compared with ratings based on in depth interviews and projective tests. The results for such in depth interviews are generally not different from responses made to single direct questions posed by an anonymous interviewer, see for example Wessman and Ricks (1966).

Reliability Doubts

Though single questions on happiness seem to measure what they are supposed to measure, they measure it rather imprecisely. When the same question is asked twice in an interview, the responses are not always identical. Correlations are about +.70, while over a period of a week, test-retest reliability drops to circa +.60. Though responses seldom change from 'satisfied' to 'dissatisfied', switches from 'very' to 'fairly' are rather common.[2] The difference between response-options is often ambiguous and respondent's notions tend to be general, thus the choice for one answer-category or the next is sometimes haphazard when answering questions on life satisfaction.

As choice is often arbitrary, subtle differences in the interrogation environment can exert a considerable effect. Variations in the places where the interviews are held, the characteristics of the interviewer, the sequence in which the questions are asked and the precise wording of the key-item can all tip the scale to one response or another. Such effects can occur in different phases of the response process; when the question is presented, during consideration of the answer and when communicating it.

Bias in Appraisal

Though most people have an idea of how much they enjoy life, responding to questions on this matter involves more than just bringing up an earlier judgment from memory. For the most part, memory only indicates a range of satisfaction. Typically, the matter is re-assessed in an instant judgment. This re-appraisal may be limited to

[2] World Database of Happiness, Correlational Findings (Veenhoven 2015d) Earlier by later happiness (H5.2.1).

recent change: Are there any reasons to be more or less happy than I used to be? It can also involve quick re-evaluation of one's life: What are my blessings and frustrations? In making such instant judgments, people use various heuristics. These mental simplifications are attended with specific errors. For instance the 'availability' heuristic involves orientation on pieces of information that happen to be readily available. If the interviewer is in a wheelchair, the benefit of good health is salient. Respondents in good health will then rate their life-satisfaction somewhat higher and the correlation with health variables will be more pronounced. Several of these heuristic effects have been demonstrated by Schwarz and Strack (1991).

Bias in Response

Once a respondent has formed a private judgment with respect to their happiness, the next step is to communicate it. At this stage reports can also be biased in various ways. One source of bias is inherent to semantics; respondents interpret words differently and some interpretations may be emphasized by earlier questions. For example, questions on happiness are more likely to be interpreted as referring to 'contentment' when preceded by questions on success in work, rather than items on mood. Another source of response-bias is found in considerations of self-presentation and social-desirability. Self reports of happiness tend to be slightly higher in personal interviews than that for anonymous questionnaires[3]; however, direct contact with an interviewer does not always inflate reports. If the interviewer is in a wheelchair, modest self-presentation is encouraged.

Much of these biases are random, and balance out in large samples. So in large samples, random error does not affect the accuracy of happiness averages. Yet it does affect correlations, random error 'attenuates' correlations. Random error can be estimated using multiple-trait-multiple-method (MTMM) studies, and correlations can be corrected (disattenuated) on this basis.

Some biases may be systematic; especially bias produced by the interrogation technique and sequence of questions. Bias of this kind does affect the reliability of distributional data, yet in principle it does not affect correlations, unless the measure of the correlate is biased in the same way, i.e. correlated error.

Comparability Across Nations

Average happiness differs markedly across nations. In the 1990s average happiness in Russia was 5.4 on a 0–10 scale, while in Canada the average was 7.7. Does this mean that Russians really took less pleasure in life? Several claims to the contrary

[3] World Database of Happiness, Correlational Findings (Veenhoven 2015d) Method of interrogation (I5.1.3).

have been advanced. I have checked these doubts Veenhoven (1993), and the results of that inquiry are summarized below.

The first objection is that differences in *language* hinder comparison. Words like 'happiness' and 'satisfaction' do not have the same connotations in different tongues. Questions using such terms will therefore measure slightly different matters. I checked that hypothesis by comparing the rank orders produced by three kinds of questions on life-satisfaction: a question about 'happiness', a question about 'satisfaction with life' and a question that invites a rating between 'best- and worst possible life'. The rank orders appeared to be almost identical in all languages. I also compared responses to questions on happiness and satisfaction in two bi-lingual countries, and found no evidence for linguistic bias.

A second objection is that responses are differentially distorted by *desirability-bias*. In countries where happiness ranks high in value, people will be more inclined to overstate their enjoyment of life. I inspected that claim by checking whether reports of general happiness deviate more from feelings in the past few weeks in these countries; the former measure being more vulnerable for desirability distortion than the latter. This appeared not to be the case.

A third claim is that *response-styles* distort the answers dissimilarly in different countries, for instance, a collectivistic orientation would discourage 'very' happy responses, because modest self-presentation is more appropriate within this cultural context. I tested this hypothesis by comparing life-satisfaction in countries differing in value-collectivism, but found no effect in the predicted direction. The hypothesis also failed several other tests.

A related claim is that happiness is a typical *western concept*; unfamiliarity with it in non-western nations would lead to lower scores. If so, we can expect more 'don't know' and 'no answer' responses in non-western nations, however, that appeared not to be the case.

Many more sources of cultural measurement bias can be involved. If so, there must be little correlation between average life-satisfaction and the actual livability of nations; in section 6 we will see that this is not the case. Using a dozen indicators of societal quality we can explain 75 % of the differences in average life-satisfaction in nations, which means that measurement error can be no more than 25 %. If we had more and better indicators of societal quality, we could probably explain some 90 % of the variation and the error-component would then be no more than 10 %. If we take into account that there is also an error component in the measures of societal quality, the estimate shrinks to some 5 %.

The issue of 'cultural bias in the measurement' of happiness must be distinguished from the question of 'cultural influence on the appraisal' of life. Russians could be truly less satisfied than Canadians, because living conditions are less good in Russia and there is much evidence that this is indeed the case. This issue is discussed in more detail in Veenhoven (2008).

In short*: *Happiness appears to be well measurable

Qualm 3: Is Happiness Relative?

Much of the research on happiness is prompted by the hope that greater happiness for a greater number can be achieved by the use of reason, such as by scientifically informed social policy. In this context researchers looked for ways to create greater happiness for a greater number, however, several theories of happiness imply that this hope is an idle one. One of these is the theory that happiness is relative.

Theoretical Assumptions

This theory holds that we assess how happy we are by comparing life-as-it-is to standards of how-life-should-be. Standards of how life-should be are seen to draw on perceptions of what is feasible and with reference to others. Standards of comparison are thought to adjust. The more money we earn and the more our neighbors have, the higher the amount of money we would deem necessary for a decent living. Together these assumptions imply that it is not possible to create lasting happiness, neither at the individual level, nor the societal level.

At the individual level, this theory predicts that happiness is a short-lived phenomenon. We would be happy when life comes close to ideal, but in coming closer to ideal we set higher demands and end up as equally unhappy as before. Likewise, social comparison can impede lasting happiness. When we have surpassed the Jones, our reference drifts upward to the Petersons, and we feel unhappy again. This theory has many variations, which are nicely combined in Michalos' Multiple Discrepancy theory of happiness (Michalos 1985).

At the societal level, the theory implies that average happiness will fluctuate around a neutral level; because individual citizens oscillate between happiness and unhappiness, the average will be in between. Social comparison is also likely to result in a neutral average; the happiness of the citizens who do better is neutralized by the unhappiness of the ones who do worse. Consequently, average happiness should be approximately the same in all countries.

Empirical Evidence

Some often-cited investigations claim support for this theory. Easterlin (1974) saw the theory proved by his observation that happiness is as high in poor countries as it is in rich countries. Brickman & Campbel (1971) assert that happiness is relative because they found that lottery-winners are no happier than paralyzed accident victims are.

Elsewhere I have exposed these sensational claims (Veenhoven 1991). Happiness appears not to be the same in poor and rich nations and economic growth is typically followed by rising happiness (Veenhoven and Vergunst 2014). Neither are accident victims equally happy as lottery winners. The differences may be smaller than one might have thought, but they undeniably exist.

I also checked some other implications of the theory that happiness is relative. One such implication is that changes in living-conditions, to the good or the bad, do not lastingly affect our appreciation of life, however, there is good evidence that we do not adjust to everything. For instance, we do not adjust to the misfortune of having a handicapped child or the loss of a spouse. Another implication I checked is that earlier hardship favors later happiness. Survivors of the Holocaust have been found to be less happy than Israelis of the same age who had not suffered at the hands of the Nazi.

All in all, there is no empirical support for the theory that happiness is relative.

Theoretical Flaws

Proponents of the theory that happiness is relative see happiness as a purely cognitive matter and do not acknowledge affective experience. In terms of Scheme 10.4 the proponents focus on 'contentment'. This raises the question of how important this cognitive component is in the overall evaluation of life. The available research findings suggest that the affective component dominates, see Scheme 10.5.

In my view affective experience signals the gratification of basic needs. Contrary to 'wants', 'needs' are not relative. Needs are absolute demands for human functioning, that do not adjust to all conditions; in fact, they mark the limits of human adaptability. To the extent that it draws on need-gratification, happiness is not relative.

Difference with Life-Aspect Evaluations

The theory that happiness is relative applies better to some domain-satisfactions; cf. the right top quadrant in Scheme 10.3. For instance, income-satisfaction appears to be largely a matter of comparison, and standards of reference on this matter have been shown to drift (VanPraag 1993). There are also indications for comparison processes in satisfaction with health and satisfaction with job, the evaluation of these specific life-domains tend to follow the right hand route in Scheme 10.5. However, evaluations of life-as-a-whole typically follow the left-hand route. Therefore, the theory does not apply to overall happiness.

***In sum*: *Happiness depends largely on need-gratifications and is as such not wholly relative*.**

Qualm 4:
Is Happiness an Immutable Trait?

Another theory that denies hope of creating greater happiness for a greater number holds that happiness is a fixed disposition. This theory figures at the individual level and the societal level.

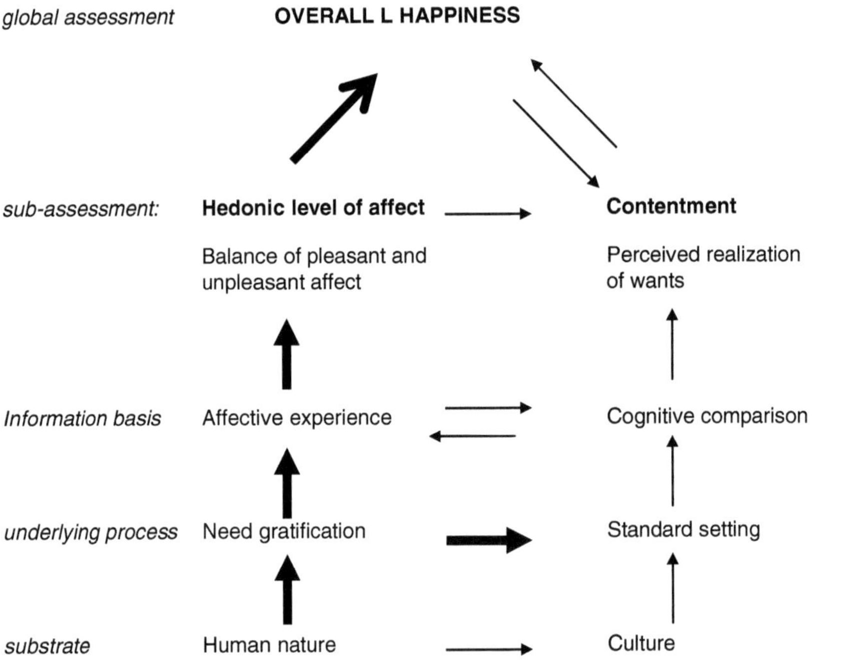

Scheme 10.5 Assessment of life-satisfaction: significance of two causal paths (Source: Veenhoven 2009)

Personal Character Trait?

The individual level variant of this theory sees happiness as a psychological trait; a general tendency to like or dislike things. This tendency can stem from an inborn temperament and from early experience. In this view, an improvement in living conditions will not result in greater happiness. The evaluative reaction will remain the same; the discontented will always be disgruntled and the satisfied will always see the sunny side of things.

Elsewhere, I have taken stock of the empirical evidence for this fixed disposition theory (Veenhoven 1994). I inspected whether happiness is (1) temporally stable, (2) cross-situational consistent and (3) inner caused. None of these appeared to be the case. Firstly, happiness does not remain the same over time, particularly not over the length of a lifetime. Individuals revise their evaluation of life periodically. Consequently, happiness changes quite often, both absolutely and relatively towards others. Secondly, happiness is not insensitive to change in living-conditions.

An improvement or deterioration in one's conditions is typically followed by a rise or decline in one's appreciation of life. These changes to the worse appear for instance as a sequel to widowhood and divorce. Thirdly, happiness is not entirely an internal matter. It is true that evaluations of life are influenced by personal characteristics; however, these inner alignments modify the impact of environmental effects rather than determine them.

National Character Trait?

The societal variant of this fixed disposition theory (folklore-theory) assumes that happiness is part of the national-character. Some cultures will tend to have a gloomy outlook on life, whereas others are optimistic. France is often mentioned as an example of the former kind, and the USA of the latter. In this view, there is also little perspective greater happiness for a greater number. Even if the quality of life in France was improved substantially, French misanthropy would prevent the French from taking more pleasure in life. Elsewhere I have examined the empirical evidence for this theory (Veenhoven 1994).

I first inspected whether the differences in average happiness in nations are unrelated to variation in objective quality of living-conditions in these nations. This is not the case. People are clearly happier in the nations that are most affluent, safe, free, equal and tolerant. Together, these societal qualities explained no less than 75 % of the variation seen in average happiness! Improvements in societal conditions tend to be followed by a raise in average happiness in nations. This is for instance visible in the rising happiness in Western Europe after World War II.

Next I regressed subjective happiness on objective livability of nations and considered the residuals. If French misanthropy reduces happiness, the French must report less happiness than their level of living would predict. In the regression chart, France must be situated below the regression line. Likewise, we can expect the USA to be situated above that line. No such pattern was found.

Lastly, I considered the happiness of migrants. I compared their appreciation of life with average happiness in their country-of-settlement and with average happiness in their country-of-origin. If happiness reflects the quality of the conditions one lives in, the happiness of migrants in a country must be close to the level of autochthons. If, however, happiness is a matter of socialized outlook, the happiness of migrants must be closer to the level in their motherland. First generation migrants in two nations were considered: in Australia, migrants from Britain, Greece, Ireland, Italy, the Netherlands and Yugoslavia; in Germany, migrants from Greece, Italy, Spain, Turkey and Yugoslavia. The trait-theory also failed this test.

In sum*: *Happiness is more a 'state' than a 'trait'

Qualm 5: Is Happines Too Idiosyncratic to Be Pursued Collectively?

The cognitive theory of happiness feeds the idea that conditions for happiness differ widely across persons and cultures. If happiness depends on getting what one wants it will be as variable as human wants are. Policies aimed at the general public will therefore often fail to meet peculiar personal demands, see Scheme 10.5. The bold arrows at the left of Scheme 10.5 suggest that conditions for happiness are typically a matter of fit with human nature, and thus, that there will be much similarity in conditions for happiness I have inspected the empirical evidence for this view elsewhere (Veenhoven 2010a). I found that the conditions that promote happiness are quite similar across the world. Likewise the consequences of enjoying life or not appeared to be almost universal. There is more cultural variation in how happiness is valued and in cultural beliefs about conditions for happiness. The greatest variation is found in how happy people are across populations.

Much Similarity in Societal Requirements for Happiness

Average happiness differs markedly across nations: the highest average on a 0–10 scale is currently (2015) observed in Denmark (8.4) and the lowest in Zimbabwe (3.2). There is a clear system in these differences. People live more happily in the most modern nations, in particular in nations characterized by economic development, freedom, rule of law, and good governance. These societal characteristics explain no fewer than 75 % of the differences in average happiness in nations.

Interestingly, the societal conditions that make people happy are not always the conditions they value. For instance, average happiness is markedly lower in nations where women are discriminated against, but this practice is widely approved in most of these countries (Chin-Hon-Foei 2007). Likewise, corruption reduces happiness, even in societies where favoritism is seen as a moral obligation.

Much Similarity in Required Living Conditions Within Nations

There are also differences in individual happiness within nations. In a happy country like Denmark, 5 % of the people still rate their happiness at 5 or lower on the 0–10 scale, and in an unhappy country like Zimbabwe, some 13 % score 8 or higher. Are the reasons for high and low scores similar across nations? I consider some living conditions for which cross-national data are available below.

Freedom
Not only is average happiness higher in free countries, within countries individuals are happier the more control they have over their life. This appears, among other things, in strong correlations between personal happiness and perceived freedom and control all over the world.

Social Rank
People are typically happier on the upper steps of the social ladder than at the bottom. This appears in findings on relative income position, occupational prestige, subjective class, identification and indexes of socio-economic status. These differences tend to be bigger at the lower end of the hierarchy, and, although the correlations with happiness differ in size, they are positive all over the world. This finding fits the view that we have an innate need for social respect. Like other animals that live in groups, we are hardwired to avoid a bottom position.

Marriage
Adults are typically happier when living with a spouse than when single. The difference is around half a point on scale from 0 to 10 and is largely independent of income, gender, and age. Again the size of the difference varies somewhat across time and nations, but the pattern is clearly universal. This finding fits the view that we are social animals and hardwired to form pairs.

Personality
Cross-national research on the relationship between happiness and personality is limited as yet, but the available data suggest that extroverted people tend to be happier across a variety of nations (Lucas et al. 2000) and that neurotics tend to be less happy in all cultures. Once more, there is a difference in the size of the effects. For instance, the effect of self-esteem appears to be stronger in individualistic cultures than in collectivist cultures (Oishi et al. 1999). Still the direction of the trend is the same everywhere.

This is not to say that all conditions for happiness are universal. One notable exception is "education." Although there is a correlation between average happiness and level of education in countries, the most highly educated individuals are not always happier. Correlation between happiness and education vary between −.08 and +.27.

In sum*: *there is much similarity in conditions for human happiness

Qualm 6: Have We Become Any Happier?

In the eighteenth century, enlightened progress optimists foresaw that social reform would result in greater happiness for a greater number. Has this promise come true? Systematic measurement of happiness started in the 1960s in some western nations, long after implementation of many of the policies based on enlightened thinking. Most people appeared to be happy when the surveys began, average happiness in nations ranging from 6 to 8 on scale 0–10 (Veenhoven 2015c). Analysis of the trend in average happiness over the next 50 years has shown that averages have increased in most countries, though not in all. See Table 10.1. The average yearly increase, on scale 0–10 was 0,012 for all analyzed nations and at this rate it will take about 80 year for average happiness to raise one full point in a nation. This is comparable to the gradual rise in longevity in modern nations.

In sum*: *Happiness is rising in contemporary society

Conclusion

The social indicator movement, since its emergence in the 1970s, has provided answers to the question of whether greater happiness for a greater number is possible. We can now answer this question affirmatively. Thanks to Alex Michalos this research strand is now well established and the way is paved for further gains in our knowledge of our quality of life in the future.

Table 10.1 Change of average happiness in 67 nations

Period	Number of nations	Yearly change
10–20 years	31	+0.010
20–40 years	27	+0.009
40 years and more	9	+0.30
All	**67**	**+.012**

Average yearly change in points on scale 0–10, split-up by length of period
Source: Veenhoven (2014)

References

Andrews, F.M. & Withey, S.B. (1976) *Social Indicators of Well-being: Americans Perceptions of Life Quality.* New York: Plenum

Bentham, J. (1789) *Introduction to the principles of morals and legislation* (Original London 1789 Payne Reprinted, London 1970 Althone Press)

Brickman, P. & Campbell, D.T. (1971) *Hedonic Relativism and Planning the Good Society* in: Appley, M.H. (Ed.): Adaptation Level Theory", Academic Press, New York, USA, 287–302

Buijs, P.M. (2007) *De eeuw van het geluk: Nederlandse opvattingen over geluk ten tijde van de Verlichting, 1658--1835* (The age of happiness: Dutch opinions of happiness during the Enlightenment, 1658–1835) Uitgeverij Verloren, Hilversum, Netherlands

Cantril, H. (1965) *The Pattern of Human Concern* New Brunswick: Rutgers University Press.

ChinHonFoei, S. (2007) *Gender equality and happiness in nations.* Paper presented at Dag van de Sociologie, Tilburg, Netherlands, June 8th-2006

Diener, E., Emmons, R. A., Griffin, S. & Larsen, R. J. (1985) *The Satisfaction With Life Scale.* Journal of Personality Assessment, 49: 71–75

Easterlin, R.A. (1974) *Does economic growth improve the human lot?* In: David, P.A, ;Melvin, W.R. (Eds.) "Nations and Households in Economic Growth", Academic Press, New York, USA, pp. 89–125

Kahneman, D., .Sarin, R. & Wakker, P. (1997) *Back to Bentham? Explorations of experienced utility.* The Quarterly Journal of Economics, 112: 375–405

Lucas, R. E., Diener, E., Grob, A., Suh, E. M., & Shao, L. (2000) *Cross-cultural evidence for the fundamental features of extraversion.* Journal of Personality and Social Psychology, 7:, 452–468

Michalos, A. (1985) *Multiple Discrepancy Theory (MDT).* Social Indicators Research, 16: 347–413

Oishi, S., Diener, E., Lucas, R. E., & Suh, E. (1999) *Cross-cultural variation in predictors of life-satisfaction: Perspectives from needs and values.* Personality and Social Psychology Bulletin, 25, 980–990

Schwarz, N. & Strack, N. (1991) *Evaluating one's life: a judgment model of subjective well-being.* In: Strack, F. ET. al. (eds.) 'Subjective wellbeing', Pergamon, London UK, pp. 27–48

VanPraag, B.M. (1993) *The Relativity of Welfare* in: M. Nussbaum, M. & Sen, A. (Eds.). The Quality of Life, Oxford: Clarendon Press. pp. 362–385

Veenhoven, R. (1984) *Conditions of happiness.* Kluwer (now Springer), Dordrecht, Netherlands

Veenhoven, R. (1991) *Is happiness relative?* Social Indicators Research, 24: 1–34

Veenhoven, R. (1993) *Happiness in nations; Subjective appreciation of life in 56 nations 1946–1992.* RISBO, Studies in Social and Cultural Transformation, Erasmus university Rotterdam, The Netherlands

Veenhoven, R. (1994) *Is happiness a Trait? Tests of the theory that a better society does not make people any happier.* Social Indicators Research, 32: 101–160

Veenhoven, R. (2000) *The four qualities of life: Ordering concepts and measures of the good life.* Journal Of Happiness Studies, 1: 1–39

Veenhoven, R. (2008) *Comparability of happiness across nations.* School of Sociology and Social Work Journal, 104: 211–234, Kwansei Gakuin University, Japan

Veenhoven, R. (2009) *How do we assess how happy we are?* In: Dutt, A. K. & Radcliff, B. (eds.) 'Happiness, Economics and Politics: Towards a multi-disciplinary approach', Edward Elger Publishers, Cheltenham UK, Chapter 3, pp. 45–69

Veenhoven, R. (2010a) *How universal is happiness?* Chapter 11 in Ed Diener, John F. Helliwell & Daniel Kahneman (Eds.) *International Differences in Well-Being*, Oxford University Press, New York, page 328–350

Veenhoven, R. (2010b) *Life is getting better: Societal evolution and fit with human nature.* Social Indicators Research 97:105–122

Veenhoven, R. (2014) *Long-term change of happiness in nations: To times more rise than decline since the 1970s.* In: Sheldon, K. & Lucas, R. (eds.), Stability of happiness: Theories and evidence on whether happiness can change', chapter 9, pp. 167–200, Elsevier
Veenhoven, R. (2015) *World Database of Happiness.* Erasmus University Rotterdam, Netherlands. Available at: http://worlddatabaseofhappiness.eur.nl
Veenhoven, R. (2015a) *Bibliography of Happiness.* World Database of Happiness, Erasmus University Rotterdam. Available at: http://worlddatabaseofhappiness.eur.nl/hap_bib/bib_fp.php
Veenhoven, R. (2015b). *Measures of Happiness.* World Database of Happiness, Erasmus University Rotterdam. Available at: http://worlddatabaseofhappiness.eur.nl/hap_quer/hqi_fp.htm
Veenhoven, R. (2015c) *Happiness in Nations.* World Database of Happiness, Erasmus University Rotterdam. Available at: http://worlddatabaseofhappiness.eur.nl/hap_nat/nat_fp.php
Veenhoven, R. (2015d) *Correlates of happiness.* World Database of Happiness, Erasmus University Rotterdam. Available at: http://worlddatabaseofhappiness.eur.nl/hap_cor/cor_fp.htm
Veenhoven, R. & Vergunst, F. (2014) *The Easterlin illusion: Economic growth does go with greater happiness in nations.* International Journal of Happiness and Development, in press
Wessman, A.E. & Ricks, D.F. (1966) *Mood and Personality.* Holt, Rinehart and Wilson, New York, USA

Part III
Monitoring Through Indicators

Chapter 11
Global Change and Quality of Life Indicators

Richard J. Estes

Introduction

Knowledge-based intervention has been a hallmark of community[1] practice since the turn of the last century. Indeed, the social survey and charity organization movements of the 1900s were a direct outgrowth of efforts on the part of community and community quality of life (hereafter CQOL) researchers and practitioners to systematically: (1) identify the nature, extent and severity of new and emerging social needs in their communities; (2) organize people and institutions to respond more effectively to those needs; and (3) establish baseline measures against which intervention successes and failures could be assessed (Bartlett 1928; Richmond 1917; Zimbalist 1977). Even the renaming of one of the field's leading journals of the day, *Charities and the Commons*, to *The Survey* illustrates the importance that practitioners assigned to the role of scientific inquiry for advancing practice. Mary Richmond's *Social Diagnosis* (1917) offered further reinforcement of the important relationship that CQOL researchers and practitioners recognized to exist between knowledge-based

---

An earlier version of this chapter appeared as Estes, R. J. (2010), Global change and indicators of social development, in Weil, M. (Editor). *Handbook of Community Practice*. 2nd Edition. Thousand Oaks CA: Sage Press. The chapter has been fully revised and updated in tribute to Alex Michalos in recognition of his exceptional contributions to the advancement of the quality of life theory and research.

[1] In this chapter "community" refers to varying units of analysis ranging from local neighborhoods, to cities and states, and to entire countries. The concept is broadly defined given the variety of approaches that have been developed to conceptualize and assess the nature of quality of life at various levels of measurement.

R.J. Estes (✉)
School of Social Policy & Practice (SP2), University of Pennsylvania,
3701 Locust Walk, Philadelphia, PA 19104-6214, USA
e-mail: restes@sp2.upenn.edu

F. Maggino (ed.), *A Life Devoted to Quality of Life*, Social Indicators Research Series 60, DOI 10.1007/978-3-319-20568-7_11

intervention and the realization of more effective outcomes. Today, of course, CQOL scholars all over the world seek to incorporate rigorous approaches to needs assessment, planning, program development, and evaluation in their work with communities (Community Indicators Consortium 2014).

This chapter discusses the contribution of social indicators, social reporting, and social indexes to advancing CQOL. Prepared as a tribute to the unique contribution made by Alex Michalos to the field of quality of life theory and research, the chapter is divided into two parts: Part I discusses the development of social indicators, social reporting, and social index construction from a historical perspective; Part II identifies the contribution of these innovations to community-focused measurement from a contemporary perspective. The concepts discussed in both parts of the chapter are illustrated with examples drawn from CQOL practice both the United States and other countries. The chapter also contains links for CQOL practitioners to some of the most valuable electronic sources of local, national, regional, and international social indicator data.

Part I: Social Indicators and Social Reporting in Historical Perspective

Social indicators, social reporting, and the development of composite measures of social progress have a long history in American social science. Indeed, the earliest efforts in all three of these fields began initially as part of the work of the Hoover *Committee on Social Trends* (Mitchell 1928) but, subsequently, continued as part of the country's effort to assess the impact of its space program on American life (Wilson 2010). President Johnson's "Great Society" initiatives of the mid-1960s, with its tightly focused emphasis on the attainment of five "great" national goals,[2] invigorated the social indicators effort and, in turn, linked the goals and processes of national development to specific measurable outcomes.

One of the earliest contributions to the development of a coherent conceptual framework for the emerging social indicator movements was that made by Raymond Bauer (1966). In his pioneering edited volume, *Social Indicators*, Bauer offered a comprehensive framework for integrating analyses that, until that time, largely had been undertaken in isolation from one another, e.g., trend analyses of changes over time in the health, education, transportation, housing, labor, urban development, and other sectors of public activity. Simultaneously, Daniel Bell (1966) published *Toward A Social Report* in which he laid out the conceptual framework for undertaking analyses of relevance to policy makers concerning national and local trends

[2]Among other initiatives, the Great Society's goals included: (a) launching the federal "war on poverty"; (b) providing significantly enhanced federal support for education; (c) establishing Medicare for the elderly and Medicaid for the poor; (d) undertaking broad-based housing reform; (e) a strong push for urban renewal; and (f) the provision of federal legal protections for African Americans deprived of voting rights by state regulations.

in social development. Wilbur Cohen (1968), Secretary of the then U.S Department of Health, Education and Welfare (USDHEW), subsequently applied the analytical principles formulated by Bauer and Bell to the Department's planning efforts (USDHEW 1969; currently the Department of Health and Human Services) in much the same way that Robert McNamara applied the principles of goal-oriented planning, cost-benefit analysis, fiscal management, and task-centered approaches to planning for the U.S. Defense Department (McNamara 1968).

Other early pioneers in these movements included the economist Donald McGranahan et al. (1972) who, in his work with the United Nations Research Institute on Social Development (UNRISD), created a system of statistical *congruencies* for identifying the discrete stages through which poorer countries move in achieving progressively higher levels of social and economic development. Campbell et al. (1976) introduced qualitative assessments of life quality, including subjective *satisfaction with life measures*, into a field, which, until then, was dominated solely by quantitative approaches to development assessment (Bell 1966,1969; Estes 1976; Land and Spillerman 1975; Morris 1977; Streeten 1981). Other important comprehensive works that would follow included the United Nations 1975, Environment Canada 2010, Unicef 2014, U.S. Central Intelligence Agency (CIA) 2014, and the many indicies developed by the United Nations Department for Economic and Social Affairs (UNDESA) 1995 both alone and in cooperation with other specialized agencies of the United Nations.

At the same time, work on the development of social indicators and national systems of social reporting was accelerating in both the United States and Europe. Most notable among these efforts was the index construction work of Drenowski and Wolf (1966). One of the early accomplishments of both the U.S. and European social indicator efforts was the establishment within the United Nations of what was to become a vast archive of now easily accessible national and international statistical data (UNDP 2014; UNESCO 2014; World Bank 2014). The contributions of investigators associated with the Club of Rome are particularly noteworthy for their contributions to physical quality of life model-building at the global level (Meadows et al. 1972; Mesarovic 1974; Tinbergen et al. 1976).

Unfortunately, the election of successive conservative governments in the United States brought the social indicator and social reporting movements to a near halt in that country, albeit work on the international dimensions of development was continued by individual American researchers (Dannerbeck et al. 2010; Estes 1984, 1988; Ferris 2010; Hagerty et al. 2002; Land et al. 2010; Miringoff et al. 1999; Sirgy 2010; Wilson 2010; Zumbo 2002). Advancements in the social indicators movements of Europe, however, continued virtually unabated with the result that, today, the contributions of European social scientists to the measurement of national and international social progress are quite substantial (Beck et al. 1998; Berger-Schmitt and Jankowitsch 1999; Galtzer et al. 1992, 2004; Noll 1996; SIPRI 2013; Veenhoven 2010; Zapf 1984).

Also of considerable importance to the history of the social indictors and social reporting movements was the establishment in 1974 of *Social Indicators Research* (SIR) under the stewardship of Alex Michalos who remained Editor-in-Chief of the journal until 2014. Between 1974 and 2014 SIR published 114 volumes of original research on social indicators, social reporting, and CQOL research. The more than 1,000 scholarly papers contained in these volumes provided the scientific basis for the field's steady conceptual development and, in time, contributed to the creation of two additional journals focused on CQOL content: the *Journal of Happiness Studies* and *Applied Research in Quality of Life*. The editorial boards of all three journals constituted a virtual "Who's Who" of the social indicators and quality of life fields (Michalos 2005, 2014).

Part II: Social Indicators and Social Reporting in Contemporary Perspective

Monitoring and assessing changes in national and international development involves three discrete arenas of research of relevance to CQOL practitioners: (1) social indicators; (2) social reporting; and (3) the construction of composite measures of social development and social well-being. Fortunately, considerable work already has been accomplished in each of these arenas of research from which CQOL practitioners worldwide can draw parallels for their locality-based community planning, research and organizational needs (CIC 2014).

Social Indicators

Social indicators are two things: (1) they are *direct measures* of phenomena they purport to measure, e.g., infant mortality rate, educational attainment level, divorce rates, the number of deaths or injuries associated with civil protest actions; and (2) they are *indirect measures* of other, always more complex, phenomena *that cannot be measured directly*, e.g., infant mortality rates often are used as a proxy measure for judging the quality of local or national health systems, divorce rates are used to indicate levels of family stability, and the number of deaths or injuries incurred in civil protest actions are used as indicators of the degree of collective and societal cohesion. Thus, as direct measures of phenomena of interest to CQOL practitioners, social indicators can serve as both direct and indirect measures of changes in socio-economic development levels over time. When selected carefully, social indicators also can serve as efficient measures of phenomena that are too complex or would be too expensive to measure directly, e.g., the comparative effectiveness of alternative service systems, hidden crime rates, patterns of human trafficking, as well as other emerging community needs, etc.

Social indicators fall into three basic categories: (1) *leading indicators* which tend to show the direction of future economic or social activity, e.g., increases in social cohesion in response to serious external threats; (2) *coincident indicators* which tend to track social and economic cycles with comparatively little time lag time, e.g., increases in crime rates during periods of growing unemployment or poverty; and (3) *lagging indicators* which measure how the economy or society *was* rather than *how it is or will be*. Lagging indicators follow after other changes in the economy or broader social system already have taken place, e.g., changes in employment levels follow changes that have already occurred in the underlying economy.

All three types of social indicators can contribute to the advancement of CQOL practice, particularly in situations for which valid, reliable and timely data are needed (e.g., needs assessment and planning) or for which the identification of pre-intervention baseline performance measures are desired (e.g., goal-setting, pre- and post-intervention assessments, cost estimations, etc.). Social indicators also are used to assess changes over time in the performances of even larger systems including census tracts, counties, states or provinces, nations, geographic sub-regions (e.g., Asia, Africa, Latin America), and the world-as-a-whole (Doh et al. 2010; Estes 2010, 2012a, b, 2014a, b; Estes and Sirgy 2014; Estes and Tiliouine 2014; Kober 2011; Moeller et al. 2008; Shek 2011; UNDP 2014; World Bank 2014).

Certain scientific criteria must be met when using social indicators for knowledge-based intervention:

1. Indicators must have a priori operational definitions. These definitions must be in place prior to the collection of data and, in any case, before the beginning of any analysis, i.e., infant mortality rates, for example, can only refer to the number of children per 1,000 born alive who die sometime between their birth and prior to reaching their first birthday (WHO 2014). Variations in this operational definition cannot exist and least of all may not vary within the same or related analyses.
2. Indicators must *validly* measure what they purport to measure, i.e., per capita income should measure all sources of income to which the individuals have access (including public transfers and income from illegal sources) and not just those income sources that are reported by employers to public tax authorities.
3. Indicators must be *reliable* such that the same measures should produce the same results no matter who is doing the measuring, e.g., studies of access on the part of women to contraception or to abortion services should produce the same results when the same concepts and the same methods are applied to the same population.
4. Indicators must be *representative* of the population(s) for which measures of a given phenomenon are being sought, e.g., the degree of social cohesion or social cleavage among the residents of a given neighborhood, community, province, or nation.
5. Indicators must be *timely*, i.e., they must reflect the times of interest to the practitioner, e.g., specific days, weeks, months, or years. Measures that are too old or otherwise untimely are of little use for purposes of assessing time-sensitive social changes.
6. Indicators must have the capacity to be *aggregated* and *disaggregated* at various levels of analysis, e.g., by year, for particular communities or neighborhoods, or for particular populations or sub-populations on which the indicators are based – gender, age, racial, ethnic, religious, nationality, political groupings, etc. (UNPOP 2014; U.S. Census Bureau 2014).

7. Indicators must be *easily interpreted.* Highly esoteric indicators that are understandable by only a small cohort of research specialists rarely have use in CQOL practice, e.g., *racial-ethnic fractionalization index scores* (CIA 2010).
8. Indicators must be *available* for purposes of analysis, i.e., practitioners must be able to secure access to the indicators of particular interest to their communities. In situations were administrative, classified, or commercial data are needed, then, prior arrangements must be made to secure access to such data (World Bank 2014).
9. To be useful in helping to guide CQOL practice, indicators must *reflect changes over time*, e.g., changes over time in the quality of plumbing, housing, emergency services, communications and other types of physical and social infrastructure available to the residents of particular communities.
10. The choice of indicators must have *policy relevance*, i.e., their collection and analysis must contain the potential for advancing different policy outcomes than those identifiable in the absence of such data.
11. At the international level, the indicators selected to guide policy-relevant CQOL practice also must have the *capacity to reflect social change(s) for different localities over time* (OECD 2014; World Bank 2014). Static indicators, or indicators that do not have the capacity to reflect change at higher levels of analysis over some designated time period are of limited use to community practitioners working on behalf of such broad-based issues as the promotion of human rights, the advancement of the status of women and children, the promotion of peace, and so on.

CQOL practitioners working in economically advanced countries are fortunate in having a vast array of high quality, socially relevant, and timely indicators available to them (U.S. Bureau of the Census 2014). The capacity for collecting still other indicators also exists and, often, existing institutional indicator collections may be enlarged once the need for new or additional indicators becomes evident (e.g., by selected governmental and non-governmental organizations as well as universities and for-profit organizations that undertake public opinion polls, neighborhood surveys, and the like). Practitioners in less economically advanced countries (as well as those working in less economically well-off communities in economically advanced societies), unfortunately, have fewer established indicator sources available to them (e.g., city planning departments and units). Typically, such practitioners also have fewer opportunities for collecting relevant data for purposes of local or neighborhood planning. Research staff members of local universities, however, often cooperate with CQOL practitioners in collecting and analyzing data in which both groups share a common interest.

Table 11.1 reports examples of major public and private social indicator collection and dissemination organizations in the United States. Parallel organizations may be found in all economically advanced countries and in regional associations of countries, e.g., the European Union, the Organization for Economic Cooperation and Development, etc. The table also identifies organizations that report a much broader range of data (e.g., the U.S. Census Bureau, the U.S. Department of Labor, and the U.S. Department of Health and Human Services, among many others).

Table 11.1 Selected public and private sources of *Social Indicators*

Organization	Title	Frequency	Comments
Selected public data sources in the United States			
U.S. Central Intelligence Agency, Directorate of Intelligence	*CIA World Fact Book*	Annually	Provides comprehensive description of changing social, political and economic situation of approximately 266 world entities
			https://www.cia.gov/library/publications/the-world-factbook/
U.S. Department of Commerce, Bureau of the Census	*Statistical Abstracts of the United States; Population Statistics of the United States*	Annually	Provides access to thousands of time-series indicators related to all aspects of social, political, economic and demographic development of the United States. Most indicators can be accessed without charge via the internet
			http://www.census.gov/compendia/statab/
U.S. Department of Commerce, Bureau of the Census	*Historical Statistics of the United States*	Annually	Provides access to thousands of time-series indicators from colonial times to the present. Data are available both at the national and state levels
			http://www.csep.ucr.edu/HSUS/HSUS.html
U.S. Department of Health and Human Services, Centers for Disease Control and Prevention, National Center for Health Statistics	*Vital Statistics of the United States*	Monthly	Contains a comprehensive set of time-series data related to birth, mortality, fetal death, marriage and divorce, etc. Data are quite detailed and can be used for national, state and local analyses. Data also are linked to dozens of other data sets assembled by the Centers for Disease Control and Prevention that are of interest to health and social scientists
	Birth and Infant Death Data Set		
	National Maternal and Infant Health Survey		http://www.cdc.gov/nchs/products/vsus.htm
	National Survey of Family Growth		
U.S. Department of Health and Human Services, Administration for Children and Families	*ACDY Data and Statistics*	Continuous	Publishes statistical national, state and country data across a broad range of service sectors including: Child Care, Child Support, Child Welfare, Head Start, Refugees, Welfare Caseloads
			https://www.acf.hhs.gov/
U.S. Department of Health and Human Service, Social Security Administration	*Social Security Programs Throughout the World*	Biannually	Publishes descriptive information concerning the existence, structure, funding mechanisms and requirements of publicly-managed social security programs worldwide
			http://www.ssa.gov/policy/docs/progdesc/ssptw/index.html

(continued)

Table 11.1 (continued)

Organization	Title	Frequency	Comments
U.S. Department of Housing and Urban Development	*HUD Statistics*	Continuous	Publishes housing related data in a broad range of categories: housing, homelessness, affordable housing, urban planning, urban development, etc
			http://portal.hud.gov/portal/page/portal/HUD
U.S. Department of Labor	*Bureau of Labor Statistics*	Continuous	The Dept. of Labor publishes a wide range of social indicators of interest to persons at various levels of social organization: *Economic Data*, *Career Guides*, *Inflation and Spending Statistics*, *Wage Statistics*, *Worker Safety and Health*, *Productivity*, *International and Comparative* data
			http://stats.bls.gov/
Selected private data sources in the United States			
Annie E. Casey Foundation	*Kids Count Data Book: State Profiles of Child Well-Being*	Annually	One of the most comprehensive statistical summaries of changing social, educational and economic conditions of U.S. children in each of the nation's 50 states, D.C. and the U.S. Virgin Islands. Data are updated regularly and are presented for the nation-as-a-whole, by state and for many local communities
			http://datacenter.kidscount.org/
National Center for Charitable Statistics (of the Urban Institute)	*Charitable Statistics of the United States*	Continuously updated	Publishes a variety of continuously updated data bases concerning all aspects of private philanthropy in the United States at the following internet address
			http://nccs.urban.org/index.cfm
National Urban League	*The State of Black America*	Annually	Contains time-series data on the changing social, political and economic status of Americans of African ancestry in the United States
			http://www.nul.org/
Selected international data sources			
Amnesty International	*Statistics on Human Rights Violations*	Continuously	Publishes both qualitative and quantitative analyses of the changing human rights situation for most countries of the world. Many of AI's most penetrating reports can be downloaded without charge from their website
			http://www.amnesty-usa.org

Stockholm International Peace Research Institute (SIPRI)	*SIPRI Yearbook (of military and defense expenditures)*	Annually	Reports nearly 100 time-series indicators on all aspects of weaponry production, sales and distribution around the world
			http://www.sipri.org
United Nations Children's Fund (UNICEF)	*The State of the World's Children*	Annually	Reports about 100 indicators on a time-series basis for all member states of the United Nations. The report's primary focus is on children and families, including changing socioeconomic status of women
			http://www.unicef.sorg/statis/
United Nations Development Programme (UNDP)	*Human Development Report*	Annually	Reports about 100 indicators on a time-series basis for all member states of the United Nations. The report's primary focus is on changing social and economic conditions in member countries, including on gender issues
			http://www.undp.org/
United Nations Educational, Scientific and Cultural Organization (UNESCO)	*Statistical Yearbook*	Annual	Reports about 150 indicators on a time-series basis for all member states of the United Nations. Focus is on educational, scientific and cultural performances of member countries
			http://unescostat.unesco.org/
United Nations High Commissioner for Refugees (UNHCR)	*Refugees and Others of Concern to the UNHCR: Statistics*	Annually	Provides a large quantity of statistical data concerning the involuntary movement of people both within and across international borders, e.g., persons displaced by war, economic disasters, natural disasters, and so on
			http://www.unhcr.org/cgi-bin/texis/vtx/home
United Nations World Health Organization	*World Health Report; The Weekly Epidemiological Record*	Annually	Reports several hundred health, morbidity and mortality indicators on a time-series basis for all member states of the United Nations
			http://www.who.int/whosis/
World Bank	*World Development Report*	Annually	Reports several hundred indicators on a time-series basis for all member states of the United Nations. The report's primary focus is on comparative economic development including trade issues
			http://data.worldbank.org/indicator

Nearly all of the data provided by these large organizations are updated annually… sometimes monthly. Some organizations update their most sensitive indicators even weekly in response to the need for more timely data of critical interest to the organization(s), i.e., the U.S. Labor Department concerning employment/unemployment trends, the U.S. Centers for Disease Control concerning the spread of infectious and communicable diseases, and so on.

Almost all of the data available from national (and regional) data dissemination organizations may be obtained without cost to the user. Given their current electronic format, in most cases these data may be disaggregated to highly specific levels of analysis of special interest of particular groups of users (e.g., by census tract, neighborhood, income groups, age groups, racial groups, and so on). In some cases, the disaggregation of complex data sets to highly specialized levels of analysis may incur a fee to the user. Unlike the majority of national data bases, however, social indicators contained in international data sets rarely can be disaggregated at a level lower than the nation-state (UNDP 2010; UNESCO 2010; World Bank 2014).

Comparable social indicator data sets are available from a variety of public and private organizations located in virtually all economically advanced countries (CIC 2010; OECD 2014; UNDP 2010). Comparable, or near comparable, data sets may exist for many larger developing countries as well (CIC 2014; World Bank 2014). Many international advocacy organizations also disseminate highly specialized cross-national indicators at regular intervals, e.g., Amnesty International (2014), Freedom House (2014), the Stockholm International Peace Research Institute (2014), and Transparency International (2014). In virtually all cases, data collected at the national and international levels may be used for cross-national comparative purposes but, always, one must check carefully for comparability of the operational definitions and data collection procedures used in obtaining such data for each nation included in the analysis.

Social Reporting

As already noted, the international social reporting movement began at the same time as the international social indicators movement. Indeed, a major motivation for collecting social indicators was to prepare national or regional social reports (e.g., Bauer 1966; Bell 1966).

In their simplest form, social reports can be little more than collections of individual social indicators put together between the covers of a book. The *Statistical Abstracts of the United States* (U.S. Census Bureau 2014) is a good example of a highly useful but primarily descriptive approach to the collection and dissemination of time-series data related to virtually all aspects of collective life in the United States. Today, nearly every country (CIC 2014) and organizations of countries (African Development Bank 2014; Asian Development Bank 2014; OECD 2014) of the world has a similar series of statistical reports that track critical social, political, and economic changes occurring in their countries. Increasingly, these indicator collections are available in both print and electronic formats and, in nearly all cases, electronic versions of these reports may be downloaded from the internet without cost to professional users.

In their more sophisticated form, national social reports include a critical analysis of the nature, sources and meaning of the broad-based changes that are taking place within a given society or subset of societies nations. Many of these reports are far-reaching in conception and frequently serve as the basis for realigning public policies toward the attainment of new societal goals. The tradition of European social reporting is particularly noteworthy with respect to its emphasis on the use of time-series data to inform social policy analysis (Hagerty et al. 2002; Moeller et al. 2008; OECD 2014; SIPRI 2013).

The situation of social reporting in the United States is at considerable variance with that found in other economically advanced countries. Although the United States collects and reports vast quantities of socially-relevant data, the country's central government does not publish a formal *state-of-the-nation* social report. Rather, a plethora of highly specialized analyses emanate from departments and agencies of the central government as well as from an array of researchers and policy analysts working in private research organizations that depend on the central government for much of their financial support, e.g., university-based research centers and independent "think tanks". Owing to the varied purposes and methodologies associated with these investigations, typically the separate results obtained from these independent studies cannot easily be integrated into the work of others. Consequently, a usually imperfect—certainly less complete and less timely—picture of critical social trends occurring in the United States emerges from such a disparate range of national analyses (e.g., changing patterns of poverty, changes in family structure and life, changes in community structure and life, increases or decreases in social solidarity, patterns of human trafficking, etc.).

A variety of responses to the absence of a national social report for the United States have emerged over the past decade and many of these approaches are quite innovative (for examples see CIC 2014). In every case, such reports tend to draw on a combination of social indicators collected at the federal and state levels in additional to original data collection undertaken at the local level. Local data collection activities typically also requires the participation of large numbers of people drawn from various sectors of the community; thus, community approaches to social indicator and social reporting tend to be highly participatory and are intended to foster a sense of "ownership" on the part of those who contribute to the effort's planning activities.

Social Index Construction at the Local Level

A number of local initiatives also have resulted in the development of composite indexes of social progress that are used to monitor changes taking place in particular sectors of development of special interest to local communities, e.g., housing, the environment, migration, poverty, etc. Two national efforts in the United States related to children include (1) Kenneth Land's *Child and Youth Well-Being Index* (CWI); and (2) the *Kid's Count Initiative* of the Annie E. Casey Foundation.

Kenneth Land's "Child and Youth Well-Being Index" (CWI)

As summarized on the project's website:

> The Child and Youth Well-Being Index (CWI) is an evidence-based measure of trends over time in the quality of life or well-being of America's children and young people. It comprises several interrelated composite/summary indices of annual time-series of numerous social indicators of the well-being of children and young people in the United States. The composite indices give a sense of the overall direction of change in well-being, as compared to two base years of the indicators, 1975 and 1985 (Land 2010).
>
> This index addresses the following questions: a) Overall, on average, how did child and youth well-being in the United States of America change in the last quarter of the 20th century and beyond?; b) Did it improve or deteriorate?; c) By how much?; d) In which domains or areas of social life?; e) For specific age groups?; f) For particular race/ethnic groups?; and g) And did race/ethnic groups disparities increase or decrease?
>
> In addressing these questions, the index…utilizes…annual time series data (from vital statistics and sample surveys) on some 28 national-level social indicators in seven quality-of-life domains, i.e., *material well-being*, *social relationships* (with family and peers), *health*, *safety/behavioral concerns*, *productive activity* (educational attainments), *place in community* (participation in schooling or work institutions), and *emotional/spiritual well-being*. Twenty-five of the CWI's time series date back to 1975 or earlier, while three are based on indicators that commenced in the mid-1980s". (Land et al. 2010)

The Duke University-based CWI is widely cited in both the national and international social reporting literatures. Findings from the CWI also have contributed to the development of new public policy initiatives relating to the advancement of life quality for the nation's many disadvantaged children and youth. CQOL practitioners may access virtually all of the project's 100-plus electronic time-series indicators from the CWI website without cost (Land et al. 2010).

The "Kids Count" Initiative of the Annie E. Casey Foundation

The Annie E. Casey Foundation publishes an annual report on the status of America's children for each state (Casey Foundation 2014). The Foundation's Kid's Count Initiative reports more than 100 indicators concerning the health, education and social status of children and youth in all 50 states of the United States. Consequently, the Casey initiative is both one of the nation's oldest, most consistent, and most comprehensive sources of data concerning changes in life quality of the nation's children. Data are aggregated at both the state and national levels and, under certain circumstances; it may be possible to obtain more detailed data for geographic territories smaller than individual states. The initiative releases both electronic and print versions of its data sets and the former are available without cost to users.

The initiative's primary purpose is to reduce poverty and social deprivation among America's 70+ million children and youth. To that end it reports regularly on the following indicators (data for the majority of which are obtained from public sources, e.g., the U.S. Census Bureau, the U.S. Center for Disease Control and Prevention, and the U.S. National Center for Health Statistics, among other sources):

- Child Death Rate (deaths per 100,000 children ages 1–14)
- Infant Mortality Rate (deaths per 1,000 live births)
- Overall Rank
- Percent Change Over Time Analysis
- Percent Low–Birth weight Babies
- Percent of Children in Poverty (income below $23,850 for a family of four in 2014)
- Percent of Children in Single-Parent Families
- Percent of Children Living in Families Where No Parent Has Full–Time, Year–Round Employment
- Percent of Teens Not Attending School and Not Working (ages 16–19)
- Percent of Teens Not in School and Not High School Graduates (ages 16–19)
- Teen Birth Rate (births per 1,000 females ages 15–19)
- Teen Death Rate (deaths per 100,000 teens ages 15–19)

Like the CWI, the trend-analyses reported by the Casey Initiative are highly influential and often serve as the basis for public policy debates. They also serve to animate the advocacy efforts of local and state-wide child focused organizations and, in doing so, foster an integration of knowledge with action.

Social Index Construction at the International Level

Considerable work also has been done on developing indexes for measuring social progress at the international level. The source of much of this work centers around the activities of various specialized agencies of the United Nations (e.g., the United Nations Development Programme [UNDP], the United Nations Research Institute for Social Development [UNRISD]) as well as that of nongovernmental organizations engaged in international development assistance, e.g., Freedom House, Save the Children, Transparency International. A large number of academics also have taken up the challenge of developing policy-relevant composite measures of changes in national and international social progress (see Estes 2014a, b for comprehensive citations lists).

In general, the international social index movement emerged side by side with the social indicator and social reporting movements. Indeed, many of the same people were involved in leadership positions for all three movements (e.g., William Behrens, Robert Cummins, Jan Drenowski, Richard J. Estes, Wolfgang Glatzer, Mabub al Haq, Kenneth Land, Donnelly Meadows, Donald McGranahan, Mihajlo Mesarovic, Morris D. Morris, Paul Streeten, Jan Tinbergen, and Ruut Veenhoven). The goals of development assistance organizations and independent investigators working on the creation of international indexes of global social progress were the same: (1) to create new tools for use in monitoring changes in social progress throughout the world over time; (2) to establish baseline measures against which future changes in development could be assessed; and (3) to serve as a basis for establishing new development goals designed to advance world and national development objectives.

Table 11.2 identifies some of the most widely used composite measures of international development that have emerged since the mid-1970s. Each of the indexes

Table 11.2 Examples of *Composite Measures* of social progress used in international and comparative research

Organization/ author	Title/name	Frequency	Comments
International			
Organization for Economic Cooperation and Development (OECD)	***Core Indicators For Measuring Development Progress***	Continuous	For nearly two decades the OECD has sought to develop a set of "core indicators" closely associated with its international development assistance priorities (OECD 1977). The organization's current set of 21 indicators are associated with a different development assistance goal: (1) reducing extreme poverty; (2) promoting universal primary education; (3) promoting gender equality; (4) reducing infant and child mortality; (5) reducing maternal mortality; (6) promoting reproductive health; and (7) protecting the natural environment (OECD 1999)
			http://www.oecd.org/statsportal/0,3352,en_2825_293564_1_1_1_1_1,00.html
Estes, Richard J.	***Index of Social Progress*** (ISP; WISP)	Published every 5 years	Developed at the University of Pennsylvania (Estes 1976), the ISP consists of 45 social indicators divided among 10 sectors of development: Education, Health Status, Women Status, Defense Effort, Economic, Demographic, Geographic, Social Chaos, Cultural Diversity, and Welfare Effort. Statistically weighted versions of the index (WISP), are used to assess the changing social capacity of countries and major world regions
			http://www.sp2.upenn.edu/restes/WSS09.html
United National Development Programme (UNDP)	***Human Development Index*** (HDI)	Annually	The HDI was introduced by the UNDP in 1990 as part of its now annual series of *Human Development Reports* (UNDP 2002). The HDI uses three indicators to assess national levels of "human development": longevity (as measured by life expectation at birth), educational attainment (as measured by adult literacy rates in combination with primary, secondary, and tertiary school enrollment levels), and standard of living (as measured by real GDP or PPP)
			http://hdr.undp.org/en/
United National Development Programme (UNDP)	***Gender-Related Development Index*** (GDI)	Annually	Introduced by the UNDP in 1995, the GDI makes use of the same indicators as those contained in the HDI. However, the GDI assigns different weights to the indicators in order to reflect "inequalities in achievement between women and men." In effect, the GDI is simply the HDI adjusted downward for gender inequality
			http://hdr.undp.org/en/

has its own following and each, in turn, has produced a body of empirical work that seeks to impact patterns of national and international development.

The Physical Quality of Life Index (PQLI)

The Physical Quality of Life Index (hereafter "PQLI") was developed in the mid-1960s by Morris David Morris and his colleagues at the Overseas Development Council (Morris 1979; Streeten 1981). Morris sought to achieve three purposes with the PQLI: (1) to refocus the international debate on poverty and development to include more than just economic outcomes; (2) to focus international attention on the primacy of *human development* as the central goal of development; and (3) to serve as a measure of changes over time in nations achieving their development priorities.

The PQLI consists of three indicators: (1) *infant mortality*; (2) *life expectation at age one*; and (3) *basic literacy*. Country performances on each indicator are combined into unweighted composite scores that range from a low of "0" for countries with the least favorable development performances to "100" for those with the most favorable. Re-applications of the PQLI allow for assessments over time of the changing capacities of governments meet the basic needs of their populations.

Despite its initial influence in the field of development monitoring, the PQLI rarely is used today both because of the elementary nature of the PQLI indicators and the ready availability of other, more robust, analytical tools.

Richard Estes' Index of Social Progress (ISP; WISP)

The Index of Social Progress (hereafter "ISP"; "WISP") initially was conceptualized by this author in 1976 (Estes 1976). In its present form, the ISP consists of 41 social indicators divided among 10 sectors of development: *Education*, *Health Status*, *Women Status*, *Defense Effort*, *Economic*, *Demographic*, *Geographic*, *Political Chaos*, *Cultural Diversity*, and *Welfare Effort*. Statistically weighted versions of the index (WISP) are used periodically to assess the changing capacity of nations, world regions, and the world-as-a-whole in providing for the basic social and material needs of their growing populations (Estes 2010, 2012a, b; Estes and Sirgy 2014, Estes and Tiliouine 2014). The data summarized in Figs. 11.1 and 11.2 represent the results of a worldwide trend analysis in social development and well-being for the 40-year period 1970–2010 (Estes 2014b). Of particularly note in the last wave of data are the dramatic advances in social development that took place in Sub Saharan Africa between 2000 and 2010 (Estes 2014a).

Figure 11.3 illustrates a graphical analysis of the "distribution" of social development and well-being across the planet. Countries presented in lighter colors have attained higher levels of quality of life and social development than those represented by darker colors. The graphs presented for a larger analysis varying considerably and reflect the changes in national regional development over a 40-year time span.

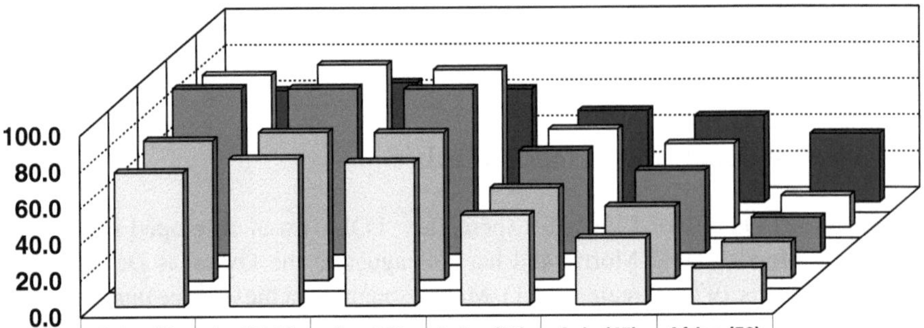

	N Am (2)	Au-NZ (2)	Eur (35)	L Am (26)	Asia (45)	Africa (50)
1970	73.9	81.0	79.0	49.8	36.6	19.8
1980	77.3	81.6	81.2	50.4	40.0	19.9
1990	91.8	91.6	91.2	57.0	45.8	19.5
2000	85.2	91.0	87.8	54.7	46.4	17.5
2011	62.5	66.8	62.9	50.9	47.7	37.6

[CONT_11_bw]

Fig. 11.1 Average WISP scores by continent 1970–2011 (N = 160). (Source: Estes 2014a, b)

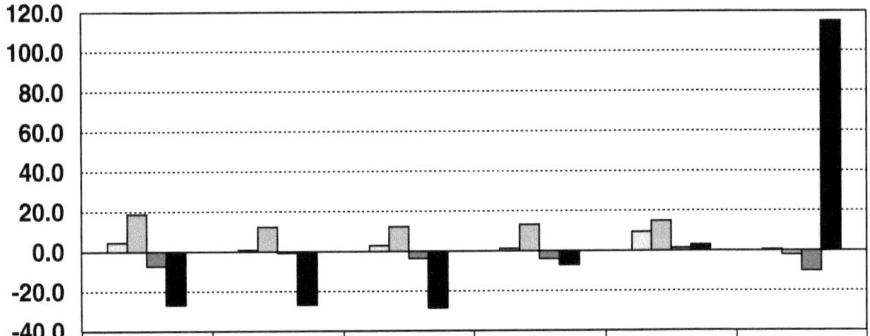

	N Amer (2)	Aus-NZ (2)	Europe (35)	L Amer (26)	Asia (45)	Africa (50)
% 1970-80	4.6	0.7	2.8	1.2	9.3	0.5
% 1980-90	18.7	12.3	12.3	13.1	14.8	-2.2
% 1990-00	-7.2	-0.7	-3.7	-4.0	1.3	-10.1
% 2000-10	-26.6	-26.6	-28.4	-7.0	2.8	114.9

[CONT_11_bw]

Fig. 11.2 Percent change in average WISP scores by continent (N = 160), 1970–2011 (Source: Estes 2014a, b)

The United Nation's Human Development Index (HDI)

The Human Development Index (hereafter "HDI") was introduced by the United Nations Development Program (hereafter "UNDP") in 1990 as part of its now annual series of *Human Development Report(s)*. The HDI builds on the conceptual legacy of both the *PQLI* and Drenowski and Scott's *Level of Living Index*.

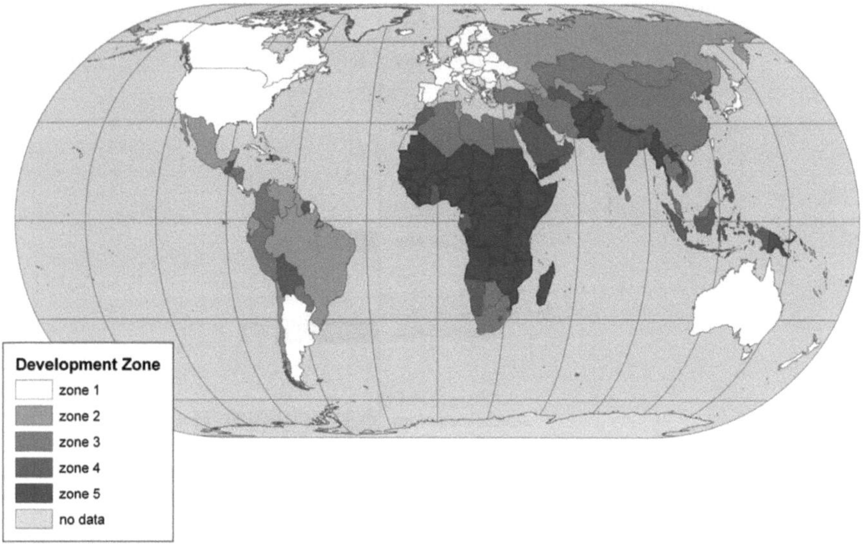

Fig. 11.3 Distribution of WISP scores by country and development zone, 2009 (Source: Estes 2010)

The HDI uses three indicators to assess national and international progress in "human development": (1) *longevity* (as measured by life expectation at birth); (2) *educational attainment* (as measured by adult literacy rates in combination with primary, secondary, and tertiary school enrollment levels); and, (3) *standard of living* (as measured by real *Gross Domestic Product* or *Purchasing Power Parity*). Country performances on each of these indicators are transformed into standardized scores and, then, using a moderately complicated system of statistical weights, are combined to produce a single composite HDI score.

Like many of its predecessor indexes, the HDI attempts to focus international attention on *both* the economic and non-economic aspects of development, e.g., the persistence of global poverty, gender inequality, the relationship between social and economic development, and the need of people everywhere to participate more fully in framing both the goals and means of development. In 1995, the UNDP released two additional indexes that focus specifically on the changing status of women worldwide, i.e., the *Gender Related Development Index* (GDI) and the *Gender Empowerment Measurement* (GEM).

Figure 11.4 summarizes changes in the rate of absolute poverty for selected regions of the world (UNDP 2013). The data reported are for 1990 and 2010 and show dramatic changes in both the incidence and percentage of absolute poverty (defined as less than \$1.25 per day) for the two decades of the United Nations' Millennium Development Campaign—MDC (United Nations 2005). In all, and as a direct result of the MDC's unparalleled global campaign commitment to the elimination of extreme poverty in the world's poorest nations (MDG Goal #1), 700 million fewer people live in poverty today than in 1990. The trends are fully captured

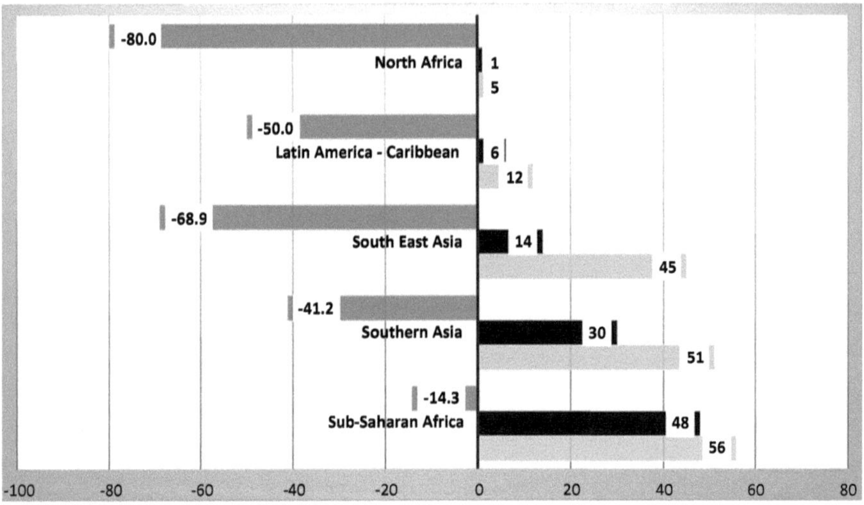

Fig. 11.4 Proportion of people living in extreme poverty and % change, 1990 and 2010 (Millions) (Source: Estes 2014a, b based on data obtained from UNDP (2013))

in the time-series national and regional HDI scores reported by the UNDP (2014, Tables 11.1 and 11.2).

Discussion

Social indicators, social reporting and composite indices of social progress can and do play an important role in CQOL research and practice. When applied correctly, these tools can be used to advance practice in at least five ways: (1) by providing an integrated conceptual framework into which diverse social, political and economic phenomenon can be incorporated; (2) by helping to identify the goals toward which development activities can be directed and the means by which these goals can be attained; (3) by identifying specific targets that are to be achieved within designated time periods; (4) by providing a baseline against which subsequent development successes and failures can be assessed; and (5) by fostering active participation as well as a sense of *ownership* among all the stakeholders involved in the development and application of more knowledge-based approaches to CQOL research and practice.

The use of social indicators, social reports and social indexes, of course, is not the answer to every information or data challenge confronting CQOL researchers and practitioners. Their judicious use, though, can help to both further rationalize our practice and, at the same time, promote progressively higher levels of goal attainment in our work with communities.

References

African Development Bank. (2014). *African Economic Outlook, 2013*. Available at http://www.afdb.org/en/.

Amnesty International. (2014). State of the world report, 2013. Available at http://www.amnesty-usa.org/research/reports/state-of-the-world-2013.

Asia Development Bank (ADB). (2014). Asian and Pacific economic development report. Manila: ADB.

Annie E. Casey Foundation. (2014). *Kids count data book: State profiles of child well-being*. Baltimore: Annie E. Casey Foundation.

Bartlett, H.M. (1928). The social survey and charity organization movements. *American Journal of Sociology*, 34(2), 330–346.

Bauer, R. A. (Editor). (1966). *Social indicators*. Cambridge: MIT Press.

Beck, W. et al. (1998). *The social quality of Europe*. Bristol: The Policy Press.

Bell, D. (1966). The reforming of general education: The Columbia College experience in its national setting. New York: Columbia University Press.

Bell, D. (1969). Toward a social report. *Public Interest* 15, 72–84.

Berger-Schmitt, R., & Jankowitsch, B. (1999). *Systems of social indicators and social reporting: State of the art*. Mannheim: ZUMA.

Campbell, A., Converse, P., & Rodgers, W. (1976). *The quality of American life: Perceptions, evaluations and satisfactions*. New York: Russell Sage Foundation.

Central Intelligence Agency (CIA). (2010). The world factbook. Washington: CIA.

Central Intelligence Agency (CIA). (2014). *World factbook*. Available at http://www.odci.gov/cia/publications/factbook/.

Cohen, W. (1968). Social indicators: Statistics of public policy. *The American Statistician*, 22(October), 14–16.

Community Indicators Consortium (CIC). (2014). About CIC. Available at http://www.communityindicators.net/.

Dannerbeck, A., Casa, F., Sadurni, M., and Coenders, G. (Editors). (2010). *Quality-of-life research on children and adolescents*. Dordrecht NL: Springer.

Doh, C.S., Rutkowski, C.P., and Park, C.M. (Editors). (2010). The quality of life in Korea: Comparative and dynamic perspectives. Dordrecht NL: Springer.

Drenowski, J., & Wolf, S. (1966). *The level of living index*. Geneva: United Nations Research Institute for Social Development.

Environment Canada. (2010). measuring sustainability: Canadian environmental sustainability indicators. Available at: http://www.ec.gc.ca/indicateurs-indicators/. Retrieved October 27, 2010.

Estes, R. J. (1976). World social welfare analysis: A theoretical model. International Social Work 19(2), 29–41.

Estes, R. J. (1984). *The social progress of nations*. New York: Praeger.

Estes, R. J. (1988). *Trends in world social development*. New York: Praeger.

Estes, R. J. (2010). The world social situation: Development challenges at the outset of a new century, *Social Indicators Research*, 98(3), 363–402.

Estes, R. J. (2012a). "Failed" and "failing" states: Is quality of life possible?" in Land, Kenneth, Alex C. Michalos, and M. Joseph Sirgy (Eds.). *Handbook of Quality of Life Research*. Dordrecht NL: Springer, pp. 555–580.

Estes, R. J. (2012b). Economies in transition: Continuing challenges to quality of life, in Land, Kenneth, Alex C. Michalos, and M. Joseph Sirgy (Eds.). *Handbook of Quality of Life Research*. Dordrecht NL: Springer, pp. 433–457.

Estes, R. J. (2014a). Development trends among the world's socially least developed countries: Reasons for cautious optimism", in Spooner, B. (Editor). *Globalization in progress: Understanding and working with world urbanization*. Philadelphia: University of Pennsylvania Press.

Estes, R. J. (2014b). Trends in world social development: The search for global well-being", in Glatzer, Wolfgang (Ed.). *The global handbook of well-being: From the wealth of nations to the well-being of nations*. (Dordrecht NL: Springer).
Estes, R. J., & Sirgy, M.J. (2014). Radical Islamic militancy and acts of terrorism: A quality-of-life analysis, *Social Indicators Research*, 117(2):615–652.
Estes, R. J., & Tiliouine, H. (2014). Islamic development trends: From collective wishes to concerted actions, *Social Indicators Research*, 116(1): 67–114.
Ferriss, A.L. (2010). *Approaches to improving the quality of life*. Dordrecht NL: Springer.
Freedom House. (2014). *Freedom in the world, 2014*. Available at http://www.freedomhouse.org/report/freedom-world/freedom-world-2014#.U7lCgthOX3g.
Galtzer, W. et al. (1992). *Recent development trends in West Germany*. Frankfurt am Main: Campus Verlag (McGill-Queens University Press).
Glatzer, W. et. (2004). *Challenges for the quality of life in the contemporary world*. Dordrecht NL: Springer.
Hagerty, M., J. Vogel & V. Moller (Editors). (2002). Assessing quality of life and living conditions to guide national policy: The state of the art. Special issue of *Social Indicators Research*, 58(1–3), 1–440.
Kober, R. (Editor). (2011). *Enhancing quality of life of people with intellectual disabilities*. Dordrecht NL: Springer.
Land, K. C., & Spillerman, S. (Editors). (1975). *Social indicator models*. New York: Russell Sage Foundation.
Land, K. (2010). The child and youth well-being index. Available at http://www.soc.duke.edu/~cwi/sectiona.htm.
Land, K. et al. (2010). Child trends data bank. Available at http://www.childtrendsdatabank.org/.
McNamara, Robert S. (1968). Robert S. MacNamara. Available at http://www.defense.gov/specials/secdef_histories/bios/mcnamara.htm.
McGranahan, D. V., Richard-Proust, C., Sovani, N.V., & Subramanian, M. (1972). *Contents and measurement of socio-economic development*. New York: Praeger.
Mesarovic, M. (1974). *Mankind at the turning point*. New York: Dutton.
Meadows, D.H., Meadows, D.L., Randers, J., & Behrens, W.W. (1972). *The limits of growth*. New York: Universe Press.
Michalos, Alex. (Editor). (2005). *Citations Classics from Social Indicators Research*. Dordrecht: Springer.
Michalos, Alex. (Editor). (2014). *Encyclopedia of Well-Being and Quality of Life Research*. 12 volumes. Dordrecht: Springer.
Miringoff, M. L., Miringoff, M.L., & Opdyke, S. (1999). *The social health of the nation: How America is really doing*. New York: Oxford University Press.
Mitchell, W. C. (1928). *Recent social trends in the United States: Report of the president's research committee on social trends*. 2 volumes. New York: McGraw-Hill.
Moeller, V., Huschka, D., and Michalos, A. (Editors). (2008). *Barometers of quality of life around the globe*. Dordrecht NL: Springer.
Morris, M. D, (1977). The physical quality of life index. Washington: Overseas Development Council.
Morris, M. D. (1979). *Measuring the conditions of the world's poor: The physical quality of life index*. New York: Pergamon Press for the Overseas Development Council.
Noll, H.-H. (1996). *Social indicators and social reporting: The international experiences*. Mannheim: ZUMA.
Organization for Economic Cooperation and Development (OECD). (2014). *Statistics and reports*. Available at: http://www.oecd.org/
Richmond, M. (1917). *Social diagnosis*. New York: Sage Foundation.
Shek, D.T.L. (Editor). (2011). *Quality of life of Chinese people in a changing world*. Dordrecht NL: Springer.
Sirgy, M. J. (2010). *The psychology of quality of life*. Dordrecht NL: Springer.

Stockholm International Peace and Research Institute (SIPRI). (2013). *SIPRI Yearbook, 2013: Armaments, disarmament and international security*. Available at: http://www.sipri.org/yearbook/2013

Stockholm International and Peace Research Institute (SIPRI). (2014). World armaments and disarmaments. Stockholm: SIPRI.

Streeten, P. (1981). *First things first: Meeting basic human needs in developing countries*. New York: Oxford University Press for the World Bank.

Tinbergen, J., Dolman, A., & Ettinger, J.V. (1976). *Reshaping the international order (RIO)*. New York: Dutton.

Transparency International. (2014). *Global corruption report, 2013*. Available at: http://www.transparency.org/publications/gcr.

U.S. Bureau of the Census. (2014). *Statistical abstracts, 2014*. Washington: U.S. Government Printing Office.

United Nations. (1975). *Toward a system of social and economic indicators*. New York: United Nations.

United Nations. (2005). The United Nations millennium development campaign. Available at http://www.un.org/millenniumgoals/.

United Nations Children's Fund. (2014). *The state of the world's children, 2013*. New York: Oxford.

United Nations Development Programme (UNDP). (2010). The human development report, 2010. New York: Oxford University Press.

United Nations Development Programme (UNDP). (2014). *Human development report, 2013*. New York: Oxford University Press.

United Nations Department of Economic and Social Affairs (UNDESA). (1995). *World summit for social development*. Proceedings available at: http://www.un.org/esa/socdev/wssd/index.html. Retrieved October 10, 2009.

United Nations Educational, Scientific, and Cultural Organization (UNESCO). (2010). World yearbook. Paris: UNESCO.

United Nations Education, Scientific, and Cultural Organization (UNESCO). (2014). *Statistical yearbook*. Paris: United Nations.

United Nations Population Division (UNPOP). (2014). *World population prospects: 2012 Revisions*. Geneva: WHO.

U.S. Department of Health, Education, and Welfare. (1969). *Toward a social report*. Washington: Government Printing Office.

Veenhoven, R. (2010). *World data base of happiness*. Available at: http://worlddatabaseofhappiness.eur.nl/. Retrieved October 27, 2010.

Wilson, J.R. (2010). NASA's positive impact on society: 50th anniversary. Available at: http://www.nasa.gov/50th/50th_magazine/benefits.html. Retrieved October 26, 2010.

World Bank. (2014). *World development report, 201*. (Oxford University Press, New York).

World Health Organization. (2014). *World health report, 2013*. Geneva: WHO.

Zapf, W., (1984). Individuelle Wohlfahrt: Lebensbedingungen und wahrgenommene lebensqualität. In W. Glatzer/W. Zapf (Ed.), *Lebensqualität in der Bundesrepublik*, (pp.13–26). Frankfurt am Main.

Zimbalist, S. (1977). *Historic themes and landmarks in social welfare research*. New York: Harper & Row.

Zumbo, B.D. (Editor). (2002). Advances in quality of life research, 2001. Special issue of *Social Indicators Research* 60(1–3), 1–334.

Chapter 12
The Spread of Social Indicators- and Quality of Life-Research in Germany and Europe: An Overview in Honour of Alex Michalos

Wolfgang Glatzer and Wolfgang Zapf

This overview is a comprehensive reconstruction of the social indicators movement from the middle of the 1960s up to the actual quality of life and wellbeing-research 50 years later. The time span regarded here corresponds roughly with the professional life of the two authors and the article is dedicated to Alex Michalos, to whom our research network thanks a lot.

From the Beginning to Intergenerational Continuity

Social indicators and quality of life research begins in the 1960s like a tiny spring that developed more than 40 years later into a broad diversified stream. The initiative was carried from the late 1960s by a group of young social scientists in North America and Europe, among them Alex Michalos and Wolfgang Zapf, who met at the beginning of the 1970s in North America and Germany. As far as Germany is concerned the first steps of social indicators research were initiated by Wolfgang Zapf. He brought from a visit to the United States some ideas from the so-called social indicators movement with him together with the stimulating book "Social Indicators" from Raymond Bauer (1966). At the Frankfurt University Zapf developed a seminar program about this topic – together with his assistant at this time Karl Ulrich Mayer – and attracted a number of students (among them Wolfgang Glatzer).[1]

[1] Glatzer was after finishing his study co-opted into the research project SPES (content see later) guided by Hans-Jürgen Krupp and Wolfgang Zapf.

W. Glatzer (✉)
Goethe-University, Im Rothkopf 8, 61440 Oberursel, Frankfurt am Main, Germany
e-mail: glatzer@soz.uni-frankfurt.de

W. Zapf
WZB Berlin Social Science Center, Reichpietschufer 50, 10785 Berlin, Germany
e-mail: wolfgang.zapf@wzb.eu

F. Maggino (ed.), *A Life Devoted to Quality of Life*, Social Indicators Research Series 60, DOI 10.1007/978-3-319-20568-7_12

During this time – the early 1970s – Wolfgang Zapf proposed to establish the "Sektion soziale Indikatoren" within the "Deutsche Gesellschaft für Soziologie" and organized in January 1972 its first session in the Werner Reimers Stiftung in Bad Homburg. Later Alex Michalos was invited to the third social indicators conference in 1973 at the Reimers Stiftung. Here Alex Michalos presented his journal "Social Indicator Research" (Michalos 1974) and met with Wolfgang Zapf and Wolfgang Glatzer. He did not forget this event as he shows in his contribution to the oral history of ISQOLS.[2] From this meeting onward the national and international social indicators network was strengthened, it has existed through the decades for more than 40 years until today. From there developed the field of social science activities described multi-named with the terms of social Indicators, quality of life and wellbeing, social reporting and social monitoring. These concepts guided for decades the professional activities of this group of social scientists.

Alex Michalos was very creative in publishing affairs and networking and shaped directly and indirectly the research and publishing activities in North America and Europe to a significant degree. In the beginning of his working career he founded in 1973 the Journal "Social Indicator Research- an internationally and interdisciplinary journal for the quality of life measurement",[3] which contains nowadays thousands of informative pages from a global scientific community. The same can be said for his preliminary final accord which he set after about 40 years of professional engagement by his tremendous work, the "Encyclopedia of Quality of Life and Wellbeing Research"(Michalos 2014). Obviously he will influence through this big opus our speaking and thinking in the future, may it be in Germany, USA or elsewhere. He created a voluminous row of books, the "Social Indicators Research Series" which contains now 55 titles on this subject for all continents.[4] Together with colleagues from the USA he cofounded the International Society for Quality of Studies (ISQOLS) which attracted quality of life and wellbeing-researcher worldwide at the many conferences.[5] He organized the ISQOLS-forerunner conference in Prince George in Canada. Though its gravity centre was in North America a number

[2] Listen at: www.isqols.org/about-isqols/oral-histoy-alex-c-michalos/

[3] Since 1984 on the side of SIR were introduced the Newsletter SINET edited since this time by Kenneth C. Land. Additional journals in the quality of life- and wellbeing-context were Journal of Happiness Studies"(since 2000) and the Journal of "Applied Research in Quality of Life"(since 2006). There is also the journal "Quality of Life Research" which is not related to ISQOLS moreover to ISOQOL, which is an alternative organization dedicated to medicine and life sciences. This list of successful publications – journals and book series - is an indicator for the worldwide increasing interest in this approach.

[4] As it is typical for the network-building of Michalos and his colleagues they pulled Wolfgang Glatzer among others into all the editorial teams of the increasing publications on social indicators and quality of life.

[5] An interesting proof for the internationally and interdisciplinary broad interest in quality of life and wellbeing topics is that two big organizations emerged: ISQOLS (International Society of Quality of Life Studies since 1996), dedicated to quality life and wellbeing, and ISOQOL (International Society for Quality of Life Research since 1994), focused on health-related quality of life, which met and worked parallel and developed their own journals (see Internet Homepages).

of congenial social scientists enlarged the indicators group in Europe, for example active personalities at this time were Rudolf Andorka from Budapest and Michael Illner from Prague. In general the American group members performed a politic of European inclusion and above in the time ahead: Wolfgang Glatzer was elected as the fifth president of ISQOLS after A. C. Samli, Ed Diener, Alex Michalos and Kenneth C. Land and all were accompanied by Joe Sirgy as executive director. European conferences happened in the course of time in Girona (2000), Frankfurt (2003), Florence (2009) and Venice (2012). The research ideas around social indicators found resonance on both sides of the Atlantic and Germany was always included as part of the broad social indicators movement.

The continuity of social indicators and quality of life research through 40 years is extraordinary, it is best visualized in the long series of books and journals. Mostly the same people met at regularly conferences and mostly the same people were elected into the positions of board and executive committee. After a long time of continuity the intergenerational change of the research context began with younger people joining the conferences and taking part in organizational matters. Recently a younger generation – mainly consisting of women – took over the responsibility in different positions: Rhonda Phillips was elected as the actual ISQOLS-president, Filomena Maggino became the new chief editor of "Social Indicators Research", GracielaTonon took over the task of the series editor of the "International Handbooks of Quality of Life Research" (Land et al. 2012). In Germany the long-time engagement of Zapf and Glatzer, who are both retired now, is concluding and younger colleagues joined their path: for example Petra Boehnke, Jan Delhey, Roland Habich, Peter Krause, Denis Huschka, Jürgen Schupp, Stefan Weick. Social indicators research is on a good way into a new era but the challenges to attain awareness for their concerns are still high (Glatzer et al. 2002).

Approaches and Arrangements of Social Indicators Research

Early Social Reporting in Germany

All modern ideas have their predecessors and studies in the style of social reports can be found, already in the nineteenth century. In the German context two interesting examples of past social reporting are "Hoher Taunus" by Gottlieb Schnapper-Arndt (1883) and "Die Lage der ostelbischen Landarbeiter" by Max Weber (1884). These investigations, who were influenced from the tradition of "social statistics", are still models in theoretical, methodological and empirical respect, and are also interesting due to their social and political engagement.

Governmental Social Reporting[6]

Since the beginning of modern social reporting, the German government contributed official studies: in the late 1960s and 1970s family reports and social reports were published and disseminated. Starting in the 1960s, Germany produced various national reports, some were repeated several times. Topics were significant population groups such as children and youth (first 1965), family (first 1968), migrants (first 1987), and the elderly (first 1993). Others were specifically related to the social policy arena, such as social security (first 1970), hidden poverty (1998), extreme poverty (2003), migration and integration (1993), as well as poverty and wealth (first 2001). Obviously the idea of social reporting found some resonance in German governments and was used in everyday politics (Glatzer/Wagner 2014).

Particularly important in the early 1970s were the reports on the state of the nation ("Materialien zum Bericht zur Lage der Nation") that were published several times from the Bundesminister für innerdeutsche Beziehungen in the years 1971, 1972, 1974. Their focus was on the separation of Germany. An interesting result from the surveys was that in the 1970s a large percentage of the German population still believed in the idea, that Germany could be unified. At that time this was a dream which became a surprising reality two decades later.

The unification of Germany in 1990 after 40 years of separation attracted a lot of social research. A governmental supported big research association was related to the unification process under the name "Commission for research on social and political change in the new states of Germany" (KSPW). The commission produced several informative volumes focussing on societal problems especially social security (Hauser et al. 1996). The concept of "transformation" was the guiding idea for the KSPW-work, which is presented in a summary publication (Bertram and Kollmorgen 2001).

In the unified Germany social reporting was continued for example with Government Reports on Poverty and Wealth; the fourth government report on poverty and wealth has been published in 2013. There was also an Enquete-Kommission "Growth, Wealth, Quality of Life" (2012) which enforced thinking about quality of life. The plans of the government aim at a Reporting and Indicator-System for Quality of Life. In this context a commission under the topic "Good life – quality of life in Germany" works with the task to elucidate people's understanding of a good life.

The "Sektion Soziale Indikatoren"

In Germany each scientific approach that wants to be recognized by the scientific community strives to establish a "Sektion" in the "Deutsche Gesellschaft für Soziologie". This also applied for a number of social scientists interested in social indicators who organized themselves as the "Sektion soziale Indikatoren" (Glatzer/Weick 2014). In

[6] This content depends on the article "German Social Reporting" from Wolfgang Glatzer and Gert G. Wagner in the Encyclopedia of Quality of Life and Well-being" (In: Michalos 2014).

January 1972 the first session took place under the auspices of the Werner Reimer Stiftung in Bad Homburg. Starting from there a number of active chairmen guided the section through the decades. Wolfgang Zapf laid the foundations and established a book series of the social indicator section, which was published in 20 volumes until recently (first book Zapf 1974). His successor was Hans-Joachim Hoffmann-Nowotny (1976–1982) who arranged a great conference in Zürich under the title "Soziale Indikatoren – Internationale Beiträge zu einer neuen praxisoriénti-erten Forschungsrichtung" (Hoffmann-Nowotny and Hans Joachim 1976): He was joined by Friedhelm Gehrmann who chaired the section from 1983 to 1988. In the following era of Wolfgang Glatzer (1989–1995) the unification of Germany took place and constituted central topics of conferences during this time. He was continued by Heinz-Herbert Noll (1996–2007) whose successors were Jürgen Schupp (2008–2012), Stefan Weick (2013–2014) and now Jan Delhey (since 2014). The activities of the section are well-documented and can be regarded on the homepage[7]: the conferences and their topics, the titles of their book series, the speaker at the sessions and the participants of all the sessions. After 40 years conferences of the Sektion sozial Indikatoren are still carried through and contribute to the inclusion of the research network.

SPES and the Sonderforschungsbereich 3

In the beginning of the 1970s at the universities of Frankfurt and Mannheim research group was developed, which combined under the guidance of Hans-Jürgen Krupp und Wolfgang Zapf social policy questions with social indicators research (Glatzer 2010, Schupp 2014). The "Sozialpolitische Entscheidungs- und Indikatorensystem" (Socio-political decision and indicator system) was one of the early projects, which was related to the measurement of outputs of societal and political processes and the microsimulation of alternative political measures. Hans-Jürgen Krupp and Wolfgang Zapf wrote an expert opinion for the German Economic Council with the title "Die Rolle alternativer Wohlstandsindikatoren bei der Begutachtung der gesamtwirtschaftlichen Entwicklung" (Krupp and Zapf 1972/2011) and presented their basic ideas in a collection of articles (Krupp/Zapf 1977). There the authors recommended Social reporting and quality of life measurement. In this broad context the first published book was the "Soziologischer Almanach" (Ballerstedt et al. 1975). It is a handbook of meaningful statistics of social and economic importance, inspired by the American "Sociological Almanac" (published 1961 by Gendell and Zetterberg). The chapters were organized in the order of significant long-term time series, selected international country comparisons, and yearly significant indicators. Additional tables illustrated the context of related problems. The Sociological Almanac was published in three editions and was a not at least a pioneer-publication in combining quantitative data and qualitative analysis.

An immediate follower of the SPES-project was the Special Research Unit 3 ("Mikroanalytische Grundlagen der Gesellschaftspolitik") who was active through two decades and produced a broad range of research results (An overview gives:

[7] www.soziologie.de/de/de/sektionen/sektionen/soziale-indikatoren/portrait.html

Deutsche Forschungsgemeinschaft 1994, Volume 1 and 2). German television reported about the basic analysis of societal conditions and processes in Germany published from Zapf (1978) with the title "Lebensbedingungen in der Bundesrepublik". The reconstruction of societal developments with the use of social indicators was integrated into a German System of Social Indicators which is after many years of elaboration still in use.[8] It is characterized by 13 life domains and presents approximately 83 key-indicators for the time after 1950. A new step joining the study on living conditions was the investigation of the perceived quality of life in Germany with the use of a new developed representative "Wohlfahrtssurvey". The first one was carried through 1978 with replications in 1980 and 1984 and than published in respect to quality of life in Germany ("Lebensqualität in der Bundesrepublik Deutschland", Glatzer and Zapf 1984).[9] Whereas the emphasis of the Lebensbedingungen-approach was on "objective" statistics, which were produced from the established statistical institutions, the Lebensqualitäts-study was created to satisfy new demands for "subjective" statistics, which expressed needs and evaluations of the people. In order to satisfy the demand for this kind of data, the "Wohlfahrtssurveys" were introduced and implemented several times (Zapf 2001) within the framework of the Special Research Unit 3.

An important extension of the data reports came with analyses and indicators based on the longitudinal data from the German Socio Economic Panel Study (SOEP) (Wagner et al. 2007). The SOEP, which was initiated by Hans-Jürgen Krupp, started by the Special Research Unit 3 in 1984, was one of the first long-running household panel studies in the world. SOEP made it possible to use longitudinal micro-data for example to analyse the duration of poverty or the amount of income mobility. SOEP-based longitudinal results became a major part of socio-economic reporting by the German Council of Economic Experts (Sachverständigenrrat 2010).

The Datenreport and Official Statistics

In Germany the goal to inform the broader public in an understandable scientific way was realized by the "Datenreport" starting in 1984. The "Datenreport," as a comprehensive social report for Germany, was a cooperative venture by the Statistisches Bundesamt (the federal statistical office) and the Sonderforschungsbereich 3 (the Special Research Unit 3) of the University of Frankfurt and the University of Mannheim. The idea for the creation of this cooperative Datenreport came von Wolfgang Glatzer, who was successful in bringing together the capacities of the welfare-survey-team with the existing reporting capacities of the Statistisches

[8] https://www.gesid-org/fileadmin/up-load/dienstleistung/daten/soz_indikatoren/SSI_en/German:System_of_Social_Indicators.pdf

[9] There was an English edition "German Social Report" (Zapf 1987), which was published as a special volume of "Social Indicators Research".

Bundesamt and – most important – with the material and immaterial support of the Bundeszentrale für politische Bildung (Zapf 2001, p-308).

The Datenreport was first published in 1985 (Statistisches Bundesamt 1985) and then repeatedly updated and improved, though the most recent, 14th edition released in 2013 (Statistisches Bundesamt/Wissenschaftszentrum Berlin 2013). Collaborators in later stages included GESIS (ZUMA), the Science Center Berlin (WZB) and, more recently, the German Institute for Economic Research (DIW Berlin). The original data reports include both an official statistical part and a non-official scientific part according to the availability of statistics. Starting with its 12th edition, the report began to adapt an integrational approach organized around life domains and societal dimensions. It is the most comprehensive data source of problem-oriented statistics for German society. Besides the traditional official statistics, subjective data about the attitudes and feelings of the population are presented in a problem-oriented manner. Some 10,000 copies are always requested by interested people.

The federal German statistical office is publishing also the "Nachhaltige Entwicklung in Deutschland" (Statistisches Bundesamt 2014), a social indicators report, that contains in four fields of action, 21 topics with 38 indicators. The goal of the report is to measure the national strategy of sustainability and was published in response to the United Nations Declaration in Rio de Janeiro. The first German report was published in 2002 and the data came from the National Accounts and the Umweltökonomische Gesamtrechnung (Diefenbacher/Zieschank 2010).

Diversified Social Monitoring

In addition to the large long-term projects mentioned before, a number of further examples in the tradition of social reporting and quality of life research exist.

A solid textbook about "Gesellschaftliche Berichterstattung" was early published (Leipert 1978) as an introduction into theory and practice of social indicators. Under the title "Deutschland im Wandel," social structural analyses were presented; they develop a comprehensive picture of Germany at the dawn of the new century (Glatzer and Ostner 1999). Twenty years after the unification, a follow-up social report for the unified Germany was published (Krause and Ostner 2010). Further social reporting can be found in the handbook of the German society ("Handbuch der deutschen Gesellschaft"), which reviews 20 areas of society (Schäfers and Zapf 1998, 2001).

Another branch are Allensbacher publications especially the "Allensbacher Jahrbücher" which provided survey data designed as subjective complements to official statistics. More than 12 volumes are presented from dozens of representative surveys. The 12th volume was – after the death of Elisabeth Noelle-Neumann, the founder of the Allensbach Institute – edited by Renate Köcher (2009).

Further, "Recent social trends" were regarded in a number of industrial countries from the "International Research Group Comparative Charting of Social Change". They were using a similar format as the Sociological Almanac for the countries Bulgaria, Canada/Quebec, France, Germany (Glatzer et al. 1992), Greece, Italy,

Russia, Spain and USA. The theoretical focus is the question for convergence and divergence in industrial societies (Langlois et al. 1994). Later this research question has been changed to the problem of social cohesion in these countries, published in the Tocqueville Review 2010.

In Germany special attention was given to the performance of the Welfare State and the quality of society on the basis of four representative "Social state surveys", carried out between 2005 and 2008 (Glatzer et al. 2009; Nuechter et al. 2010). European comparative studies show, that quality of life varies significantly according to the different types of welfare states in Europe.

Social Reporting in Germany is conducted by multiple agencies. An independent "Rat für Sozial- und Wirtschaftsdaten" is regarding and organizing the complex field of data production in Germany (RatSWD 2010). The German Council of Economic Advice, joined by a task force of the Franco-German Ministerial Council, designed an indicator tableau according to the ideas of the Stiglitz-Sen-Fitoussi-commission. For the three domains of material wealth, quality of life, and sustainability, a detailed proposal was presented (Sachverständigenrat 2010).

European Activities in Social Reporting and Quality of Life-Research

European countries were continuously present among the social reporting actors, but followed preferable their egocentric approaches, Germany among them. Nevertheless social scientists from European countries came together and discussed their individual approaches.[10]

At the same time European states were connected up to a certain degree as members of supranational organizations like the United Nations and the OECD, in their activities. Regarding Europe, the European Union created all time arrangements for quality of life and wellbeing research and included in the course of its growth more and more countries from originally 7 up to 28.

One of the most ancient long term approaches in Europe is represented by the Eurobarometer. It exists since 1973 and published recently it's 80th volume.[11] Although the Euro-barometer conception has a traditional orientation towards "opinion research", it is nevertheless a huge source of quality of life- and wellbeing-data. For example the recent volumes contain unique data about European identity and attitudes towards migrants, they ask for the effects of the actual financial and

[10] One example is the conference 1994 in Stockholm (Stockholm Seminar on Social Statistics, June 6–7). The contributions to "Social Statistics" in the sense of social reporting were presented from various countries from Italy to Finland. That this conference took place in Sweden was due to the fact, that Sweden and the Nordic countries were at this time leading with autonomous ideas of social reporting (level of living surveys). All in all there were in Europe numerous country-specific activities of social reporting. Main points of discussion were always the technical problems, the samples and their validity and the specialities of the countries which should be included.

[11] http://ec.europa.eu/public_opinion/cf/index.cfm?lang=en

economic crisis on people's wellbeing. The data is presented in the Eurobarometer interactive search system. The Eurobarometer offers the possibility to review in its survey documentation the change of interesting topics in the course of decades.

Aiming at monitoring political and societal progress or regress a Social Indicator System for Europe was constructed in the last two decades.[12] "The *European System of Social Indicators"* is based on a theoretical framework and system architecture which is oriented towards continuous monitoring and analysing the individual and societal well-being of European citizens in terms of quality of life, social cohesion and sustainability, as well as of changes in the social structure of European societies (Noll no date). The EU-27 member states of its time are covered but also Norway and Switzerland, who are two European non-EU countries, and also Japan and the United States, who are two interesting reference societies. There are time series data available, often broken down by socio-demographic and regional variables, since the 1980s for roughly 650 indicators concerning most of the projected 13 life-domains. Access is organized through the online system SIMon at GESIS: http://www.gesis.org/en/social-indicators/products-of-the-zsi/simon-social-indicators-monitor/. "Thereby it represents not only an instrument for scientists to analyse societal developments in Europe but also an information tool for politicians on the attainment of goals like the improvement of living conditions in Europe, the reduction of disparities between countries, or equal opportunities for all population groups within a society" (Berger-Schmitt 2001).

As a main center of European quality of life research Eurofound was established in 1975 as a tri-patriarchic European Foundation agency, whose task is to provide knowledge for social and work related policies (Eurofound 2013). The research team relates itself to the conceptual work of "Beyond GDP" from the European Commission and the Stiglitz-Sen-Fitoussi-report which centers on the well-being of people. Three regularly repeated surveys are related to the planning and establishment of better living and working conditions.[13] Of primary interest is here "The European Quality of Life Survey (EQLS), implemented in 2003, 2007 and 2011–2012, which provides a comprehensive portrait of living conditions in European countries. It contains a broad range of indicators on different dimensions of quality of life, both objective and subjective" (Ahrendt et al. 2015). The results are published in Ahrendt et al. 2015. There was already a coordinated project with a Special Eurobarometer on Poverty and Social Exclusion in autumn 2009 and 2010.

In addition a special European Survey, the "Perception survey in 79 European cities" was conducted with 41,000 interviews in 2012 (European Union 2013). Earlier surveys were carried through 2004, 2006 and 2009. The interesting points are the huge disparities between the cities, the negative effects on wellbeing, which

[12] https://www.gesis.org/soziale-indikatoren/produkte-des-zsi/european-system-of-social-indicators/

[13] In addition to the Eurpean quality of life survey there were carried through the European Company Survey (ECS) and theEuropean Working Conditions Survey (EWCS) which has become a well-established source of information about working conditions and the quality of work and employment.

are accounted to the economic crisis, and the problems of urban development within an integrated approach.

In Eurostat, the statistical office of the European Union, various European statistical projects are carried through among them "EU-SILC". It is dedicated mainly to the investigation of Income and Living Conditions (ec.europa.eu/Eurostat/web/microdata/european_union_statistics _on_income_and_living_conditions). Main topics are detailed explorations of income, also the investigation of housing and health. A more recent concern is the study of poverty and the account of an "at risk of poverty rate". Social exclusion and social cohesion are among the reference points. These statistics should be especially of use for European social policy and have a relationship to the Laeken-indicators". These 18 indicators refer to social participation in the countries and were postulated as goals from the European Council 2001. EU-SILC is carried through since 2003/2005 as a household survey with questionnaires for the household and the household members.

If the time span since the 1960s is regarded, a tremendous expansion of social indicators-, quality of life- and wellbeing-research has taken place in European contexts. There was a continuous side by side of university research, national agencies and supra-national actors (Weick 2014). Whereas the innovations at the beginning seemed to come more from individual researchers, the establishment of continual research is up to now, much more successful on the supranational level. There is currently on the EU-level a high performance of social indicators, nevertheless improvements in detail and coordination of the many facets should be discussed further.

Resumée

It was always difficult to attain a comprehensive overview of activities on social indicators and quality of life-research. The question was already asked years ago: "Whatever happened to social indicators?" (Andrew et al. 1989), but many initiatives were flourishing and were often not related to another.[14] The main fact is obvious: there were few actors in the middle of the 1960s in this field, but stimulation and empowering led to a multi-variety of actors 50 years later on all levels from universities, private institutes nations and not at least supranational organizations (Glatzer et al. 2015). Their main legitimation is expressed several times in the sentence "Democratic societies do not function properly without a solid basis of reliable and objective statistics" (Eurostat: ec.europa.eu/Eurostat/about/overview).

Obviously social indicator research in the sense of a broad spectrum of activities and its off-springs spread in 50 years around the world. The spread of the research approach took place in kind sense of quantity and diversity. New research directions were differentiated: quality of life-research and wellbeing-research, social reporting

[14] Another balance was given in "an overview of the international development in macro social indicators" 35 years ago (Glatzer 1981).

and social monitoring. The spread did not occur in the shape of a train of barges, it was a self-directed organization at many centers in many societies. The main appeal of the research program of this type of social sciences, was to establish a better communication between science, people and politicians. Main part of the scientific concern was the improvement of adequate knowledge regarding our societies.

Many colleagues from North America and Europe contributed through the past 50 years to the success of establishment and institutionalization of related research approaches. Alex Michalos was an efficient and friendly main contributor. He supported the initiatives in the beginning at the change from the 1960s to the 1970s and was through the decades continually contributing to the improvement and consolidation of the research direction. He was a master of conflict management and social integration.

He could use favorable conditions for the success of his activities: primarily there were cooperative colleagues in the USA and in Europe and later on all continents, interested in the same ideas and ready to invest working capacities in this field. That the personal relationships have partly continued for about more than 50 years, is an additional indicator for "the strength of weak ties". Beyond this, it seems to have existed something like a general sounding board, which indicated that time was ready for these ideas and is still ready for them today.

References

Ahrendt, Daphne; Dubois, Hans; and Mezger, Erika (2015). An Overview of Quality of Life and Wellbeing in Europe. In: Glatzer (2015)

Andrews, Frank M. et al (1989). Whatever happened to Social indicators? A Symposium. In: Journal of Public Policy 9/4,p. 399–450

Ballerstedt, Eike; Glatzer, Wolfgang unter Mitwirkung von Mayer, Karl Ulrich; Zapf, Wolfgang (1975): Soziologischer Almanach. Frankfurt/New York, Herder & Herder, 531 p. (3rd ed. 1979)

Bauer, Raymond (ed.) (1966). Social Indicators. Cambridge: Mass. London

Berger-Schmitt, R. (2001): Towards a European System of Social Reporting and Welfare Measurement. EuReporting Working Paper No. 16. Retrieved from http://www.gesis.org/fileadmin/upload/dienstleistung/daten/soz_indikatoren/eusi/paper16.pdf

Bertram, Hans; Kollmorgen, Raj (eds.) (2001): Die Transformation Ostdeutschlands. Berichte zum sozialen und politischen Wandel in den neuen Bundesländern. Opladen. Leske & Budrich, p. 485

Bundesminister für innerdeutsche Beziehungen (1971): Materialien zum Bericht zur Lage der Nation. Berlin

Deutsche Forschungsgemeinschaft (ed.) (1994). Mikroanalytische Grundlagen der Gesellschaftspolitik. Akademischer Verlag; Berlin, Band I und II

Diefenbacher, H.; Zieschank, R. (2010). Measuring Welfare in Germany. A suggestion for a new welfare index. Federal Environment Agency: Dessau-Roßlau, URL http://www.umweltdaten.de/publikationen/fpdf-l/3903.pdf, viewed 24.04.2012

Eurofound (2013). Third European Quality of Life Survey – Quality of Societies and Public Services. Publications Office of the European Union: Luxembourg

European Union (2013). Quality of Life in Cities – Perception Survey in 79 European Cities. Publications Office ofthe European Union: Luxembourg

Enquete-Kommission Wachstum, Wohlstand, Lebensqualität (2012), Arbeitsbericht der Projektgruppe 2 „Entwicklung eines ganzheitlichen Wohlstands- bzw. Fortschrittsindikators", in: Kommissions-Drucksache 17(26)72 des Deutschen Bundestags, Berlin

Glatzer, Wolfgang (1981): An Overview of the International Development in Macro Social Indicators. In: Accounting, Organisation and Society Vol. 6, No.3, pp 219–234

Glatzer, Wolfgang; Zapf, Wolfgang (1984): Lebensqualität in der Bundesrepublik. Objektive Lebensbedingungen und subjektives Wohlbefinden. Frankfurt/New York: Campus

Glatzer, Wolfgang/Hondrich, Karl Otto/Stiehr, Karin/Wörndl, Barbara (1992): Recent Social Trends in West Germany 1960–1990. Frankfurt/Main, Campus; Montreal et al: McGill Queens University Press, 549 p

Glatzer, Wolfgang/Ostner, Ilona (Hg.) (1999). Deutschland im Wandel - Sozialstrukturelle Analysen. Leske & Budrich, Opladen.

Glatzer, Wolfgang; Habich, Roland; Mayer, Karl Ulrich (2002) (eds.): Sozialer Wandel und gesellschaftliche Dauerbeobachtung. Leske und Budrich, Opladen

Glatzer, Wolfgang/Becker, Jens/Bieräugel, Roland/Hallein-Benze, Geraldine; Nüchter, Oliver/Schmid, Alfons (2009): Reichtum im Urteil der Bevölkerung. Legitimationsprobleme und Spannungspotentiale in Deutschland. Opladen & Farmington Hills.

Glatzer, Wolfgang (2010) Dauerbeobachtung der Gesellschaft – Der Sonderforschungsbereich 3 und seine langfristigen Auswirkungen. In: RatSWD Working Paper Nr. 133

Glatzer, Wolfgang/Weick, Stefan (no date). 40 Jahre Sektion "Soziale Indikatoren" in der Deutschen Gesellschaft für Soziologie - Vermessung und Analyse der modernen Gesellschaft. At www.soziologie.de/fileadmin/user_upload/Sektion_Soziale_Indikatoren/Geschichte_der Sektion_Sozialindikatoren.pdf

Glatzer, Wolfgand/Wagner, Gert G. (2014). German Social Reporting. In: Michalos (2014)

Glatzer, Wolfgang/Camfield, Laura/Moller, Valerie/Rojas, Mariano (Ed.) (2015. Global Handbook of Quality of Life - Exploration of Well-Being of Natioans and Continents. Springer: Doordrecht, Heidelberg, New York, London

Hauser, Richard; Glatzer, Wolfgang; Hradil, Stefan; Kleinheinz, Gerhard; Olk, Thomas; Pankoke, Eckhart (1996): Ungleichheit und Sozialpolitik. Berichte zum sozialen und politischen Wandel in Ostdeutschland. Opladen, Leske + Budrich

Hoffmann-Nowotny, Hans Joachim (ed.) (1976). Soziale Indikatoren – Internationale Beiträge zu einer neuen praxisorientierten Forschungsrichtung. Huber: Frauenfeld und Stuttgart

Krause, Peter/Ostner, Ilona (Hg.) (2010). Leben in Ost- und Westdeutschland. Eine sozialwissenschaftliche Bilanz der deutschen Einheit 1990–2010. Campus: Frankfurt am Main

Köcher, R. (2009) (ed). Allensbacher Jahrbuch der Demoskopie 2003–2009. Band 12. Die Berliner Republik. De Gruyter, Berlin/New York

Krupp, Hans-Jürgen/Zapf, Wolfgang (1972/2011): Die Rolle alternativer Wohlstandsindikatoren bei der Begutachtung der gesamtwirtschaftlichen Entwicklung. Reprint in Rat für Sozial- und Wirtschaftsdaten, Working Paper No. 171. Berlin: http://www.ratswd.de/eng/index.html.

Krupp, Hans-Jürgen/Zapf, Wolfgang (1977): Sozialpolitik und Sozialberichterstattung. Frankfurt/New York, Campus

Land, Kenneth C./Michalos, Alex C./Sirgy, M. Joseph (eds.) (2012): Handbook of Social Indicators and Quality of Life Research. Dordrecht, Netherlands: Springer Publishers

Langlois, Simon/with Caplow, Theodore/Mendras, Henri/Glatzer, Wolfgang (1994). Convergence or Divergence? Comparing Recent Social Trends in Industrial Societies. Campus/McGill-Queen's University Press: Frankfurt am Main/Montreal

Leipert, Christian (1978). Gesellschaftliche Berichterstattung. Eine Einführung in Theorie und Praxis sozialer Indikatoren. Springer: Berlin, Heidelberg, New York

Michalos, Alex M. (1974): "Social Indicators Research" - An international and interdisciplinary journal for quality of life measurement. In: Zapf (1974)

Michalos, Alex M. (2014). Encyclopedia of Quality of Life- and Wellbeing-research. Springer Netherlands

Noll, H.H. (no date): Towards a European System of Social Indicators : Theoretical Framework and System Architecture. Retrieved from http://www.gesis.org/fileadmin/upload/ dienstleistung/ veranstaltungen_fortbildungen/archiv/soz_ind/sek01_noll.pdf

Nuechter, Oliver/Bieräugel, Roland/Glatzer, Wolfgang/Schmid, Alfons (2010): Der Sozialstaat im Urteil der Bevölkerung. Frankfurter Reihe "Sozialpolitik und Sozialstruktur" Band 5, Opladen und Farmington Hills, Barbara Budrich

RatSWD (2010). Building on Progress. Expanding the Research Infrastructur for the Social, Economic, and Behavioral Sciences, Vol. 1 +2, Budrich UniPress Ltd.: Opladen Farmington Hills

Schäfers, Bernhard; Zapf, Wolfgang (1998): Handwörterbuch zur Gesellschaft Deutschlands. Opladen, Leske + Budrich, p. 797, (2nd ed. 2001)

Schnapper-Arndt, G. (1883). Fünf Dorfgemeinden auf dem Hohen Taunus - Eine socialstatistische Untersuchung über Kleinbauernthum, Hausindustrie und Volksleben. Leipzig: Duncker & Humblot. Reprint 1975: Hoher Taunus: eine sozialstatistische Untersuchung in 5 Dorfgemeinden. Allensbach: Verlag für Demoskopie.

Statistisches Bundesamt (Hrsg.)In Zusammenarbeit mit dem Sonderforschungsbereich 3 der Universitäten Frankfurt und Mannheim) (1985): Datenreport 1985 - Zahlen und Fakten über die Bundesrepublik Deutschland. Bonn: Bundeszentrale für politische Bildung

Statistisches Bundesamt/Wissenschaftszentrum Berlin für Sozialforschung (2013): Datenreport 2013 - Ein Sozialbericht für die Bundesrepublik Deutschland. Bonn: Bundeszentrale für politische Bildung

Statistisches Bundesamt (2014). Nachhaltige Entwicklung in Deutschland - Indikatorenbericht 2014. Wiesbaden

Sachverständigenrat (2010) für die Beurteilung der gesamtwirtschaftlichen Entwicklung): Monitoring economic performance, quality of life and sustainability. Wiesbaden: http://www.sachverstaendigenrat-wirtschaft.de/fileadmindateiablage/Expertisen/2010/ex10_en.pdf

Schupp, Jürgen (2014): 40 Jahre Sozialberichterstattung und Lebensqualitätsforschung in Deutschland – Rückblick und Perspektiven. In: SOEP-papers 680

Wagner, Gert G., Joachim R. Frick, and Jürgen Schupp (2007), The German Socio-Economic Panel Study (SOEP) – Scope, Evolution and Enhancements. Schmollers Jahrbuch 127.1: 139–169

Weber, Max (1884): Die Lage der ostelbischen Landarbeiter. Tübingen, Mohr (Paul Siebeck)

Weick, Stefan (2014). Europe. In: Alex Michalos (2014)

Zapf, Wolfgang (ed.) (1974). Soziale Indikatoren – Konzepte und Forschungsansätze I. Herder & Herder: Frankfurt/New York (until volume 20)

Zapf, Wolfgang (1978) (eds.): Lebensbedingungen in der Bundesrepublik. Sozialer Wandel und Wohlfahrtsentwicklung. Frankfurt/New York: Campus, 946 p

Zapf, Wolfgang (1987): German Social Report - Living conditions and Subjective Wellbeing 1978–1984. In: Social Indicators Research. Vol. 19 No. 1, 171 p

Zapf, Wolfgang (2001): Die Wohlfahrtssurveys 1978–1998 und danach. In Becker, Irene; Ott, Notburga; Rolf, Gabriele (2001): Soziale Sicherung in einer dynamischen Gesellschaft. Campus: Frankfurt am Main

Chapter 13
Challenges, Needs and Risks in Defining Wellbeing Indicators

Filomena Maggino

A Challenge: Complexity

Complex Definition

The main complexity in developing indicators of wellbeing concerns the definition of "wellbeing". This exercise, as stressed by many, should take into account the multidimensionality of that concept. Actually, the wellbeing of a nation involves several concepts, which can be defined by different dimensions and sub-dimensions.

The conceptual approaches trying to define the idea of "wellbeing" are many. They can be classified according to different criteria.

(A) **Definitions related to "structures of values"**
The concepts classified according to this criterion can be distinguished with reference to different structures of values adopted. In this sense, three different philosophical approaches can be identified (Diener and Suh 1997), synthesized in Table 13.1:

(B) **Definitions referring to "observational perspectives"**
The concepts classified according to this criterion look at reality from different perspectives of observation. Wellbeing can be seen in terms of (i) process, (ii) conditions or (iii) goals.

   (i) *Process*. According to this approach, individual and collective well-being is related to some (more or less virtuous) processes, which can be described in terms of

F. Maggino (✉)
Dipartimento di Statistica, Informatica, Applicazioni "G. Parenti" (DiSIA), Università degli Studi di Firenze, Viale Morgagni 59, 50134 Firenze, Italy
e-mail: filomena.maggino@unifi.it

F. Maggino (ed.), *A Life Devoted to Quality of Life*, Social Indicators Research Series 60, DOI 10.1007/978-3-319-20568-7_13

Table 13.1 Well-being definitions classified in terms of "structures of values"

What is wellbeing related to?	What should be observed	Observational strategies?		What measures?
		What?	At what level?	
Functioning and capability to select goods and services that one desires	**Income**, considered the main mean to achieve an acceptable standard of living	Wealth (observed or estimated)	Individual (micro) → income	Economic indices
			Community (macro) → GDP	
Normative ideals	Set of characteristics inspired by normative aims, grounded in moral **values** or policy **goals**	Living conditions	Individual (micro) → work, …	Social indicators
			Community (macro) → social cohesion, democracy	
Subjective experiences	Individual's cognitive and affective reactions to one's own life (or specific domains)	Subjective perceptions and attitudes	Individual (micro) → satisfaction	Subjective indicators

- *Development* (often referring to qualitative dynamic change of an economic system)
- *Growth* (referring to quantitative expansion on the scale of physical dimensions of economic system)
- *Progress*, indicating generally "moving forward" (from Latin "*progressus*", *going forward*, *advance*).

Those concepts include the reverse and opposite processes ("de-development", de-growth, recession (Horn 1993).

(ii) *Conditions*. According to this approach, wellbeing of societies is seen as a function of:

- *availability of economic resources* (manpower, equipment, budget)
- *income and wealth distribution* (and its social implications)
- *welfare* and its relationships and impacts on economics.

This perspective requires that each individual:

- identifies oneself in his/her own community
- acquires collectively the knowledge, values and skills for sharing and expanding the community's resources for the benefit of all its members without being at the expense of other communities or of the environment (Horn 1993). In other terms, the conditions should be sustainable.

(iii) *Goals*. This perspective moves the attention from processes and conditions to goals (sustainability, quality of life, and so on).

(C) **Definitions referring to "points of observation"**

The concepts classified according to this criterion (Berger-Schmitt and Noll 2000) are distinguished with reference to the point of observation, which can be centred on (i) individuals (*quality of life*, *QoL*) or (ii) communities (*quality of societies*).

Definitions of wellbeing conceptualised implicitly or explicitly at individual level consider individual resources, objective needs), capabilities, subjective well-being, basic needs, objective living conditions.

Definitions focused on communities refer to liveability and quality of nations, integration, solidarity (social cohesion, social exclusion, social capital), social quality, human development.

(D) **Definitions classified in terms of "different theoretical views of Quality-of-Life"**

According to this criterion (Sirgy 2011), the different conceptual approaches to the concept of good society are distinguished with reference to the different theoretical perspectives through which QoL is seen.

(a) **Socio-economic development**

According to this approach, social development follows the achievement of a satisfactory level of economic development. Two emergent concepts are related to

- **Capital**: in particular, there are five major capitals: (a) financial or economic capital, (b) human capital, (c) social capital, (d) built capital, and (e) natural capital. Particular attention has been dedicated to the social capital dimension, seen as more significantly related to subjective well-being than economic indicators.
- **Stocks and flows**: as known, stocks constitute capital account whereas flows make up the current account. These concepts have been translating also into psychological terms: stocks are the strength of one's personality, health, social networks, leisure skills and equipment, work skills and equipment, education and general knowledge, and socioeconomic status. Flows are satisfaction or dissatisfaction experienced in relation to daily activities in the context of various life domains (finances, leisure, family, job, friendships, and health). Thus, a person characterized as having a high QOL is likely to possess good stocks and experiences flows.

(b) **Personal utility**

According to this approach, QoL is related to the subjective experience of individuals, observed in terms of evaluations, perceptions, and expressions of satisfaction of their living conditions. There are numerous conceptual models classified with reference to how subjective well-being is explained. The explanations can be related to individual's

(i) *personality traits* (top-down approach);
(ii) *evaluations and values* (bottom-up approach, comparison approach, multiple-discrepancy approach, purpose and meaning in life);

(iii) *feelings and emotions* (hedonic psychology approach, positive/negative affect, positive emotions theory)
(iv) *perceptions and functionings* (flow and engagement approach, eudaimonistic[1] identity theory)
(v) *mixed approach* (moods–and-disposition approach, cognitive-and-affective components approach, up-down approach).

(c) **Just society**
According to this approach, the QoL of a community is that in which its members enjoy a high level of social justice, when two distinct principles are met:

1. equality in the assignment of basic rights and duties, which can be viewed in terms of at least six dimensions: (i) right to meet basic needs, (ii) right to safety, (iii) right to employment, (iv) right to a healthful environment, (v) duty to pay taxes, and (vi) duty to vote.
2. inequalities are justified to benefit the least advantaged members of the society (children, women, minorities, the poor, the disabled).

(d) **Human development**
QoL is related to satisfaction of people's developmental needs, which refer to a hierarchy of

- Lower-order needs such as health, safety, and economic needs (lower-order needs); generally, they can be viewed in terms of nine dimensions: (a) environmental pollution, (b) disease incidence, (c) crime, (d) housing, (e) unemployment, (f) poverty and homelessness, (g) cost of living, (h) community infrastructure, (i) illiteracy and lack of job skills.
- Higher-order needs such as social, esteem, actualization, knowledge, and aesthetics needs; generally, they can be seen in terms of nine different dimensions: (a) work productivity and income, (b) consumption of non-basic goods and services, (c) leisure and recreational activities, (d) educational attainment, (e) community landscape, (f) population density and crowdedness, (g) arts and cultural activities, (h) intellectual activities, and (i) religious activities.

To achieve a high level of QoL, community members have to satisfy both lower- and higher-order developmental needs.

(e) **Sustainability**
Sustainability has been defined by the World Commission on Environment and Development as the effort to meet the needs of the present without

[1] Eudaimonia or eudaemonia or eudemonia, is a Greek word commonly translated as "human flourishing", considered as an accurate translation.

compromising the ability of future generations to meet their own needs. Two different perspectives of sustainability can be seen:

- environmental sustainability (environmental wellbeing)
- environmental and human sustainability (sustainable community, sustainable development, and sustainable growth) by considering sustainability in terms of the interrelationship between the human and environmental dimensions.
  - "sustainable communities" are those that enhance the economic, environmental, and social characteristics of a community. The three sets of QoL characteristics (economic, environmental, and social) are also referred to as "three E's of Sustainability" (economy, environment, equity).
  - "sustainable development" is a combination of human well-being and environmental well-being. Since, there is no good human condition in a bad environment, indicators of human well-being should include also indicators concerning environmental well-being.

(f) **Functionings**

Individual life is a combination of doings and beings—referred to as *functionings* (activities and situations that people consider as important in their lives, e.g., health status, level of education, and current employment status). QoL is assessed with reference to the individual freedom to choose among the various *functionings*. This freedom to choose is referred to as *capabilities*, defined as the ability to achieve *functionings*. In other words, *functionings* represent the goals of human living, while capability indicates the freedom or choice that one has to experience the end results of *functionings*.

From a *functionings* perspective, well-being can be developed in terms of a summary index of people's *functionings*, e.g., education provides freedom to earn a living and pursue a desired lifestyle. Thus, the desired lifestyle can be viewed as the outcome or functioning, whereas education is the means for achieving it (i.e., capability). Many health-related indicators projects are now using the concept of functioning to guide their efforts in constructing indicators.

Towards a Comprehensive Definition

From the previous synthesis, it is easily deducible that each of the identified approaches is not able to fully describe *wellbeing*. In fact, they focus upon certain aspects only and do not consider the reality in its complexity. It is difficult to identify a comprehensive and shared definition of wellbeing. In order to overcome partialities and incompleteness, a multidimensional conceptual framework should be adopted,[2] able to conciliate

(i) the individual level (*quality of life*, to be observed and monitored at individual/micro level)
(ii) the community level (*quality of society*, to be observed and monitored at societal/macro level).

Both levels are defined by objective and subjective aspects and are observed through objective and subjective measures and indicators.

Quality of Life

The definitions of "quality of life" are many and can be classified according to different perspectives (Sirgy 2011). Any approach highlights how defining a group of characteristics concerning individuals' life is important. They should be "intrinsically as objective expressions of a good life, or instrumentally, to achieve valuable subjective states or other objective goals" (Stiglitz et al. 2009) and should allow people to have resources. The possibility to adequately exploit opportunities contributes to the betterment of quality of life. For example, concept of "security" can be seen in objective terms but also in its dynamics related to subjective perceptions.

Among the many approaches, the model proposed by Zapf (1975, 1984), showing two macro components, *living conditions* and *subjective wellbeing*, represents one of the most adopted and accepted.

Living Conditions

The relevant aspects of living conditions refer to objective living conditions and the subjective aspects of living conditions.

Objective living conditions relate to the different situations (observed in the perspective of outcomes) which each individual is involved in. In other words, objective living conditions refer to resources, capabilities, standards of living, external circumstances.

The subjective aspects of living conditions can concern different dimensions, like

- self-determination (expressed in terms of perceived autonomy),
- freedom to choose one's lifestyle,

[2] A possible multidimensional conceptual definition could be the following: *A good and healthy society is that in which each individual has the possibility to participate in the community life, develop skills, abilities, capabilities and independency, adequately choose and control his/her own life, be treated with respect in a healthy and safe environment and by respecting the opportunities of future generations.*

- spirit of initiative (in the meaning of capacity/possibility to contribute to building common wellbeing),
- sense/scope in one's own life,
- perceived adequacy.

Subjective Wellbeing

One of the most accepted and adopted definitions of *subjective wellbeing* conceives it as a composite construct described by two distinct components, cognitive and affective (Diener and Emmons 1984; Diener 1984).

The cognitive component is related to the process through which each individual retrospectively evaluates (in terms of "satisfaction") her/his life, as a whole or in different domains. The subjective evaluation is made by taking into account personal standard (expectations, desires, ideals, experiences, etc.). Consequently, the level of satisfaction is expressed as a function of the reached objectives, fulfilled ambitions, comparing ideals, experiences, other persons. In other words, satisfaction with life is the result of a cognitive process, allowing the individual to evaluate her/his present situation with reference to *standards* (Nuvolati 2002) individually defined.

The affective component refers to the emotions experimented by individuals during their daily lives and relates to the their present situation. The emotions can be positive (*pleasant affects*) or negative (*unpleasant affects*), which are considered conceptually distinct and influenced by different variables (Bradburn 1969; Diener and Emmons 1984; Argyle 1987). Observing this component is particularly important since it allows us to obtain information about the temperamental structure used by each individual in facing the everyday life.[3]

The combination of the two components allows subjective well-being to be assessed. Some authors proved that individual choices in the long term are influenced by both components (Kahneman and Krueger 2006).

Summarizing, the concept of subjective wellbeing can be framed through the following dimensions:

- the "cognitive" dimension

  satisfaction with life as a whole
  satisfaction with different life domains[4]

- the "affective" dimension

[3] According to some authors, like Veenhoven, affects' determinants are universal and consequently not produced by individual response-styles or cultural differences.

[4] One of the first attempts aimed at identifying the more relevant life domains is Andrews and Withey's study (1976). By admitting that individual *concerns* can be infinite, they focus on those domains which seem to be relevant and meaningful for individuals and their QoL. Different studies identify different lists of domains, even very different from each other (e.g., *Extended Satisfaction with life scale*, Allison et al. 1991).

positive *affect* (happiness,[5] serenity, etc.)
negative *affect* (concern, anxiety, stress, etc.)
affect related to particular situations or activities (family, work, etc.).

Quality of Society

From the point of view of the society, wellbeing involves concepts like economic and social cohesion, integration of individuals and groups, social capital, referring to dimensions observed at both macro and micro level, like:

- social engagements and political activities (through associations, organizations, …),
- social and political participation,
- social relations (informal networks),
- quality of relations (shared values, conflicts, solidarity),
- performance of institutions.

By exploring the subjective aspects of wellbeing, we can identify:

- *Trust*, expressed in terms of (i) *interpersonal trust (*in family, relatives, friends, neighbours, colleagues, other social groups, …) and (ii) *systemic trust* (State, national government, parliament, politics, institutional figures, public administration, political parties, judiciary system, the police, public education system, public health system, financial and credit system, enterprises, media/information system, associations, international organizations, religious organizations, etc.)
- *Identity*, expressed in terms of *perceived sense of belonging* to one's town, region, country, etc.
- *Perceived social structure*, with reference to (i) *social exclusion* (weather one feels or not to be part of the society), and (ii) *solidarity* (ones' consideration/concern for other social groups' living conditions).

[5] Particular attention should be devoted to the term "happiness", which assumes different meanings according to different authors. Many scholars refer "happiness" to the affective component of subjective well-being (Nuvolati 2002; Diener et al. 2008). Others consider happiness as a synonymous of life satisfaction Veenhoven (1994).

Besides the different conceptual views, the statistical evidences can tell different stories. The highest rank correlation value between "*level of satisfaction with life as a whole*" and "*level of happiness*" by country in round 4 of the European Social Survey data is 0.6 (registered for the United Kingdom sample), revealing not only that the two components are not coinciding but also that a linguistic problem underlies the definition of happiness.

Just an example concerning that. "Happiness" (one of the dimensions of the subjective wellbeing) is translated in Italian "felicità". Actually, if we look at the linguistic roots of them we could realize that they are dealing with two different worlds, since the former comes from "to happen" and latter from the Latin "felix" which can be translated as "chance".

In the rest of this work this definition of subjective wellbeing will be adopted, in which happiness represents just one of the aspects (the positive affect).

- *Values*, ach subject can be expressed through the importance that each individual assigns to different life domains with reference to anyone's life and one's own life. While in the former case, the expression of individual structure of values is explored, in the latter case, the individual "investment" in different life domains is observed.

Comparing different realities (represented by countries or by areas inside one country) does not necessarily imply using the same variables and – consequently – the same indicators but requires differentiated choices (Stiglitz et al. 2009). In fact, variables' choice is function of time since it depends on shared values that can change from time to time. Consequently, transferring a certain quality-of-life concept developed in a different context could be misleading.

The Quality of Wellbeing

The relationship between the individual (subjective and objective) wellbeing and the society's wellbeing should be considered by exploring two issues. On one hand, even though the concept of "community wellbeing" could be covered by referring to aggregation of individual outcomes, the simple sum of all individuals' wellbeing composing that community cannot represent in itself the community wellbeing, which should include also other different characteristics. On the other hand, the discussion concerns if pursuing community's wellbeing requires a compromise between individuals' wellbeing. In other words, it should be verified whether any individual wellbeing is pursued at the expense of other individuals' wellbeing.

Observing society's wellbeing requires checking also its quality. In an attempt to define the quality of wellbeing, two particular conceptual perspectives should be considered, the fairness in its distribution (*equity*) and the limit in its promotion (*sustainability*).

Fairness in the Distribution of Wellbeing (Equity)

The fair distribution could be referred to concepts like *social inclusion/exclusion, disparities and inequalities*, related to welfare distribution within a society and assessed by checking both

- inequalities among individuals, groups, organizations,
- disparities among geographical areas, regions and so on.

However, it is possible to identify the equity dimension also at individual level (*equity of wellbeing at micro level*). In this perspective, we can identify two levels of equity,

- *external*, observed by comparing different social groups (identified through different perspectives, age, gender, races, citizenship groups, and so on), and
- *internal*, referring to the balance among the different life aspects in each individual.

Table 13.2 "Sustainability": capitals, perspectives and level of observation

		Perspectives ↓			
		Present generations' ...	Future generations' ...		
Capitals →	Physical	...behaviours affecting individual health		micro	← Level of observation
	Social	...behaviours affecting social relations and networks		micro & macro	
	Economic	...processes affecting welfare		micro & macro	
	Human	...processes affecting individual skills, training, education		micro	
	Natural	...processes affecting natural resources		macro	

External equity could be assessed also in terms of individual perceptions. The perceived equity can be referred to subjective evaluations expressed with reference to different levels and living conditions and contexts. For example:

- *Perceived equity/inequality in living conditions by comparing one's conditions with reference persons' conditions* (better or worse)
- *Perceived equity/inequality in living conditions by comparing one's conditions with other social groups' conditions* (better or worse)

Sustainability of Wellbeing

The wellbeing of a society should be monitored also with reference to its limit. The idea of *limit* can be seen as related to the concept of *sustainability of wellbeing*, not easy to be defined. It could refer to the possible erosion/durability/improvement/deterioration of those conditions (interpretable in terms of capitals) with reference to present generations' future and future generations.[6]

In this perspective, sustainability of wellbeing can be defined by referring to the capitals which should be preserved (five dimensions) and to two perspectives (Table 13.2)[7]:

Another way to look at the sustainability of wellbeing is through the concept of **vulnerability**. This concept requires the identification of, on one hand, the *risks factors* of the present level of wellbeing and, on the other hand, the *resilience*

[6] For example, any attempt aimed at improving connections between cities (in terms of travelling time) faces limits. Time spent to go from one city to another can be reduced thanks to new technologies and improvements in territorial structures. However, the commuting time that can be reduced should be balanced with the capitals (such as the territory) that need to be consumed and sacrificed for that reduction. In other words, the question is: what is the price to be paid in order to reduce the commuting time by a few minutes? Perhaps the technological efforts could be oriented towards how to reduce the amount of people that need to commute each day.

[7] According to the World Bank's four-capital approach, for example, sustainable development should enhance and preserve social, human, produced and natural capital of present generations and provide future generations with them.

factors (resources and capabilities) which can be activated in order to face possible future needs and risks. In both perspectives, the observations (but also the activations) can be accomplished at micro and macro level with reference to time and space. The concept that can relate risk and resilience is precaution (not only in terms of prevention).

Whatever approach to limits is adopted, its monitoring would require ad-hoc measures as well as a different analytical approaches of those already monitored (Stiglitz et al. 2009; Giovannini et al. 2012).

Also sustainability can be explored in terms subjective aspects; in fact, we can

- analytically explore the sustainability of subjective aspects of wellbeing (e.g., sustainability of subjective wellbeing)
- measure the subjective aspects of sustainability, referring to retrospective comparisons and prospective evaluations, for example:
  - *Perceived sustainability in terms of expectations*:
    - present one's living conditions in comparison with future ones (possible improvement/worsening)
    - present nation's conditions in comparison with future ones (possible improvement/worsening)
  - *Expectations in one's level of standard of living* (improvement/worsening)

Additional Definitions: Contextual Characteristics and Life Domains

The Socio-economic Structure

Besides the defined concepts, an additional dimension allowing the description of the whole society should be described and monitored, the socio-demographic-economic structure. In this perspective, a particular role is played by the structure and dynamics of the population, seen as a producer of constraints.

The Life Domains

Assessing national wellbeing and its equity and sustainability needs social and political consensus on the definition of the concepts (quality of life, equity and sustainability) but also on further key topics like *life domain* (Noll 2004).

Life domains represent segments of the reality in which each individual lives and the relevant concepts and dimensions have to be observed, monitored, and assessed. Typically, they are households and families, housing; health, transport, environment, work (labour market, working condition), and so on.

Actually, a shared list of domains showing explicit priority does not exist, also because the list strictly depends on value judgments, valid and acceptable in a certain place or time (Noll 2004). However, many scholars noticed that many domains recur in empirical studies (Felce and Perry 1995; Nuvolati 1997; Johansson 2002; Stiglitz et al. 2009), highlighting how human conditions lead individuals to face challenges that are common all over the world and that require collective solutions. Generally, the differences concern the importance assigned to each domain.

Complexity in Selecting Indicators

Defining a concept is always a demanding exercise, especially when the concept is complex and multidimensional, like wellbeing. This introduces a further complexity concerning the selection and development of the indicators which should be consistent to the adopted concepts.

Investigating different aspects related to wellbeing requires the definition of basic elementary indicators, defined for each conceptual dimension and each domain.

In order to select and manage indicators, different issues need to be addressed, especially when this has carried out into a complex system allowing the accomplishment of functions like monitoring, reporting and accounting.[8] Below, some of those issues will be explored.

1. **Perspectives of observation**
   We can refer to indicators by distinguishing them according to different *perspectives of observation* . In a general view, we could identify the following perspectives:
   - *Conglomerative* and *deprivational* perspectives; measures of the former perspective increase when wellbeing increase and decrease when wellbeing decrease; measures of the latter perspective measures only the welfare of the worst-off.[9]
   - *Input (resources) and outcomes (results) perspectives.* It is difficult to distinguish the two situations; in fact, some aspects could be classified at the same time (or in subsequent times) as input or output; families' lower expenses for foodstuffs could represent an output indicator but also an input indicator for the consequences that such change can produce.
   - *Positive and negative perspectives*: negative indicators can be managed or interpreted so that they can represent positive measures (e.g., in the health

[8] Michalos identified 15 different issues related to the selection of social, economic, and environmental indicators. As Michalos asserts, these issues, are collectively yielded over 200,000 possible combinations (Sirgy et al. 2006).

[9] Anand and Sen (1997), arguing that the conglomerative and deprivational perspectives are not substitutes for each other, proposed a *complementary* approach. The adoption of the complementary approach allows us to construct indices of social and economic well-being that should reflect the aggregated and disaggregated approaches. According to this methodology, conglomerative and deprivational indices should be constructed separately side-by-side along the lines of the United Nations Development Programme indicators (Sharpe and Salzman 2004).

domain, measures of morbidity and mortality may crowd out positive measures of well-being).

- *Benefits and costs*: different measures of value or worth yield different overall evaluations as well as different evaluations for different people.
- *Status and trend perspectives*. Status indicators measure a certain phenomenon in a particular moment; they allow for cross-comparisons between different realities. These indicators can produce cross data that need to be carefully managed since the different realities cannot always be directly compared; this is particularly true in the case of subjective characteristics observed in different geographical, social, cultural, political, environmental, and administrative conditions. Trend indicators measure reality along time; they require data collected through a longitudinal design (for example, repeated surveys on particular populations). These indicators can produce *time series* that need to be carefully managed since the observed moments could turn out to be incomparable and/or the defined indicators could reveal to be non-applicable after some time.

2. **Levels of observation**

   We can refer to indicators also by distinguishing them according to different *levels of observation* **.**

   - Indicators are said *micro* when the values refer to individuals or groups, while they are said *macro* when the values refer to communities, regions, countries, etc. It should be stated that values referring to macros do not necessarily correspond to the sum of micros. At the same time, values referring to each micro do not necessarily reflect what emerges at macro level.
   - *Internal* and *external*, duality sensitive to individual observation; in fact, the concepts defined at individual level can be observed at both "external" (e.g., objective living conditions) and "internal" (e.g., subjective evaluations or perceptions) level.

3. **Nature of the observed characteristics**, which can be

   - *Objective and subjective*, referring to two aspects of the reality integrating each other
   - *Quantitative and qualitative*, implying a consistent choice of the indicators. Actually, the transition from the quantity to the *quality paradigm*[10] implies a consistent choice of the indicators: this means, for example, turning an indicator of quantity like "life expectancy" into an indicator of quality like "healthy life expectancy."

In using dichotomies such as *objective – subjective* and *qualitative – quantitative* it should be clarified the context in which they are used:

- are we talking about defining the concepts?

[10]The dichotomy quality/quantity introduced here refers to the technical expression of indicators and not to their meaning.

- are we talking about components of the concept?
- are we talking about defining the method of measurement and analysis?

Let's see the differences in using the dichotomy *objectivity – subjectivity*:

- *In defining concepts.* In this case, we are referring to the conceptual framework defined in order to observe and to interpret the reality. The conceptual framework is always yielded by a **subjective** hypothesis and a subjective process related to the researchers' view of the world.

- Concerning this, as Michalos (1992) noticed, the models defined to observe a reality are only apparently neutral. Actually, the conceptual model represents only a "small window" through which only some facets of the reality can be seen (reductionism); in this sense, the view is politically and socially distorted and can condition knowledge, evaluations, choices, actions, and policies. In this sense, subjectivity expresses the unavoidable working hypothesis helping in understanding the reality. The researcher, through the dialogue with the working hypothesis, can change the perspective in a continuously evolving knowledge path. In any scientific field, a meaning does not exist without "subjectivity". This dimension is present also in the ambit of hard sciences, where it helps in structuring the observed reality. In this perspective, data represent the "text" to be read by the researcher in search of a sense. This process cannot be considered arbitrary, since the sense cannot be "invented" regardless of the relationship with the reality.
- *As components of the concept/reality.* In this case the adjectives refer to the kind of information which has been defined in the ambit of a conceptual framework and subsequently objectively measured and analyzed. In order to make the distinction between objective and subjective characteristics more clear from the operative point of view, we can refer to the source – called unit – on which the characteristic of interest is measured. The units can be represented by individuals, institutions, social groups, services, administrative areas, geographical areas, nations, and so on. Consequently, we can distinguish between:

  - *objective information*, collected by observing reality
  - *subjective information*, collected only from individuals and their assertions.

As known, defining what we are going to measure represents the first step of the measuring process. This distinction can be developed into other resulting definitions:

- *objective indicator*, based upon explicit criteria, shared by external observers
- *subjective indicator*, based upon subjective evaluations and implicit criteria which can vary from individual to individual.

Subjective indicators aim at measuring and quantifying individual components involving different elements – as conscience, cognition, emotion, attitude, and opinion – that are related to contingent and mutable situations. Consequently, measuring subjective aspects needs many elements to be considered and requires an interdisciplinary approach, able to consider and understand the different levels at which each individual react to the submitted question. The different levels involve personality, values, interests, motivations, intellectual and expressive dispositions, memory, experiences, social attitudes as a member of a limited group or of a community, and so on.

- In the measuring process. The methodologies adopted to observe and study the characteristics defined in the ambit of the conceptual framework have to be objective. In other words, the methodological objectivity concerns the capacity of a procedure to measure without alteration due to external factors and to be free from effects due to the observer; this notion spreads from the procedure of measurement to the data analysis to the interpretation of the results.

- In this context, the distinction between objective and subjective is considered equivalent to the distinction between quantitative and qualitative. Of course, this is not correct. The two dyads can be summarized as follows:

  – "**objective – subjective**" refers to what we are going to observe
  – "**quantitative – qualitative**" refers to the methodological approach applied in order to observe the previous dimensions.

4. **Level of dis/aggregation**

   In defining indicators, it should be considered also the difficulties related to the availability of indicators (over time and across space) and in harmonizing different data sources and levels of observation.

   - **Times frame**, which is not necessarily equal for all selected indicators but should be adequate to the dynamics of the observed phenomenon. Moreover, in policy perspective, the dynamics should consider also the optimal duration to understand resource diminution as well as impacts of changes.
   - **Area sizes**, which should be adequate to the phenomenon under observation; e.g., the best size to understand air pollution may be different from the best size to understand crime. Moreover, it is important to take into account some territorial peculiarities. E.g., certain facilities are necessarily located and distributed across territories in an unequal way (hospitals, schools, theatres, museums, libraries).

5. **Criteria**

   - **Goals** (direction to be adopted by the society). Goals are not only time and space dependent but rely on political views. In this perspective, the role that international organizations can play is definitely important in defining the goals to be pursued. It is important to set clear and shared goals (in the *wellbeing for all* perspective), by giving philosophical and political debate (understandable for all) more space. These topics are related to indicators definition, especially with reference to their benchmarks.
   - **Identifying benchmark**. The definition and selection of an indicator should be accompanied by the identification of its benchmark, which represents a reference point allowing the present situation to be evaluated and assessed. In this perspective, a benchmark may represent the point from which measurements can be made.

Comparing with a benchmarking is a systematic process, useful for monitoring and encouraging actions and improvements. It[11] allows priorities to be established, better practices to be defined, impacts to be evaluated, and awareness among the stakeholders to be aroused.

In fact, the benchmark, interpreted in terms of reference point, can assume different shapes (Śleszyński 2012):

1. reference point (or critical value),[12] representing quantitative information established thanks to scientific research or to desired norms;
2. signpost arrow, indicating the comparison with reference to previous performance (betterment or worsening);
3. best practice, representing a model to be followed;
4. goals, defined through a consensual process, by referring to cultural paradigms or normative demands, or through expert groups' pressure or public opinion movement.

In any case, benchmark values require a consensus to be reached. This is particularly true in case of subjective wellbeing indicators.

6. **Levels of communication**
   The indicators can be distinguished according to their **levels of communication** with reference the target group which the final indicator will be communicated. In this perspective, indicators can be classified in:

- *cold indicators*: in this case, the indicators show a high level of complexity and difficulty;
- *hot indicators*: in this case, the indicators are constructed at a low level of difficult;
- *warm indicators*: in this case, the indicators show a good balance between comprehensibility and complexity.

The level of communication concerns also the approach to media and/or formats (reports, graphs, ...) and requires particular skills.

7. **Purposes**
   The indicators can be distinguished according to their **purpose**, which can be:

- *descriptive*, when the indicators are aimed at describing and knowing a particular reality. These indicators are said to be informative and baseline-oriented; in other terms, they allow changes along time, differences between geographical areas, and connections between social processes to pointed out;
- *explicative*, when the indicators are aimed at interpreting reality;

---

[11] The use of benchmarks plays an important role in the ambit of a program development. Used in combination with the program objectives they provide the basis for program accountability.

[12] A reference point can be actually represented by a reference group (e.g., percentage of people with a high level of satisfaction with life as a whole).

- *predictive*, when the indicators help to delineate plausible evolutional trends that is possible to describe in terms of development or decrement; these indicators require strong prediction models and continuous observations along time;
- *normative*, when the indicators are aimed at supporting, guiding, and directing decisions and possible interventions (policies) concerning problems to be solved. The normative function needs the definition of particular referenced standards defined in terms of time, territory, etc.; the reference values allow evaluating the attainment of defined goals;
- *problem-oriented*, when the indicators are defined as a function of a specific hypothesis of research and analysis aimed at identifying contexts, kinds, severities of specific problems (for example the lack of quality-of-life conditions among immigrants);
- *evaluating*, that can be distinguished in

practical: indicators interfacing with observed process (e.g. in an organization), *directional*: indicators testing if the observed condition is getting better or not, *actionable*: indicators allowing change effects to be controlled.

8. **Governance contexts**
   The indicators can be distinguished according to the **context** in which they are created, used, and interpreted. In this perspective, we can identify different contexts. For example:

Public debates: in this case the indicator/s have the function of informing, stimulating, forming and developing particular sensitiveness;

Policy guidance: in this case the indicators/s can support particular policy decisions;

Administrative guidance: in this case the indicator/s can support the evaluation of the different impacts of different alternatives.

In these contexts it should be taken into account that different stakeholders often have very different views about what is important to be monitored and how to evaluate whatever is monitored.

Choices and options selected for each issue have implications for the other issues. The issues are not mutually exclusive and are not expected to be exhaustive as other can be identified. Some of them are merely a technical problem to be solved by statisticians or information scientists. On the other hand, the construction of indicators of well-being and quality-of-life is essentially a political and philosophical exercise, and its ultimate success or failure depends on the negotiations involved in creating and disseminating the indicators, or the reports or accounts that use those indicators (Michalos, in Sirgy et al. 2006).

Table 13.3 Dimensions of indicator quality

AN INDICATOR SHOULD BE	Clear, appropriate, exhaustive, meaningful, accurate, well-designed	WITH REFERENCE TO ITS CAPACITY AND POSSIBILITY TO	**Define and describe** (*concepts, definitions and scopes*)	(I) METHODOLOGICAL SOUNDNESS
	Measurable, stable		**Observe** unequivocally and stably (in terms of space and time)	
	Reliable, valid, repeatable, robust, rigorous, precise, exact, faithful		Record by a **degree of distortion as low as possible** (explored through statistical and methodological approaches)	
	Transparent, with ethical standards		**Adhere** to the principle of objectivity in the collection, compilation, and dissemination	(II) INTEGRITY
	Consistent, pertinent, coherent		**Reflect adequately the conceptual model** in terms of aims, objectives and requirements underlying its construction (knowing, monitoring, evaluation, accounting, …)	(III) SERVICEABILITY
	Relevant		Meet current and potential users' needs. It refers to whether all indicators that are needed are produced and the extent to which concepts used (definitions, classifications etc.) reflects user needs. The identification of users and their expectations is therefore necessary.	
	Practicable, inspectable, up-to-datable		**Be observed** through realistic efforts and costs in terms of development and data collection (for example, short time between observation and data availability)	
	Well-timed, timely, periodic		Reflect the length of time between its availability and the event or phenomenon it describes	
	Regular, punctual		Reflect the time lag between the release date of data and the target date when it should have been delivered	
	Comparable, discriminant, Disagregable, thrifty		**Be analyzed** in order to record differences and disparities between units, groups, geographical areas and so on, by employing the available information as much as possible	
	Credible, accessible, interpretable, comprehensible, simple, manageable		**Be spread** that is, it has to be easily findable, accessible, useable, analyzable, and interpretable in order to gain also users' confidence (*brand image*)	(IV) ACCESSIBILITY

Quality of Indicators

Many international institutions, like World Bank and Unesco (Patel et al. 2003) and Eurostat (2000a, b) tried to identify the attributes of **quality** that indicators (and approaches aimed at their management) should possess and need to be considered vin the process of developing of new indicators or selecting available indicators (Table 13.3):

I. **Methodological Soundness**

This characteristic refers to the idea that the methodological basis for the production of indicators should be attained by following internationally accepted standards, guidelines, or good practices. This dimension is necessarily dataset-specific, reflecting different methodologies for different datasets. The elements referring to this characteristic are (i) concepts and definitions, (ii) scope, (iii) classification/sectorization, and (iv) basis for recording. Particularly important is the characteristic of **accuracy and reliability**, referring to the idea that indicators should be based upon data sources and statistical techniques that are regularly assessed and validated, inclusive of revision studies. This allows accuracy of estimates to be assessed. In this case accuracy is defined as the closeness between the estimated value and the unknown true population value but also between the observed individual value and the "true" individual value. This means that assessing the accuracy of an estimate involves analyzing the total error associated with the estimate: sampling error and measurement error.

II. **Integrity**

Integrity refers to the notion that indicator systems should be based on adherence to the principle of objectivity in the collection, compilation, and dissemination of data, statistics, and results. The characteristic includes institutional arrangements that ensure (i) professionalism in statistical policies and practices, (ii) transparency, and (iii) ethical standards.

III. **Serviceability**

Serviceability refers mainly to comparability. In fact, it aims at measuring the impact of differences in applied concepts and measurement tools/procedures:

- over time, referring to comparison of results, derived normally from the same statistical operation, at different times;
- between geographical areas, emphasizing the comparison between countries and/or regions in order to ascertain, for instance, the meaning of aggregated indicators at the chosen level;
- between domains. This is particularly delicate when involving subjective measurement (e.g. cultural dimensions).

IV. **Accessibility**

Accessibility relates to the need to ensure:

(i) cvlarity of presentations and documentations concerning data and metadata (with reference to information environment: data accompanied with appropriate illustrations, graphs, maps, and so on, with information on their quality, availability and – contingent – usage limitations);

(ii) impartiality of access;
(iii) Pertinence of data;
(iv) Prompt and knowledgeable support service and assistance to users.

In other words, it refers also to the physical conditions in which users can obtain data: where to go, how to order, delivery time, clear pricing policy, convenient marketing conditions (copyright, etc.), availability of micro or macro data, various formats (paper, files, CD-ROM, Internet, and so on), etc.

Prerequisites of Quality

Although they do not represent a dimension of quality in itself, prerequisites of quality refers to all those (institutional or not) preconditions and background conditions allowing quality of statistics.

In other words, indicators construction is not simply a technical problem but should become part of a larger debate concerning how to construct indicators obtaining a larger legitimacy to be promoted. These prerequisites cover the following elements:

(i) legal and institutional environment, allowing
   (a) conceptual framework to be defined
   (b) coordination power within and across different institutions to be framed
   (c) data and resources to be available for statistical work
(ii) Quality awareness informing statistical work.

The process allowing the construction of indicators leads to a conceptual matrix in which each raw represents a conceptual dimension/sub-dimension, while each column represents a life domain. Indicators are realized in each cell. Each combination raw/column is not necessarily observed through indicators.

A Need: Making Relative

Relative Concepts

The indicators selection implies a reflection about the objectives of their adoption (monitoring, comparing and benchmarking among territories, supporting and evaluating policy decisions, etc.).

In particular, that reflection requires considering two related indicators' characteristics: *consistency* with reference to concepts and *adequacy* with reference to the observed reality.

Adequacy stresses the idea to observe and monitor in a relative way. Even though the definition of well-being may find a wide agreement, its operationalization (in terms of indicators) should take into account that different areas could adopt different indicators in order to measure the same concept.

This represents a delicate issue especially when there is a need of comparison. What it should be clarified is that comparing different realities (cultures, values, countries, regions or areas) does not necessarily imply using the same variables but could require differentiated choices (Stiglitz et al. 2009). In fact, variables' choice depends on shared values, which are functions of time and place. Consequently, transferring a wellbeing concept developed in a certain context could be misleading. With this respect, a good example is the variable "leisure time" whose definition can be different also from one individual to another. So, the process of comparing different areas would refer to the concept and not to single indicators (comparing synthetic indicators).

Relativization also involves the measuring and monitoring of the wellbeing concept and should urge better policies. This can be illustrated with a simple and simplified example: how to interpret a region's high value produced by the ratio *number of hospital bed/dimension of population*? At a first glance, a high level could reveal a region paying attention to needs and requirements of population's health. A later look could be alarming: Does the high number of available hospital beds fit a real need of that territory? If so, the interpretation could lead to a particular evaluation of policy decisions. The territory's need, for example, could be related to particular pathologies. The policy action could have been directed towards other domains (e.g., environment). Therefore, proposing city mobility compatible with a healthy environment allows air quality and life style to be improved allowing a healthy life and hopefully a lower need of hospital beds.

Making Relative Through Analyses

Monitoring wellbeing through indicators requires controlling values and levels through different perspectives allowing variations to be detected and different things to be revealed. This can be done through

- *Distributions analysis*, in order to avoid average figures which can conceal variation; choices must be made about appropriate representations of distributions.
- *Correlation analysis*, in order to explore also hypotheses concerning possible causal relations; this is crucial also in policy perspective: before intervention, one must know what causes what, which requires relatively mainstream scientific research, which may not be available yet.
- *Break downs analysis, according through population composition* (e.g., analyses by language, sex, age, education, ethnic background, income, etc.).
- *Trend analysis*, which can reveal different tendencies and evolutions (linear, non-linear, chaotic, and s on).

A Risk: Reductionism

As we have seen, the complexity of the system of indicators may require approaches allowing more synthetic views. In this perspective, as we will see, statistics offer many analytical instruments to adopt.

The guiding concept is **synthesis**. From the methodological point of view, synthesis concerns different aspects of the system (Maggino 2009):

- *Synthesis of units* (cases, subjects, etc.), which aims at aggregating the value of one of more indicators observed in micro units to be compared at macro level (social groups, age groups, geographic areas), with reference to (synthetic or not) indicators. This kind of synthesis is generally accomplished by applying very simple even statistical instruments (e.g., average), which turn out to be very unsatisfying since they do not allow the phenomenon's distribution to be correctly represented. A possible (not necessarily the best) solution is to report, for example, the percentage of a subgroup or a dispersion index (standard deviation or interquartile range).
- *Synthesis of basic indicators* which can be carried out at both micro (individual level) and macro level (regional, national, group level).

The systematic identification of elementary indicators, in terms of concepts and domains, allows a downright **system of indicators** to be constructed (more complex than a simple **set of indicators**, which are not always related to a conceptual framework). In other words, the consistent application of the hierarchical design produces a complex structure.

In order to obtain a meaningful and interpretable picture, data should be managed in some way. In other words, the system of indicators may require the indicators to be reduced in order to allow more comprehensive measures. This issue is referred as *reductionism*. Reductionism cannot be avoided, since it is actually impossible pull an image and a story from a pure observation of the reality and completely grounded on it. On the other hand, it is dangerous to concentrate just on a few elements and statistically infer the sufficiency of the reduced observation from them.

Reductionism applied to indicators can find essentially two solutions: (i) reducing the number of indicators, (ii) synthesising indicators.

The former approach needs a solid conceptual support. From the statistical point of view, the only evidence supporting the exclusion of one between two indicators is interrelation A high level of relation between two indicators allows us to consider just one of them, assuming that indicators showing high relation are actually measuring the same concept's component. However, this assumption is not necessary always true. The degree of freedom for such decisions is in the reality: the relationship between two indicators (e.g., number of firemen and amount of damages in a fire) can be high but mediated by a third one (e.g., dimension of the fire). If the nature of the third indicator changes, the relationship between the other two indicators changes or disappears, even though they will continue to describe, autonomously, the reality. If, by observing the previous high correlation, we excluded one of the two indicators, doing without one of them could deny ourselves precious pieces of the whole picture (as represented by the indicators). This means that having a solid conceptual model allowing indicators concepts' relationships to be identified and interpreted.

The latter approach consists in combining the indicators in a meaningful way.

Final Remarks

Dealing with wellbeing of societies by taking into account its multidimensionality not only involves philosophical/political issues but concerns each individual's and community's real life. Consequently, the three concepts are taken into account at both individual and community level. The family's decision to have a vacation (or not) or the community's decision to have a new tram line (or not) should take into account issues related to quality of life, cohesion and sustainability.

The different levels (individual, family, local, national …) interact and lead to fruitful and positive changes only if the decision-making process is supported be a **monitoring system**, seen as a continuous observation of the well-being allowing changes to be observed, effects of policies to be evaluated, and future activities to be planned.

However, the monitoring should be grounded on a solid democratic system and transparent media system as well as on the education of the citizens. In this, important roles are played by the education and research system (school, university, etc.) and the official statistics, two strategic and institutional sectors, both meeting social consensus.

As said, a complex approach is needed in order to measure and monitor wellbeing.

Complexity requires many indicators, designed and organized in consistent conceptual structure. The obtained system provides all the cognitive instruments allowing decisions to be taken more consciously. In any case, those decisions appertain to policy.

In this frame, we could image the policy maker like a pilot sitting at the flight desk (Maggino 2009). Statistics has the task of defining, constructing and developing the instruments located in the cockpit. However, that activity needs to take into account that it needs:

- A clear definition of destination (referring to *goals*)
- A democratic process allowing the community to take a shared decision concerning destination (referring to democracy)
- A deep knowledge of pre-conditions (referring to resources, …)
- A constant monitoring of flight conditions (corresponding to the monitoring process)
- A continuous transmission and sharing of information on flight conditions (systematized in what can be named communication and information system)

- A cultural environment available to support scientific research (basic and applied) to improve the whole system's conditions
- A system allowing the community to face and manage emergencies (definable in terms of welfare and social security, etc.)

If even just one of these items is missed, achieving a good society is seriously damaged.

References

Allison, D. B., Alfonso, V. C., & Dunn, G. M. (1991, January) "The extended satisfaction with life scale", *The Behavioral Therapist*, 15–16.

Anand, S., Sen A. (1997) "Concepts of Human Development and Poverty: A Multidimensional Perspective" *Human Development Papers 1997*, UNDP.

Andrews, F. M. & Withey, S. B. (1976) *Social Indicators of Well-Being: Americans' Perceptions of Life Quality*, New York, Plenum Press.

Argyle, M., (1987). *The Psychology of Happiness*, Methuen, London (trad. it. *Psicologia della felicità*, Cortina Editore, Milano).

Berger-Schmitt R. and H.-H. Noll (2000) *Conceptual Framework and Structure of a European System of Social Indicators*, EuReporting Working Paper No. 9, Centre for Survey Research and Methodology (ZUMA) – Social Indicators Department, Mannheim.

Bradburn N.M. (1969) *The Structure of Psychological Well-being*. Aldine, Chicago.

Diener E., E. Suh (1997) "Measuring quality of life: economic, social, and subjective indicators", *Social Indicators Research*, vol. 40, 189–216.

Diener E. and Emmons R.A. (1984). "The independence of positive and negative affect". *Journal of Personality and Social Psychology*, 47 (5).

Diener, E., Lucas R.E., Schimmack U., Helliwell J. (2008) *Well-Being for Public Policy*, Oxford University Press, Oxford.

Eurostat (2000a) *Definition of quality in Statistics*, Eurostat Working Group on Assessment of Quality in Statistics, Eurostat/A4/Quality/00/General/Definition, Luxembourg, April 4–5.

Eurostat (2000b) *Standard Quality Report*, Eurostat Working Group on Assessment of Quality in Statistics, Eurostat/A4/Quality/00/General/Standard Report, Luxembourg, April 4–5.

Felce D., Perry J. (1995). "Quality of Life: Its Definition and Measurement". *Research in Developmental Disabilities*, 16 (1), pp. 51–74.

Giovannini E., A. Morrone, T. Rondinella, L.L. Sabbadini (2012) "L'iniziativa CNEL-ISTAT per la misurazione del Benessere Equo e Sostenibile in Italia" in *Autonomie locali e servizi sociali*, n. 1, Il Mulino, Bologna.

Horn R.V., (1993) *Statistical Indicators*, Cambridge University Press, Cambridge.

Johansson S. (2002). "Conceptualizing and Measuring Quality of Life for National Policy". Social Indicators Research, 58.

Kahneman, D. and Krueger, A. B. (2006) "Developments in the measurement of subjective well-being" *Journal of Economic Perspectives*, 20(1).

Maggino F. (2009) *The state of the art in indicators construction in the perspective of a comprehensive approach in measuring well-being of societies*, Firenze University Press, Archivio E-Prints, Firenze.

Noll H.-H. (2004) *Social indicators and indicators systems: tools for social monitoring and reporting*, paper presented at OECD, World Forum "Statistics, knowledge and policy", Palermo, 10–13 November 2004.

Nuvolati G. (1997). Uno specifico settore di applicazione degli indicatori sociali: La qualità della vita. In: Zajczyk F. *Il mondo degli indicatori sociali, una guida alla ricerca sulla qualità della vita*. La Nuova Italia Scientifica, Roma, pp. 69–94.

Nuvolati G. (2002). *Qualità della vita e indicatori sociali.* Seminar held at the PhD degree programme "Scienza tecnologia e società", aprile, Dipartimento di Sociologia e di Scienza Politica, Università della Calabria. Available on http://www.sociologia.unical.it/convdottorati/nuvolati.pdf

Patel S., M. Hiraga, and L. Wang (World Bank) D. Drew and D. Lynd (Unesco) (2003) *A Framework for Assessing the Quality of Education Statistics*, Development Data Group and Human Development Network, World Bank, Washington, D.C.

Sharpe A., J. Salzman (2004) *Methodological Choices Encountered in the Construction of Composite Indices of Economic and Social Well-Being*, Center for the Study of Living Standards, Ottawa.

Sirgy M.J. (2011) "Theoretical Perspectives Guiding QoL Indicators Project", *Social Indicators Research*, vol. 103, 1–22.

Sirgy M.J., A.C. Michalos, A.L. Ferriss, R.A. Easterlin, D. Patrick and W. Pavot (2006) "The Quality-of-Life (QOL) Research Movement: Past, Present, and Future", *Social Indicators Research*, vol. 76, n.3, 343–466.

Śleszyński, J. (2012) *Prospects for synthetic sustainable development indicators*, paper presented at the conference "Quality of Life and Sustainable Development", September 20–21, Wroclaw (Poland).

Stiglitz J. E., A. Sen & J.-P. Fitoussi eds (2009) *Report by the Commission on the Measurement of Economic Performance and Social Progress*, Paris. http://www.stiglitz-sen-fitoussi.fr/en/index.htm

Veenhoven, R. (1994) "Is happiness a trait? Tests of the theory that a better society does not make people any happier" *Social Indicators Research*, 32(2).

Zapf W. (1975) "Le système d'indicateurs sociaux: approches et problèmes", *Revue Internationale des Sciences Sociales*, Vol. XXVII, n. 3.

Zapf W. (1984) "Individuelle Wohlfahrt: Lebensbedingungen und Wahrgenommene Lebensqualität", in W. Glatzer e Zapf W. (eds.) *Lebensqualität in der Bundesrepublik*, Frankfurt a. M. – New York, Campus, pp. 13–26.

Part IV
Territories and Quality of Life

Chapter 14
Quality of Life Research in Asia

Takashi Inoguchi

QOL research in Asia was limited until recently to demographically small societies, such as Hong Kong (Chua et al. 2014) and Singapore (Tan and Tambyah 2014). Then the research focus shifted to South Korean (Shin and Spina 2014; Park 2014) and Taiwanese (Hsiao and Wan 2014; Yao 2014) QOL, followed in the 2000s to Chinese (Xing 2014) and Japanese (Inoguchi 2014a, b; Iwai 2011) QOL, then Macau (Davey and Rato 2014) and Malaysian (Abdullah 2014) QOL came to the fore. In the 2010s all of Asia appeared on the research radar. Daniel Shek in Hong Kong spearheaded it. In Singapore S.J. Tan and S.K. Tambyah have been steady and vigorous in developing QOL research in Singapore. Moving to Taiwan and South Korea, we have seen Grace Yao, Michael Hsiao, Chong Min Park and Doh Chull Shin become pace setters of sorts in terms of subject focus and methodological advance.

While those research areas have remained active in the 2000s and 2010s, Japanese and Chinese QOL research has also become activate. Noriko Iwai (2011) spearheaded a collaborative four-society QOL research project on East Asia that concentrates on Japan, China, Taiwan and South Korea. The four research teams are from Osaka University of Commerce, Chinese Renmin University, Korea University, and Taiwan Chengchi University. Then Takashi Inoguchi pioneered a research project on the QOL of all societies in Asia, meaning East, Southeast, South and Central Asia, with the two notable exceptions of North Korea and Timor Leste and with the notable inclusion of adjacent societies of Australia, Russia and the United States.

T. Inoguchi (✉)
University of Niigata Prefecture, Niigata, Japan

University of Tokyo, Tokyo, Japan
e-mail: inoguchi@ioc.u-tokyo.ac.jp

F. Maggino (ed.), *A Life Devoted to Quality of Life*, Social Indicators Research Series 60, DOI 10.1007/978-3-319-20568-7_14

In terms of academic discipline of major authors, Asia is no exception to diversity. Daniel Shek is a social psychologist, S.J. Tan and S.K Tambyah (2014) are experts of marketing and business research. Grace Yao is a psychologist. Michael Hsiao is a social anthropologist. Chong Min Park is a social psychologist. Doh Chull Shin is a political scientist. Noriko Iwai is a psychologist. Takashi Inoguchi is a political scientist. Thus quality of life research in Asia is no exception in the richness of disciplinary mingling.

In terms of analysis, the more recent academic undertakings in this area have explored subjects beyond what first generations of QOL scholars touched on and have yielded enormously revealing and stimulating results. Hsin-Huang Michael Hsiao and Po-san Wan (2014) have analyzed "public attitudes toward the state in Asia-Pacific region". Yoshinori Kamo and Makiko Hori (2014) have analyzed "marital and family satisfaction in 32 countries". Shinya Sasaoka and Katsunori Seki (2011) have analyzed democracy and quality of life in Asian societies. Doh Chull Shin and Nichaolas Spina (2014) have analyzed faith in democracy. Seoyong Kim (2014) has analyzed cultural capital and quality of life in Korea.

Then, I give a summary portrait of what is the AsiaBarometer survey and what aims and with what scope and methods. I focus on wide-raging analyses of the AsiaBarometer survey data to highlight the project's profile and some analytical thrusts into such topics as trust, democracy, civilizational clash and societal types.

AsiaBarometer Survey's Profile "AsiaBarometer" in Wiley-Blackwell Encyclopedia of Sociology, 2nd Edition (Inoguchi forthcoming)

The AsiaBarometer Survey conducted over 50,000 face-to-face interviews in 29 Asian societies and 3 Western countries. Its objective was to examine and better understand the quality of life in Asia. Survey topics ranged from personal health to trust and confidence in social institutions to political orientation to international relations. Given the varied and diverse social, economic, and political conditions of the region, the secondary questions provide useful insight to the nature of response when viewed through a wider lens to society and overall quality of life. Through its investigation, the survey and the ensuing analyses also made achievements in the areas of methodology, theoretical impact, and substantive contributions.

In the area of methodology, the survey researchers could pursue four types of comparative analyses: comparison within each participant society, comparison within and between Asia's different sub-regions, and comparisons between Asian and Western countries. A significant accomplishment is that although 27 or the 29 Asian countries have non-democratic systems, the government's agreed to the survey because the focus was on the daily life of ordinary citizens. In terms of theoretical contribution, the survey enabled the researchers to test theories, such as modernization, globalization, clash of civilizations, and the Asian value hypothesis.

For substantive contributions, the survey focuses on three key areas. (1) The happiest people are not the high-wage earners of democratic Japan, South Korea, and Taiwan, they are, in fact, the least happy group of respondents. The happiest people are in the poor regions of South Asia, which suggest that family, religion, and community are critical components of happiness. (2) Five key typologies of society are identified through the analysis of materialism, post-materialism, and public sector dominance. (3) Influences that are deeply rooted and affect social relations then impact quality of life. These influences include interpersonal trust and confidence in social institutions. Historical experiences and accumulated patterns of political culture are at the center of these influences.

Analytical Thrusts into Trust, Democracy, Clash of Civilizations and Societal Types

Asia, Quality of Life (Inoguchi 2014a, b)

Quality of life in Asia is one of the areas on which the AsiaBarometer Survey focuses (Inoguchi and Fujii, 2013). Asia covers a wide expanse of countries with very different economic, political, and social conditions. The region also includes five of the eight civilizations that Samuel Huntington identifies—Hindu, Chinese, Islamic, Christian, and Japanese—in his volume Clash of Civilizations and the Remaking of World Order (1996). To cover such an expanse of societies makes the AsiaBarometer Survey the most comprehensive survey in the world.

In the AsiaBarometer, the respondents are asked to rank different parts of their life, and the top-five domains or lifestyle aspects are in descending order of importance, health, home, diet, job, and family. Placing physical conditions (health, home, diet) over job and family is understandable. Other domains that ranked in the top-five lifestyle aspects for a few societies include income, absence of crime, medical care, and being devout. To gain more insight and a more nuanced appreciation of these societies, the survey examined the domains of family, job, and being devout as they relate to the family dimension, occupational dimension, and spiritual dimension.

The family dimension figures most prominently in Japan and Korea, followed by Brunei, Malaysia, Singapore, and Sri Lanka. In this second set of societies, they are located in maritime regions with have experienced immigration, resulting in the cohabitation of varied races. In these circumstances, family is the smallest unit of human existence. The occupational dimension is strongest in Vietnam and Kazakhstan, followed by China and Japan. Of these four countries, three can be classified as Northeast Asian (Kazakhstan is the exception), known for being diligent, and three are or have been communist (Japan is the exception). The spiritual dimension is greatest in Myanmar (Buddhist) and Bangladesh (Islam), followed by Afghanistan, Pakistan, and Indonesia (all Moslem). There is a high correlation to this finding with a low level of per capita income, regardless of religion.

The AsiaBarometer also attempted to measure happiness. A difficult concept to define and measure in one language, the survey also faced the challenge of articulating the concept with a constant meaning through many languages and cultures. The English question as respondents: "On the whole, do you think you are very happy, quite happy, neither happy nor unhappy, quite unhappy, or very unhappy?" To quantify the responses, the survey used a percentage difference index (PDI) to obtain the average for each society. To obtain a PDI average, the first two positive responses are added together, then the two most common negative responses are added together, and finally the negative responses are subtracted from the positive ones. The five happiest countries in the survey are Brunei, Maldives, Malaysia, Bhutan, and Sri Lanka; the five unhappiest places are Tajikistan, Kazakhstan, Cambodia, Kyrgyzstan, and Afghanistan. The happiest regions are Southeast Asia, followed by South Asia; the unhappiest regions are East Asia, followed by Central Asia. According to Human Development Index (HDI) scores, the PDI scores of Southeast and South Asia are higher than what HDI indicators suggest, and conversely, the PDI scores of East and Central Asia are lower than what HDIs suggest. In large part, the self-assessment of happiness for Southeast and South Asians appears to be based on religiosity, that is Buddhism, Hinduism, and Islam. For East Asians, who seek social harmony and collectivism, neuroscientists place anxiety as a central trait for this regional group 9 (Chiao and Blizinsky 2010). For central Asians, who still have nomadic tribes, a predominant quality is suspicion that is triggered by scarce water and grass resources (Matsui 2011).

Interpersonal Trust and Quality of Life: A Cross Sectional Study of Japan (Tokuda et al. 2008)

The connection between positive attitudes and quality of life (QOL) or subjective well-being is important. Psychosocial factors, such as interpersonal trust, optimism, and sociability, impact QOL. As a case study, Japan provides insight into the link between interpersonal trust and QOL. In Japan, subjective well-being is poor and interpersonal trust is relatively low.

Many factors are behind subjective well-being: genetics, demographics, lifestyle, environmental factors, and socioeconomic factors (income, education, occupation). Research has shown that moving from an impoverished situation to the middle class improves QOL but a higher income after that does not impact QOL. Also, being gainfully employed adds to subjective well-being.

The focus of academic inquiry has now shifted to psychosocial factors. A significant positive predictor of QOL is interpersonal trust. Trust can be defined as a belief that others can be relied on to act with good will and with sincerity. Trust an indispensable component in developing an integrated personality that deals successfully with social adjustment. The opposite qualities of mistrust, hostility, suspiciousness, and cynicism are negative attributes associated with poor psychological well-being. Mistrust is the belief that others will put themselves first and will even victimize others to achieve their goal. Mistrust also negatively impacts the creation and use of social support networks. A vicious cycle can develop between the mistrusting individual and the rest of society: one where mistrust prompts adverse reactions from others, thereby justifying beliefs with the potential to spiral into paranoia, which also brings a higher risk of suicide.

Industrialized societies are showing an increasing trend toward social disconnection and poor subjective well-being. Japan is no exception. The AsiaBarometer Survey shows that Japan has comparatively low levels of interpersonal trust. Also, the international values survey also registers Japanese as poor in subjective well-being or the most unhappy among industrialized societies.

Methods

Study Participants and Data Collection

The 2008 study used face-to-face interviews to survey 1000 persons from Hokkaido to Kyushu. Participants ranged in age from 20 to 69 years. The data collection included demographics, marital status, socioeconomic factors, health-related QOL, and interpersonal trust. The survey also covered political, environmental, and social issues as connected to the AsiaBarometer Survey.

Age groups were broken down into decades, 20–29, 30–39 all the way to 60–69 years. Education was categorized into three levels: high (post-secondary education), mid (high school completion), and low (elementary or junior high completion). Occupation was categorized as: self-employed, homemaker, employed or unemployed. Students, retirees, and unemployed were placed in the last grouping of unemployed.

The Japanese version of the WHOQOL-BREF served to assess QOL. The WHOQOL-BREF has 26 items that cover four domains that include physical, psychological, social and environmental QOL. The only item excluded from this undertaking was sexual satisfaction. The concern was that it might provoke an emotion response. The scores were transformed into a scale of 1–100.

To measure interpersonal trust, the survey focused on trust in people, human fairness, and human nature. Question posed: "Would you say that (1) most people can be trusted; or do you think (2) you can't be too careful in dealing with people?" Respondents chose on a scale of 0–10. If they chose the first part of question, then they received a score of 10 (highest level of trust), and if they chose the second part of the questions, then they received a score of zero (lowest level of trust).

The survey question to assess human fairness asked: "Do you think that (1) most people would try to be fair; or do you think that (2) they would try to take advantage of you if they got the chance?" To assess human nature, the survey asked: "Would you say that (1) most of the time people try to be helpful; or that (2) they are mostly looking out for themselves?" The same method to score respondents' responses to the first question about trust in people was followed in these two questions.

Statistical Analysis

SPSS 15.0J was used in all statistical analyses. Two-tailed p-values _0.05 were treated as statistically significant.

The three trust scales were positively correlated with all QOL domains. Adjusting for age, gender, size of residence, income, education, and occupation, we constructed multiple linear regression models for QOL and the main component score of the trust scales.

Results

The socioeconomic features of the survey participants are: mean age 45 years; 49 % female; 78 % married; 34 % lived in the Kanto region; 33 % had an annual household income under five million Japanese Yen (2008 average exchange rate to 1 US dollar was 100 JY); and 7 % indicated a low level of education, that is, junior high or less.

In a general examination of trust scales according to socioeconomic factors, trust is greater among women than men, the oldest age group (60–69 years) is more trusting than those in the youngest age group (20–29), and a higher income impacts trust positively. In reviewing each of three scales of trust investigated, women have greater trust in all three than men. In comparing age groups, participants over 60 years have a better assessment of human fairness and nature, whereas those in their twenties have a low level of trust in human nature. Income is also a factor. Of those with an income of eight million JY, trust in people and human nature is higher. In terms of occupation, specifically the employed groups, homemakers show greater trust in human nature. Size of residence and education levels does not display any meaningful difference in trust scales.

The mean scores of QOL domains by sociodemographics show that: women have a higher social QOL than men; greater environmental QOL is indicated in the 60–69 age bracket and a lower environmental QOL for those in the 40–49 age bracket; participant residing in cities of 100,000 have a greater environmental QOL and those residing in metropolises have a lower environmental QOL.

In terms of income, the participants with a five million JY household income have a lower physical QOL and those with an eight million JY household income have a better physical and environmental QOL. A similar picture appears for education levels, that is, those with a junior high level or less have a lower physical and psychological QOL. Occupation does not have a significant impact on QOL domains.

The correlation coefficients between QOL and trust scales as well as among trust scales are significant. Moderate positive correlations exist between all QOL domains and the three trust scales and a high positive correlation among the three trust scales.

In multiple linear regressions for QOL domains of sociodemographics and interpersonal trust, a positive and significant association exists. This analysis shows that higher interpersonal trust are linked to greater scores in the QOL domains (physical, psychological, social, and environmental).

In considering the other variables of gender, age, size of residence, and income that are associated with the QOL domains, the results show that: women are have a greater social QOL than men; those in the 40–49 and 50–59 age brackets have lower physical and social QOL than those in the 20–29 age bracket; those in the 50–59 age bracket also have lower social QOL than the youngest survey participants. In a comparison of city size with the major metropolises as the standard, participants residing in a city over 100,000 people have a greater environmental QOL; those living in a city of 100,000 or less have greater psychological and environmental QOL. In terms of income, those with a household income of eight million JY have a greater physical, psychological, and environmental QOL than those in households of five million JY. Educational levels and occupation make no significant difference in al QOL domains.

Discussion

In this case study of Japan, research shows that participants who have a greater sense in interpersonal trust are more likely to have greater QOL in all domains than those participants who have a lower sense of trust. The results confirm other studies that show that greater interpersonal trust is linked to better individual health assessments. The present task is to conduct a controlled interventional study that confirms that such a causal relationship exist between interpersonal trust and QOL. The objective is to move toward designing public health policies that promote improved interpersonal trust, and ultimately, improved global QOL.

In examining the relationships between sociodemographic factors and QOL, some findings bear speculation on the reasons behind them. For example, environmental and physical QOL is better in moderate sized cities than in larger metropolitan areas. Such cities may have less air and water pollution, noise, traffic volume, and living cost than their larger counterparts. Moderate sized cities may also provide better access social and commercial services, such as public transportation, theatre, and shopping malls.

Other studies in Europe also confirm this study's finding that higher income is associated with greater physical, psychological, and environmental QOL. Those in a higher income group are usually less inclined to partake in high-risk behavior, such as drugs and alcohol, are more likely to have regular health check-ups, and may have a better job that allows control and decreases the potential for accompanying stress. Hence, the "healthy" Japanese probably resides in a moderate sized city, is female, is either in her 20s or 50s, has a high-income household, and has a high level of interpersonal trust.

Greater interpersonal trust may prompt a better QOL for multiple reasons. First, trust of others is related to more robust connections with friends, family, and society, providing an overall sense of community support. The social ties and network also contribute to a sense of well-being. The concept of well-being is associate with pleasure, engagement, and meaning in life. Engagement with others is the most critical component. Second, interpersonal trust can also contribute to greater health of neighbors and communities, which leads to greater support and sources of mutual respect. Third, innovative ideas spread easier when others trust each other and share in the diffusion of innovative ideas in the health field. Fourth, access to resources, services, and amenities is better when community interpersonal trust is high because of a higher level of local groups lobbying on behalf of the community.

Further research is required as the current study has inferential limitations. A long-term study is needed in this experimental study to strengthen the current findings by accumulating evidence to support causality. Our conclusion is that interpersonal trust is related to better QOL for Japanese. Strengthening interpersonal trust on a larger level is difficult, but the first step is to identify the qualities of civic associations and public policies that are more likely to promote common interests and that will lead to greater interpersonal trust.

Social Capital in East Asia: Comparative Political Culture in Confucian Societies (Inoguchi et al. 2007)

Does globalization weaken or strengthen traditional types of social capital? As a concept, social capital often refers to the social infrastructure of business, politics, and community (Coleman 1990; Lin 2001; Putnam 2000; Stolle 2007; Inoguchi 2007). Social capital performs a critical role in bringing together the business community and in bringing together the political community. It is a necessary component in networks that face barriers and bottlenecks as they move forward. Social capital also allows actors in business, politics, and other areas to act with confidence in times of uncertainty or risks.

At the crux of social capital and social infrastructure is a set of agreed norms and common networks. Defining and measuring the extent of social capital is difficult because human actions are not limited to certain community interactions or groups. The most accepted definition of social capital centers on interpersonal relations. Social capital is the variable that determines how smooth and efficient interpersonal relations flow. It can be viewed as a collective good that promotes understanding, efficiency, and effectiveness within business, politics, and community.

Just as defining social capital is challenging, measuring the concept is equally problematic. How to measure something that is difficult to define? We argue that the line of inquiry into social capital is limited by the emphasis placed on interpersonal relations that then extends into research probing human nature and tolerance. The line of inquiry comes from the relative homogeneity of Western societies in terms of Christianity, democratic values, and free capitalist market practices. Western literature on social capital appears to frame its research questions around human nature and its ability to be good or evil. Instead, we propose that by examining Asia and its diversity of religions (Buddhism, Hinduism, Christianity, Islam), political systems (of 29 surveyed countries, only nine are qualified as democracies by Freedom House), and economic systems (only six governments have adopted a floating exchange rate system), the line of inquiry into social capital goes beyond interpersonal relations, human nature, and the subsequent presumption of a relative homogenous population.

In Asia, the Confucian tradition is a strong influence. It teaches that the starting point is the individual and her values, and that it starts at the individual level and builds to the greater world level. Confucian teachings stress that peace and stability starts with the individual who nurtures her own development of a virtuous self that leads to peace and stability in the family, then radiates outward toward the state and world. The focus is on the virtuous self and the development of being a good-natured individual, which then extends to the assumption that others are similar in nature. It is through this discussion that a commonality with social capital is made.

Our objective is to examine the relationship between globalization and social capital through the lens of traditional Confucian teachings. Does globalization reinforce or weaken social capital in Asia? For insight into this research question, we review data from the 2006 AsiaBarometer Survey that includes seven "Confucian" societies: China, Hong Kong, Japan, South Korea, Singapore, Taiwan and Vietnam.

To pursue this line of research we look at four questions from the 2006 AsiaBarometer Survey. The first two questions are numbered 11 and 13 in the survey. The first question is about a general sense of trust, whereas the second question is about goodwill toward others. Both questions deal with interpersonal relations but are approached from opposite sides of receiving and giving.

Question 11: Generally do you think people can be trusted or do you think that you can't be too careful in dealing with people (that it pays to be wary of people)? Possible responses: (1) Most people can be trusted; (2) Can't be too careful in dealing with people; (9) Don't know.

Question 13: If you saw somebody on the street looking lost, would you stop to help? Possible responses: (1) I would always stop to help; (2) I would help if nobody else did; (3) It is highly likely that I wouldn't stop to help; (9) Don't know.

The next two questions are numbered 37 and 44 in the survey. While the first set of questions focused on trust, which is an important element in ensuring that interpersonal relations work efficiently and smoothly, the second set of questions acknowledges that personal connections are also significant in navigating daily obstacles. This question also explores perceptions about fairness of rules and trade in a globalized world. The last question probes how Confucian virtues of benevolence, care for others, mindfulness, and thoughtfulness, which keep a society functioning, are prioritized in a globalized world that emphasizes competition. If competitiveness is sought, then that requires a strength and self-sustainability that conflict with mindfulness toward others.

Question 37: What should a person who needs a government permit do if the response of the official handling the application is: "just be patient and wait"? Possible responses: (1) Use connections to obtain permit; (2) Nothing can be done; (3) Wait and hope that things will work out; (4) Write a letter; (5) Act without a permit; (6) Bribe an official; (9) Don't know.

Question 44: Here is a list of qualities that children can be encouraged to learn at home. Please select two you consider to be the most important. Qualities are: (1) Independence; (2) Diligence; (3) Honesty; (4) Sincerity; (5) Mindfulness; (6) Humbleness; (7) Religiosity; (8) Patience; (9) Competitiveness; (10) Respect for senior persons; (11) Deference for teachers; (12) Don't know.

Data

Three types of variables are recognized: dependent, independent, and control. Dependent variables are the responses to the questions that reflect: general trust toward others; willingness to help others voluntarily; reliance on personal connections to resolve public dealings; and the value placed on teaching the personal traditional trait of mindfulness to children at home.

The independent variables are divided into individual-level predictors and societal-level predictors. Individual-level predictors include: attitudes toward globalization; familiarity with modern technology that connects people at a distance, i.e, Internet; interactions with foreign people; and English proficiency. Societal-level predictors include an index of economic freedoms from the Heritage Foundation that are scaled from 0 to 100 with 100 being the maximum freedom and Internet users per 1000 people. The higher the values, the more globalized a country is viewed. The economic freedoms are: business freedom, trade freedom, monetary freedom, freedom from government, fiscal freedom, property rights, investment freedom, financial freedom, freedom from corruption, and labor freedom (www.heritage.org).

Control variables are important as they could affect the respondent's social capital. At the individual level, we controlled for gender, age, marital status, education, income, and religious membership. At the societal-level, we controlled for fragmentation due to ethnicity, language, and religion and the extent of political rights and civil liberties (Alesina et al. 2003).

Results and Discussion

We used a two-level logit regression with a random intercept model. The results show that globalization has a positive impact on the general sense of trust. The coefficients are all positive and statistically significant. The respondents are 1.14 times more likely to select "Most people can be trusted" than to select "Can't be too careful in dealing with people" and "Don't Know."

Globalization appears to increase goodwill and volunteerism. The coefficients are all positive and statistically significant. Respondents indicated that they are 1.14 times more inclined to select "I would always stop to help" than the other choices.

Globalization also strengthens social capital as defined in the Western social science literature as related to interpersonal relations and human nature. Results also show that globalization undercuts social capital in the area of transparency and competitiveness. This tide of global connectedness also threatens the values of familialism and communitarianism. Respondents are 0.90 times less likely to choose "Mindfulness" over other choices, which indicates that globalization undermines the Confucian traditional value of mindfulness.

Trust, goodwill, familialism, and mindfulness are all about the traditional side of social capital. Trust and goodwill refer to interpersonal relations and human nature. Our results show that even with the tide of globalization, traditional types of social capital will continue. In contrast, familialism and mindfulness will disappear in the face of increasing globalization and the related values of competition, transparency, and accountability that accompany its development.

The follow-up question to these findings is why does globalization have this effect. Increased interactions and dealings with people in different countries allow genuine growth in human relations and understanding. In the process, preconceived ideas of others fall to the wayside. Trust is a by-product of globalization. People learn to appreciate the strengths and weakness of their country and other countries and learn that different comparative advantages of countries lead to trade. The accumulation of knowledge about other cultures and traditions on an international level leads to the accompanying development of goodwill, volunteerism, and cooperation.

In the immediate surroundings of family, daily problems may best be managed by family or close friends, a tradition referred to as familialism or family-related communitarianism. In a more negative form, it is nepotism or clientelism. Yet away from this intimate setting, the approach changes to one of caution, vigilance, and prudence. Increasing globalization means that for global trade to flourish the trust of business partners and customers must be earned through practices of fairness, equal access, and accountability. Francis Fukuyama (1997) notes that when trust is high, business benefits as transactions are quicker, less costly, and more dependable. Conversely, if trust is low, then business transactions suffer and become slower, more costly, and less dependable.

Mindfulness may result in a good society, but in a globalized world of rapid financial markets and competitive markets, other values of strength, competitiveness, and self-sustainability trump the traditional Confucian value of mindfulness toward others.

Democracy and Quality of Life in Asian Societies (Sasaoka and Seki 2011)

Does democracy affect quality of life? Many academics have studied this relationship. In particular, they try to determine if democracy leads to a good quality of life. The type of political regime determines the political rights and civil liberties of its citizens, which in turn can impact how citizens' view their opportunities in life, their satisfaction and subjective happiness with life. Political rights and civil liberties also determine the citizens' ability to participate in the political arena and to have their voices heard in the formation and reform of policies, especially in the context of enhancing public welfare. If these rights and liberties are compromised, then public frustration levels rise. Hence, the nature of the regime, in our focus—democracy—plays a significant role in the development of the individual's quality of life.

Cross-national studies indicate that democracy does have a positive effect and that it does not have a positive effect on the quality of life. The contradictory research results suggest that it depends on the type of variable applied in the studies. In the first set of studies, both objective and subjective indicators of quality of life are examined. The objective indicators measure quality of life through indices of human basic needs that are derived from indicators in the Physical Quality of Life Index and Net Social Progress. The subjective indicators of quality of life are from an international public opinion survey (ISSP 2007). This research also uses Freedom House scores, Polity IV score, and Bollen's democracy index to measure "objectively" a regime's degree of political democracy.

In the second group of cross-national analyses that reaches the opposite conclusion—democracy does not impact quality of life—scholars (Inglehart and Klingemann 2000) also use the Freedom House score to measure political democracy. However, for an indication of quality of life, this group turns to the World Values Survey (WVS) for its index of subjective well-being, which they use as an indication of happiness. The research concludes that democracy is not the critical component to improved happiness. Another study (Veenhooven 2000) that uses the Freedom House score to assess "freedom," not democracy, also relies on average poll data on happiness to indicate quality of life. The study's conclusion is that from a country-level perspective, freedom does not influence happiness in poor countries, but does positively influence happiness in developed, well-off societies.

The difference in research conclusions is due to the nature of the variable used. Four approaches are distinguishable: Approach 1 employs country-level variables as both the independent and dependent variables; Approach 2 employs the individual-level data as the dependent variable and the country-level data as the independent variable; Approach 3 is similar to approach 2 but reverse—the individual-level data is the independent variable and the country-level data is the dependent variable; Approach 4 employs individual-level data as both the dependent and independent variables. The existing literature as discussed in the above examples employs the first two approaches. To make the research findings more robust empirically, the causal relationship between democracy and quality of life must be confirmed by the analyses of the individual-level data. Moreover, because the research findings on this topic suggest different conclusions, we must test which hypothesis is valid. At the outset, we recognize that the relationship revealed through individual-level variables is not the same as that revealed through country-level variables. To bridge this difference, we use hierarchical modeling in our analysis to allow us to review the relationship between individual-level variables and, at the same time, consider country-level variation.

Democracy and Quality of Life in Asia

Asia is a good region to further probe the relationship between democracy and quality of life: four groups of regimes characterize regional governments, and regardless of the regime type, all pursue the public's well-being through policies centered on improvement of macro-economic conditions, increased infrastructure, increased household incomes, and improved livelihoods. The four groups are: (1) well-established democracies—Japan and India; (2) authoritarian regimes—China, Vietnam, Laos, Singapore, and Central Asian states; (3) "third-wave" democracies that transitioned to a liberal democracy in the 1980s—South Korea, Taiwan, Indonesia, the Philippines, and Mongolia; and (4) the regimes that go back and forth between democracy and autocracy—Thailand, Malaysia, Nepal, Bangladesh, and Myanmar.

Measurement Issues

Academics rely on the subjective assessment of happiness to measure quality of life (Dorn et al. 2007). Happiness levels are attributed to country-level economic performance (objective indicators) and personal feelings (subjective indicators).

It is also well established that citizens are not less happy because they live in a less prosperous country (Wangchuch 2007; Motobayashi 2006).

To measure democracy we rely on both objective and subjective measurements of the function of democracy. Objective measurements identify the regime as either democratic or non-democratic; subjective measurements are rendered by the citizen's own perception of democracy, that is, how the political regimes relates to her subjective happiness.

The Hypotheses

To verify that the citizens' perception of democracy impacts their sense of happiness we hypothesized:

Hypothesis 1a. The more satisfied the citizens are with the state of political rights they enjoy, the happier they are.
Hypothesis 1b. The more satisfied the citizens are with the state of civil liberties they enjoy, the happier they are.

The logic is that the more satisfied citizens are with political rights and civil liberties, that is the democratic system, the happier they be as opposed to those who are dissatisfied in these categories.

To test whether a regime types is the sources of happiness for its citizens, we examined country-level data of regime type as an independent variable.

Hypothesis 2: The citizens are in a democracy rather than a non-democracy.

If hypothesis 2 is true, this suggests that the policies pursued by a democratic government make its citizens happy.

Methods

For our data, we turned to the AsiaBarometer Survey from which we selected 39 surveys of 20 countries. The sample size was 25,661 respondents. We examined data from Bangladesh (2005), Bhutan (2005), Cambodia (2004, 2007), China (2003, 2006, 2008), India (2003, 2005, 2008), Indonesia (2004, 2007), Japan (2003, 2004, 2006, 2008), Kazakhstan (2005), Kyrgyzstan (2005), Malaysia (2003, 2004, 2007), Mongolia (2005), Nepal (2005), Pakistan (2005), the Philippines (2004, 2007), Singapore (2004, 2006), South Korea (2003, 2004, 2006), Sri Lanka (2003, 2005), Tajikistan (2005), Thailand (2003, 2004, 2007), and Uzbekistan (2003, 2005).

We used Hierarchical Modeling and followed a two-step estimation to run the model. The model specifications allowed for a varying intercept.

Variables

Dependent Variable

The dependent variable is general happiness. Respondents were asked to identify their level of happiness on a five-point scale from very happy to very unhappy.

Individual-level Independent Variables

A. Perception of Democracy. In this study, the perception of democracy is the principal explanatory variable. To measure it, respondents were asked to rate how satisfied they are with political rights and civil liberties, specifically the right to vote, the rights to participate freely in organizations, and the right to gather and demonstrate. The responses, on a four-point scale, ranged from very satisfied to very dissatisfied.

Individual-level Control Variables

To the model we included six control variables: satisfaction with government performance, standard of living, gender, age education level, and religious affiliation.

Country-level Independent Variables

A. Democracy. As a dichotomous choice of regime type—democracy or non-democracy—we used conventional sources (Polity IV data) to classify political regimes. A regime is categorized democratic if the Polity IV score is more than seven (Epstein et al. 2006: 555).

Findings and Discussion

Based on our statistical analysis, we can make two conclusions. First, a strong explanatory factor of happiness is the individual-level of satisfaction with the two main components of democracy—political rights and civil liberties. In addition to the role played by the citizen's socioeconomic status, that person's assessment about of politics also plays a critical part in augmenting the individual sense of happiness. Second, the country-level regime type is not statistically significant to impact the level of happiness. This result remains unchanged even when individual-level satisfaction about democracy is excluded. Our findings suggest that, at least in Asia, the regime type is a minor secondary consideration in increasing happiness, and that the critical element is the satisfaction levels of its citizens with the function of the political regime and with the political rights and civil liberties offered to them.

From this study, we can infer that, in Asia, the happiness of citizens is more closely connected to how well the government performs than in whether the government can be categorized a democracy. From this perspective, democracy as it manifests itself in political rights and civil liberties does affect the subjective quality of life in Asia.

Legitimacy and Effectiveness in Thailand, 2003–2007: Perceived Quality of Governance and Its Consequences on Political Beliefs (Mikami and Inoguchi 2008)

The Thai political system and its citizens experienced great political turmoil in the period leading up to, and with, the coup d'état against Thaksin Shinawatra on September 19, 2006. Given the political roil, we want to investigate two research questions. The first line of inquiry seeks to understand how the Thai people assessed the quality of governance during the Thaksin administration and with the provisional military government. The second prong of investigation seeks to evaluate the impact the populist style of the Thaksin government had on the political beliefs and attitudes of the Thai society and the impact the military coup had on these public beliefs and attitudes.

Why did democracy fail in Thailand in 2006? Some suggest that the quality of democracy was poor due to indulgent political elites, whereas others suggest that the emphasis on economic development placed the 1997 reforms in a tenuous position, and yet others suggest that the Thai democracy was fragile with a relatively high percentage of Thais favoring military rule. Although these factors help to explain the failure of Thai democracy in 2006, the other research question, which is equally important, is how did these tumultuous events affect popular political attitudes.

Data from the AsiaBarometer Survey in 2003, 2004, and 2007 shed insight from a bottom-up perspective on how those who are governed in Thailand think about their national politics. Institutionalized and regular collection of data about Thai political culture is very limited. For instance, the World Values Survey does not include Thailand as a target country. Consequently, the Thai data found in the AsiaBarometer Survey is rare.

In the next few sections, we present: an overview of Thai political history, in particular, the development of Thaksin's party, Thai Rat Thai (TRT), and its 2001 winning of the popular election; an outline of the five conceptual components of public perception and their internal relationships and how they can be measured through the AsiaBarometer Survey; and proposal of several hypotheses about the Thai situation, followed by a testing of these hypotheses. The findings indicate that from the public's perspective, the political setting deteriorated a great deal more between 2004 and 2007 than between 2003 and 2004, although the populist policies of Thaksin significantly biased the situation. In the ensuing period after the Thaksin government fell, the beliefs and attitudes of the Thai public were in a state of flux. These results impact the prospects for democratic consolidation in Thailand.

Background: Contentious Interpretation of the Thaksin Era and the Coup in 2006

The modern Thai political system has two principal actors lead the country: the first is the King who is politically active compared to other constitutional monarchies in the world; and the second is the military, which has played a political role since 1932. The military's hold on the political leadership strengthened with the 1947 coup. Thereafter, the military has controlled, either directly or indirectly, all successive civilian governments. In contrast, the monarchy has intervened only in times of crisis, such as 1951 and 1973.

During the government of Prem Tinsulanonda (1980–1988), Thai politics underwent a silent transformation to a technocratic system of governance, in which bureaucratic experts were in charge of policy formation. The military only retained veto power. Bureaucratic authoritarianism served Thai politics well, but the no-confidence vote against Prime Minister Prem, in 1988, led to Chatichai Choonhavan being the first democratically elected prime minister in 12 years. Despite the 1991 coup, democracy has maintained a popular basis and political hold on the Thai political system. The 2001 election marked the start of Thaksin's political ascent. TRT, the once fragmented political party, gained an unprecedented absolute majority in the lower chamber. The party and Thaksin's power grew as TRT regularly absorbed smaller parties, and by the 2005 general election, TRT secured about 70 % of the seats.

The political strength of Thaksin disappeared rapidly with the revelation of tax evasion in the sale of his family business. With growing public demonstrations, Thaksin called a snap election, but his strategy backfired when 38 seats did not win the necessary share of votes in uncontested districts. The ensuing constitutional crisis led to the military coup.

One possible interpretation is that the military had witnessed the emergence of the democratic system and its ups and downs through different leaders, and had decided that the unsteady hand of democracy had to end. Another interpretation is that the departure from democratic norms started with Thaksin's government. Hence, the 2006 coup is not democracy being destroyed, but it being restored. The military's explanation is that they had to step in because of Thaksin's abuse of power and corrupt practices. The military's claims can be substantiated with: the government's neutral monitoring of key institutions through personnel placement, such as the Election Commission, the Constitutional Court, and the Bank of Thailand; the imposition of an emergency law that threatens basic human rights; attempts to stifle the media and government criticism. Also, the expansion policy of TRT through the absorption of opposition parties did a disservice to electorate choices.

The military has taken its own questionable actions after the coup, such as the abolishment of the democratic constitution, dissolution of legislative branches, and restriction of political activities. Yet the King, the Privy Council, and the People's Alliance for Democracy supported the military's decisions.

The presentation of these events supports the interpretation that the coup did not overthrow a democratic government, but a populist authoritarian regime. Hence, the coup was a prelude to a more consolidated period of democracy in Thai history. All the interpretations have merits but rather than judge from the top down, it is our intention to focus on the people and how they view the more recent political events and how these events have affected their political attitudes.

Hypotheses: Components of Public Perception and Their Internal Relationships

In studying political attitudes, we are specifically examining the public assessment of policy output, satisfaction with policy formation and implementation processes, a sense of political effectiveness, trust in political institutions, and a commitment to a democratic system. In examining these five concepts, we approach them as five components that make up a value system and that have internal relationships.

The starting point of our analysis is that people's assessment of the political processes should reflect, in some way, the nature of their government. For instance, public perceptions about domestic human rights conditions are influenced by the overall repressive measures of government. The more educated the public, the more critical the assessment. For these reasons, this concept is the main component in measuring Thai governance. Yet as a subjective indicator of policy processes, the personal level of support for a political regime biases the assessment. Those who are not as robust in their support for democracy may ignore undemocratic aspects and over-evaluate the quality of governance. Satisfaction with policy-making processes may be conflated with satisfaction of policy, which could also be influenced by whether the individual has benefitted from implemented government policies.

In the Thai study, the Thaksin administration targeted the poor in its populist campaign, and so households with lower incomes are expected to have a higher level of satisfaction with actual policies, and this in turn may cause an exceptional level of satisfaction with policy processes.

Satisfaction levels in policy output and processes can engender trust in political institutions. A causal relationship also exists between satisfaction with policy output and a sense of personal impact in the political system. The higher the level of satisfaction with policy output, the more the individual is convinced that they have the ability to impact national politics. Not all components influence each other. For instance, the assessment of political processes and the individual feeling of political effectiveness are independent of the other, that is, expressing a preference and government receptiveness are not connected. Similarly, political effectiveness and trust in political institutions also do not interact with each other. Trust in political institutions depends on government performance, and even those with a strong belief in political effectiveness may distrust political institutions if they fail to work efficiently. Institutional trust does not indicate a commitment to democracy or the democratic process. Institutional trust does not apply to only democratic institutions. We view commitment to democracy or a leaning toward authoritarianism as a trait that is determined by early life experiences or a traumatic event, in the case of Thailand, the 2006 coup.

In examining the survey data, we look at the structured mean of a component and the difference, if any, between the survey years. For example, we find that the structured mean of the assessment of policy processes for 2007 to be statistically and significantly lower than that in the 2003 and 2004 surveys. This suggests that after the coup, the quality of Thai governance declined. To assess changes in political beliefs, we examine the structured means of political effectiveness and trust in political institutions. If the structured means are not statistically different, then this suggests that for the regular Thai person, it does not matter who is in power.

To test these hypotheses, we use structural equation modeling.

Results and Discussion

A. Policy output. The military government did not fare well in the public evaluation of its policy outputs, especially when compared to the Thaksin administration. The positive assessment of Thaksin's policies could be explained by his populist policies, but the surveys show that in 2003 and 2004, more than 80 % of the respondents highly evaluated the economic policies of the elected government. In contrast, the military government did not receive a positive evaluation on any single issue, and the 2007 assessment of economic policies decreased by more than 50 %. The results are proof of Thaksin's achievement.
B. Policy formation and implementation processes. Again, the military government did not do well in this assessment area. The majority of Thai respondents indicated that they were relatively satisfied with the civil liberties of both civilian and military governments, although satisfaction levels were dropping in almost all areas of political processes. Between 2003 and 2004, the category that asked about "freedom of speech" and right to criticize the government dropped significantly, reflecting Thaksin's policy of interference in the media. In terms of freedom to participate in organizations, the public perception remained somewhat unchanged in the three surveys, indicating a certain liberalness to the military government.
C. Sense of political effectiveness. The Thai people's sense of personal effectiveness in politics was enhanced during Thaksin's period in office. The percentage of respondents who concurred with pessimistic statements about power and

their own personal role decreased. The policies of the TRT to give money to villages to promote economic diversification, to provide a plan for medical care, and to give farmers a 3-year moratorium on debt probably contributed to the public's sense of power to change politics. The 2007 survey saw the levels of 2003 return in the area of political doubt and disinterest.

D. Trust in political institutions. Another consequence of the TRT policies is an elevated sense of trust in institutions in the first two surveys and a drop in the last survey. In contrast, trust levels for the media and nongovernmental organizations remained constant, suggesting that the drop in political trust is a direct reaction to the coup.

E. Commitment to a democratic system. The Thaksin administration appears to have impacted people's regime preference more than the coup did. The surveys reveal that prior to the coup, there was a significant spike in loose support for one-man rule and a military government. A technocracy appears to be the only regime type to suffer a drop in popular support after the coup. The results suggest that support for a leadership with few constraints was preferable, especially to those who benefitted from Thaksin's policies, and yet a segment of the population was more cautious about the unfettered style of Thai politics. The tense atmosphere prior to the coup appears to have made an indelible impact on regime preference.

The next step is to apply the hypothesized structural equation model to these five indicator variables that we have just discussed. The results corroborate the results. First, the 2003 survey shows that the authoritarian tendency among the Thai public is statistically and significantly lower than that found in the 2004 and 2007 surveys. This implies that the stronger psychological impact on regime preference came from Thaksin's populist policies, and not the military coup. Second, the assessment of political processes declined with each later survey, so the average assessment is lower in 2007 than 2004, and the 2004 average assessment is lower than 2003. This indicates that the public already felt that the quality of governance was declining during the Thaksin administration. For policy output and trust of political institutions, the 2004 survey revealed the highest degree of satisfaction for the former and the strongest average trust for the latter. For a sense of ineffectiveness, the 2007 survey displayed a statistically and significantly higher than average level compared to the 2004 survey. Between the 2003 and 2004 surveys, there was not any significant difference in averages for a sense of political ineffectiveness. This result suggests that Thai people felt more politically effective during the Thaksin government than under military rule.

In the next step, we examined the causality between the latent variables. Our conclusions show that the interrelationship between components was as we anticipated: authoritarian inclinations cause respondents to overestimate political processes; higher education leads to a more critical assessment; satisfaction with policy input was dependent on income level; satisfaction with policy output reduces sense of ineffectiveness and increases trust in political institutions; and trust in institutions is also enhanced with a higher degree of satisfaction with policy processes.

In sum, the empirical data gave us some insight into the political beliefs and attitudes of the Thai people during this transitional, and somewhat tumultuous, period in their political history. The high ratings for the Thaksin government came from the government's populist policies. When these policies were removed from consideration the Thai public viewed the quality of governance offered by the Thaksin administration and by the military as similar. Populist policies also impacted positively the level of trust toward political institutions. Commitment to a particular regime also weakened between 2004 and 2007. Thai politics continues to be volatile and in a state of flux. The need for additional social surveys in Thailand remains high.

Is Globalization Undermining Civilizational Identities? A Test of Huntington's Core State Assumptions among the Publics of Greater Asia and Pacific (Collet and Inoguchi 2012)

Introduction

> It is my hypothesis that the fundamental source of conflict in this new world will not be primarily ideological or primarily economic. The great divisions among humankind and the dominating sources of conflict will be cultural… The fault lines between civilizations will be the battle lines of the future.—Samuel Huntington 1993: 22

Huntington's thesis, 20 years on, continues to generate discussion and academic research. Yet concerns remain about the empirical basis of his assertions about cultural differences and about whether his approach to world politics has merit. What defines post-Cold War conflict? According to Huntington, the source of conflict is fortified religious identities, revived traditions, and incompatible values. Many scholastic studies have focused on this explanation. In contrast, few studies have investigated his contention that conflicts arise from civilizational identities that are forged at the "micro-level" through increasing cultural affiliation with core states.

Our research seeks to fill this gap. Our study is built around two questions. (1) What is the extent to which publics demonstrate culturally based affinities toward core states? (2) As Huntington argues, is religiosity a primary factor behind these affinities or does globalization and nationalism mitigate its impact? Positive evidence to this line of inquiry would suggest that the distinction between "friend" and "foe" may have a civilizational consciousness and that globalization is having a boomerang effect of producing a cultural resurgence, the basis of the clash of civilizations thesis.

The Asia-Pacific region is at the center of this investigation. It is an understudied area in the probing of Huntington's provocative work. Termed the "cauldron of civilizations" by Huntington, the region is home to 60 % of the world's population, six of the ten most spoken languages, and seven of the nine world's civilizations as defined in Huntington's framework. The ensuing analysis draws on data from the AsiaBarometer Survey of 28 Asian countries, the United States, and Russia.

The Debate Continues

The events of September 11th and the U.S. foreign policy of intervention in Iraq, Afghanistan, Pakistan and the ISIS (the Islamic State in Iraq and al-Sham) stimulate debate about this conceptualization of international affairs and conflict. The citation count for Huntington's thesis is well over 17,000 on Google Scholar. The discussion and debate has two sides. The first focuses on the concept of civilization as a unit to frame post-Cold War politics. The second focuses on the empirical/evidentiary component of the concept's expectation for conflict.

Three assertions underline Huntington's theory. (1) Religious differences have become the source for conflict, replacing the differences and tensions that came from a bipolar world in Cold War politics. Today, in Huntington's analysis, local conflicts with wider connections characterize conflicts (1996: 268). (2) The conceptualization of core states that serve as a "wider connection" and source of civilizational identity of culture to member states (1996: 135). The core states dominate at the macro-level and stand as a beacon at the micro-level, attracting those who are culturally similar and repelling those who are culturally different (1996: 155). Core states promote and reinforce civilizational identities, and so are essential to a civilizations-based world politics. (3) Globalization strengthens the power of core states as they provide a civilizational identity based on a resurgence of tradition and religiosity. Huntington does not view modernization as a Westernizing or homogenizing force, but rather views the economic, political, and military successes that accrue from this process as prompters for cultural confidence and cultural assertiveness. On the individual level, modernization prompts alienation as traditional social bonds are broken and religion can fill the space and provide answers.

Globalization strengthens civilization alignment. Increased travel and exchanges highlights differences, and brings a deeper sense of civilizational identity and consciousness, highlighting a dichotomy of "us" and "them" (1996: 129).

Many are critical about Huntington's "essentialism," categorization scheme of placing civilizations as regional über-states, and portrayal of a likely war between the "West," "Islam," and "Confucian" societies. Other critiques include: the apparent simplification in understanding identity, failure to account for transnational political identities, and neglect of nationalism and its subordination to religiosity.

Of the scholars who shared in Huntington's conceptualization of civilizations as political units, little is said about the role of core states, implying that the formation of civilization identities is taken somewhat for granted. Also, some treat inter-civilizational interaction as peaceful, not conflictual in nature. For this group of scholars, civilizations are malleable and weakly institutionalized social orders. Other studies are more nuanced, showing that modernization can lead to conflict, states with similar cultures tend to belong to the same international organizations, the chance of going to war is greater for the West as it tends to behave collectively as a civilization, and conflicts based on cross-cultural and religious conflict are increasing. In general, Huntington's clash thesis does not explain the past well, but sufficient evidence is available and sufficient speculation about future shifts in world politics, especially between the West and Islam, allows his ideas to maintain relevance.

Comparative studies after September 11th have failed to show that the United States, as the perceived core state of the West, has been significant in defining civilizational identities. The anti-U.S. sentiments that appeared after the U.S. Iraq invasion were equally palpable in Western Europe and the Middle East. Regardless of cultural zones, foreign assessment of the United States is similar. However, studies that examine foreign views of other core states are limited, although comparative surveys suggest that Islam and Confucian societies display inter-civilizational heterogeneity. The outstanding question is whether other core states are able to engender similar sentiments—both pro and con—to that of the United States and whether they are enduring and culturally based. The theoretical significance to this line of inquiry relates to civilizational identity.

Hypotheses

We have five hypotheses.

H1. In-civilization (member-state) publics will affiliate more strongly with the core state of their civilization than out-civilization publics.

The logic is that those publics in Asia that have more Western influence are more likely to view the United States as a positive and that Sinic publics are more likely than others to view China as a positive. The lack of a core Islamic state renders affiliation an open question, and so it then follows that:

H1a. Citizens in predominantly Islamic states in Asia will identify more closely with Iran and be more inclined to see it as a political influence than those in Sinic or Western-influenced civilizations.

Religion is at the center of Huntington's thesis. Religion strengthens cultural differences and civilizational identities, and so by extension the perception of core states should be affected by the degree of commitment to religion. Those most committed to religion are usually the ones most sensitive to menacing contrary values and will then view that core state as the best means to protect the integrity of the values.

H2. As religiosity within given member state publics increases, perceptions of in-civilization core states will improve and perceptions of out-civilization core states, ceteris paribus, will decline.

H3. As nationalism within given member state publics increases, perceptions of in-civilization core states will increase and perceptions of out-civilization core states, ceteris paribus, will decrease.

The final hypothesis addresses the anticipated impact of globalization.

H4. As exposure to foreign cultures within given member state publics increases, perceptions of in-civilization core states will increase and perception of out-civilization core states, ceteris paribus, will decrease.

Data and Findings

We again return to the AsiaBarometer Survey as our data source used to test our hypotheses. For this data set, we looked at 4 years of the survey from 2005 to 2008. In 2005, the countries surveyed included: Kazakhstan, Kyrgyzstan, Tajikistan, Turkmenistan, and Uzbekistan (predominantly Islamic states of the former Soviet Union) as well as Afghanistan, Bangladesh, Bhutan, India, Maldives, Mongolia, Nepal, Pakistan, and Sri Lanka. In 2006, the countries surveyed included: Japan, China, South Korea, Hong Kong, Singapore, Taiwan, and Vietnam. In 2007, the survey covered: Cambodia, Indonesia, Laos, Malaysia, Philippines, and Thailand. In 2008, the survey returned to China, Japan, and India and extended its coverage to Australia, Russia, and the United States.

Interestingly, the surveyed countries include 11 predominantly Islamic societies, 7 Buddhist societies, 5 Sinic societies, 4 Western societies, 2 predominantly Hindu societies (India and Nepal), an Orthodox society (Russia), and Japan—representing a combination of 7 of Huntington's civilizations. The wide array of countries surveyed and the topics measured makes the AsiaBarometer a good tool to test Huntington's core state assertions. The limitations of a comprehensive comparative study remain, such as cross-cultural/national measurement equivalence, inconsistencies given the nature of the regime, and the anomalies that may arise in single-year studies.

Dependent Variable

The dependent variable is core state influence. The AsiaBarometer Survey asked, "Do you think the following countries have a good influence or bad influence on your country?" Respondents rated countries on a five-point ordinal scale from "bad influence" to "good influence" with the option of "neither good nor bad influence." Countries of influence include the United States and China in all 4 years and Iran as a regional influence in 2005 and 2006.

For U.S. influence in Asia, a wide range of opinion exists: of Asian countries, Cambodia and the Philippines have the most positive attitude, China views it as mostly bad, Japan is ambivalent; of Islamic states, most are neutral, Malaysia and Indonesia are negative, Afghanistan and Tajikistan are positive; Australia is ambivalent; and Russia has the most unfavorable attitude. For Chinese influence in Asia, responses again range: Mongolia and Japan have the most negative attitude; South Korea and Vietnam have both substantial and ambivalent attitudes; the United States and Taiwan tend to view it as bad; Australia and Russia are ambivalent; Islamic Asia has a more favorable attitude than other Sinic societies; and Pakistan and Afghanistan have more positive and consistent attitudes. For Iranian influence in the region: China is ambivalent; other Asian states are more critical of Iran than China, especially Hong Kong and Singapore; predominantly Islamic societies have the most favorably attitude; and Kazakhstan and Uzbekistan are more critical than their religious peers.

A. Core State Perceptions: Are They Zero-sum? For Huntington's assumptions about core states to have empirical traction, the expectation is that societies respond in a zero-sum pattern of identifying with the core state of their civilization and, in turn, reacting adversely to competing core states. In a scatter plot of country-level mean perceptions, such a pattern is not detectable. Only when perceptions of Chinese are regressed on the perceptions of Iran is a standard level of significance reached.

Independent Variables

In our study, we focus on three independent variables: foreign exposure, ability to recite from memory national anthem (yes or no response), and religiosity (frequency of daily prayer or meditation with one indicating never and five indicating every day). For foreign exposure we asked respondents about six areas for international interaction and then applied it to an additive index. Respondents were asked whether they have: a family member or friend living abroad; traveled internationally at least three times over the past 3 years; foreign friends in home country; watched foreign-produced TV shows; communicate with people in other countries through Internet or email; and job interactions with organizations or people in other countries.

The means of the three independent variables are plotted to flesh out the interplay between them in the Asia-Pacific region. In the Sinic civilizational grouping, societies generally feature low religiosity and high levels of nationalism. Of the respondents to show a low level of foreign exposure, notable inclusion is China, Japan, and Thailand with Singapore being the standout exception. In the predominantly Islamic societies, results have a wider range. In terms of religiosity or nationalism, low levels are found in Turkmenistan, Kazakhstan, Kyrgyzstan, and Tajikistan, whereas levels for both are high in Maldives, Malaysia, Indonesia, and Bangladesh. Afghanistan is strong in religiosity and weak in nationalism. Pakistan is similar, in that religion is placed over country. Uzbekistan is in the middle. In general, the Islamic respondents have low levels of foreign exposure with the relative exception of Maldives and to a lesser extent Uzbekistan.

Comparative findings for other societies include: the United States is more religious and nationalistic than Australia: Russia exhibits low religiosity and nationalism, whereas China has low religiosity but high levels of nationalism; Philippines, Indonesia, Malaysia, and India display strong religiosity and nationalism.

Core State Affinities: Is There a Micro-level Basis for a Civilizational Framework?

Next we examine the percent change in odds of seeing core states as "good" influences by civilization vis-à-vis the reference group (Islamic for the United States, Western for China and Iran). With regard to U.S. influence, Westernized states in Asia have a stronger affinity for the United States than the Islamic reference group, but Buddhist and Sinic states outside of China have an even stronger U.S. affinity than the Westernized states in Asia. Respondents in China and Russia, in comparison to the Islamic reference group, are less inclined to consider the U.S. influence good.

With regard to Chinese influence, Sinic respondents display no noticeable difference from the Western reference group, but Islamic respondents display double the highest probability toward Chinese influence. Buddhist societies rank second in having favorable perceptions of Chinese influence. Respondents in Japan have the lowest impression of Chinese influence.

With regard to Iranian influence, respondents in Islamic societies are 156 % more likely than those in Westernized Asia to positively consider Iranian power. Respondents of Chinese, Buddhist, and Hindu societies are more positive about Iranian influence than the Western reference group. Sinic societies are not as strong in viewing Iranian influence positively, but they still meet a standard level of significance. Respondents in Japan view Iranian power less favorably than the reference group.

Explaining Core State Influence

A. The United States. Religiosity impacts perceptions of U.S. power in Asia. In China and Russia, religiosity and nationalism interact, causing positive perceptions about U.S. influence that are generated by religiosity to decline as levels of nationalism rise. In Japan, increased religiosity negatively impacts the probability of viewing U.S. influence as good. In Australia, as a predominantly Christian society, it is not surprising that increased religiosity positively impacts the assessment of U.S. power. Of the Islamic states, in 8 of the 11 societies, religiosity does not impact view of U.S. power. Foreign exposure also plays a positive role in improving perceptions about U.S influence.
B. China. In general, religiosity does not have a large impact on perceptions of Chinese influence. Singapore, Tajikistan, Maldives, and Bangladesh are the exception. For the first three states, increased religiosity affects negatively respondents' opinion about Chinese power. In Bangladesh, the effect of higher religiosity is opposite. In contrast, nationalism does impact respondents' feeling about Chinese influence. In Singapore, increased nationalist sentiments lowers opinions about Chinese power, whereas the opposite is the case among respondents in Hong Kong, Taiwan, and Bhutan. Exposure to foreign interactions also improved impressions about Chinese influence. Indonesia is the one exception in this instance.
C. Iran. Religiosity positively impacts perceptions about Iranian influence in several Islamic societies. Nationalism is not a factor in this line of analysis. The one exception to this pattern is China. In terms of foreign exposure, the pattern for Iran is opposite that of the U.S. and Chinese case. As foreign exposure grows, respondents in India, Hong Kong, Singapore, Kazakhstan, Kyrgyzstan, and Uzbekistan show a decline in opinion toward Iranian power.

Discussion and Conclusion

Based on Huntington's clash of civilization theory, several assumptions need to be empirically true. Societies belonging to different civilizational groupings should have a sense of "us" versus "them" and the dichotomy should be defined along geopolitical terms. For Huntington, this is the foundation of civilizational identities that extends into how international affairs are structured. According to this understanding of world politics, societies have a stronger affinity to the core states of their civilizational grouping and a more negative assessment of core states that belong to other "rival" civilizational groupings. These bonds should be strengthened further by religiosity. And our third variable of globalization, measured in foreign exposure, should reinforce this sense of "us," as Huntington's resurgence model would underscore negative perceptions of core states of out-civilizations.

Our results indicate that the reality of the Asia-Pacific region is more complex than Huntington's model would suggest. Some survey results from predominantly Islamic states (Indonesia, Malaysia, and Pakistan) support civilizational divisions between the United States, China, and Islamic states. Religiosity is a primary cause, although nationalism also plays a part, as does the interaction between the two. Our analysis also reveals that among the central Asian Islamic societies, Iran has the potential to be a core state. Religiosity is significant in improving the perception of Iranian influence in 50 % of the Islamic societies surveyed. We also find evidence to support some of Huntington's assertions about a Confucian-Islamic connection, in that several of these societies perceive China more favorably than the United States. China's views of Iran also serve to reinforce such a connection. Increased religiosity in Australia and Russian affect positively support for U.S. influence. These findings add weight to some aspects of Huntington's assertions regarding the evolution of the West.

Our research shows that the influence of core states is not a zero-sum game among civilizational groupings, that is, affinity for core states of an in-civilization does not translation into increased adverse feelings toward core states of an out-civilization. In reviewing how societies react to U.S., Chinese, and Iranian influence, some predominantly Islamic states view the United States and Iran as neutral or good influences; only Malaysia and Pakistan favor China over the United States; South Korea and Taiwan lean toward the United States over China; and Japan definitely supports U.S. power. Antagonism between China and Japan, regional territorial disputes with China, and nationalism sparked by these disputes cast doubt on the possibility of a cohesive Sinic civilization led by Beijing.

The effect of globalization presents the main challenge to Huntington's thesis. The overall pattern is that increased foreign exposure prompts perceptions of foreign state influence to improve. This is particularly noteworthy in some of the contentious inter-civilizational dyads, such as between the Chinese and Americans. Indonesia is the exception to this pattern and does reinforce Huntington's predicted resurgence. In the case of Iranian influence, foreign exposure undermined positive perceptions, especially in central Asia. The findings suggest that in the place of imminent conflict between the United States and China, competition in soft power and development initiatives are increasing between these two powers, leaving space for potential improvement in U.S.-Sino relations at the micro-level.

The deterministic value Huntington places on religion as a key in identity formation is overstated. Civilizational identities have multiple influences leading them in different directions. Foreign exposure, rather than reinforce increasing religiosity and nationalism, serves to bolster outside perceptions of states and pull them away from the collision of values and culture that Huntington predicts. The potential of modernity to impact future identities, as Shmuel Eisenstadt suggest, should not be overlooked. The approach that appears as empirically plausible, if scholars in international relations and comparative politics choose to pursue the civilizational paradigm, is the one that Peter Katzenstein proposes—a middle ground that conceptualizes them as "weakly institutionalized orders." Core states may participate in defining politics at the macro-level, but globalization has blurred their role in defining publics at the micro-level.

Multiple Modes of Well-Being in Asia: Typologies of Asian Societies via Satisfaction About Life Domains (Inoguchi 2014a, b)

Introduction

Asia, as a demographically dense and vibrant economic region of the world, also has a varied sense of well-being among its many societies and their populations. In this segment, I argue that Asia has multiple modes of well-being. To apply this concept, I use data from the AsiaBarometer Survey (2003–2008), which involved over 50,000 respondents in 29 states or autonomous regions (e.g. Hong Kong). Based on this data, I propose a typology of societies in Asia. I factor-analyze responses of each society with five societal types that uses two heavily loaded dimensions after varimax rotation: materialism (quality-of-life sustaining), post-materialism (quality-of-life enriching), and public sector dominance (quality-of-life enabling).

Well-Being

Well-being is a personal and subjective assessment of how you feel about yourself in society. Therefore multiple modes of well-being is a natural phrasing to qualify how a person feels about her or his existence in a society and what she or he may be prioritizing in this assessment, such as happiness, health, prosperity, or accomplishment. The data from the AsiaBarometer Survey that was used in evaluating well-being asked respondents to indicate their level of satisfaction along a five-point scale regarding 16 lifestyle domains. The rationale is that if a life domain provides a level of satisfaction, then the dopaminergic system of the body is activated. In so doing, this indicates a priority of life and/or a contributor to well-being.

A critical feature of multiple modes of well-being is that it can be identified beyond the national level to the individual level. That this concept can be assessed at the individual level allows it to undergo strict scientific empirical testing. In this analysis, multiple modes of well-being is also examined as possessing a pluri-potent quality, that is, it has multiple potentials in its growth. Although borrowed from biology and usually applied to the growth of cells, pluri-potent fits this stream of analysis that includes: individual well-being, group well-being, national well-being, supra-national well-being (regional well-being, well-being by religion, well-being by beliefs, well-being by gender, well-being by race, well-being by class, well-being by income level, well-being by educational level, well-being by language, etc.).

The AsiaBarometer Survey asked: "Please tell me how satisfied or dissatisfied you are with the following aspects of your life." Respondents answered on a five-point verbal scale of "very satisfied," "somewhat satisfied", "neither satisfied nor dissatisfied", "somewhat dissatisfied," and "very dissatisfied," with a "don't know" category. The lifestyle domains probed are:

1. Housing
2. Standard of living
3. Household income
4. Health
5. Education
6. Job
7. Friendship
8. Marriage
9. Neighbors
10. Family life
11. Leisure
12. Spiritual life
13. Public safety
14. Condition of the environment
15. Social welfare system
16. Democratic system

Method

To manage national diversities, my team factor-analyzed each country with a varimax rotation, the pattern of life domain satisfaction. In the period from 2003 to 2008, each country had one to three surveys administered. The data was pooled and variations among the years are averaged. This method allows factor-analysis results to be more robust compared to those results that are based on a 1-year survey.

In this work, three factors emerged: materialist, post-materialist, and public sector dominance. Each of the three factors is influenced by different life priorities. The materialist factor is determined by priorities, such as housing, standard of living, household income, health, education, and work. The post-materialist factor is decided by priorities in the area of friendship, marriage, neighbors, family life, leisure, spiritual life, and public safety. For the public sector dominance factor, this is shaped by conditions of the environment, social welfare system, and democratic system. These three factors also refer to three different quality of life factors (QOL). Materialist is also called the QOL-sustaining factor; post-materialist is the QOL-enriching factor; and the public sector dominance is also known as the QOL-enabling factor. A factor analysis for all 29 Asian countries shows the first factor's eigenvalue as 5.4, the second factor's value as 1.0, and the third factor's eigenvalue as 0.5. For Asia, the materialist factor ranks first with the other two QOL factors playing a secondary role.

In this study, each factor is assigned a letter that is capitalized if the factor is dominant and lower cased if the factor is secondary. In the case of dominance, the materialist factor is A, the post-materialist factor is B, and the public sector dominance is C. In the case of being an auxiliary factor, the materialist factor is a, the post-materialist is b, and the public dominance factor is c. The national diversity of the study is high. Many factors, both at the individual level and beyond individual control, determine how respondents prioritize their life. Hence, the materialist factor is not always the most significant, just as the post-materialist factor is not always second in value, and the public sector dominance is not third in this hierarchy. Not all countries indicated a strong dominance of the materialist factor. By examining the first two factors that are deemed important by a country, that is using the eigenvalue for each country, the following life priority types can be expressed: Ab, Ac, Ba, Bc, and Ca.

Typology of Asian Societies Based on Life Priorities

The collective view of ordinary people, followed by factor-analyzed data, provides a typology of societies.

A. Materialism is the most significant factor. In its pure form, it promotes a strong society.
B. Post-materialism is the most significant factor. In its pure form, it promotes a society that partially colonizes the state.
C. Public sector dominance is the most significant factor. In its pure form, it promotes a state that constructs and suppresses society.

The five types of society are:

Ab The dominant factor is materialism and the secondary one is post-materialism. This type combines a weak state and a strong society.
Ac The dominant factor is materialism and the secondary one is public sector dominance. This type combines a strong state and a strong society.
Ba The dominant factor is post-materialism and the secondary one is materialism. This type combines an enmeshed state and a strong society.
Bc The dominant factor is post-materialism and the secondary one is public sector dominance. This type combines a colonized state and a strong society.
Ca The dominant factor is public sector dominance and the secondary one is materialism. This type is a strong state.

This set of typologies can be further refined with the consideration of geography and history. In total, ten types of society exist in Asia.

Ab1 Japan, Indonesia, Taiwan: maritime peripherals in the Western Pacific
Ab2 Afghanistan: border state of South Asia
Ab3 Uzbekistan, Tajikistan: core states of Central Asia
Ac1 China, South Korea: core states of continental East Asia
Ac2 Cambodia, Laos, Myanmar: river-based continental Southeast Asia
Ac3 Bangladesh, India, Nepal: core states of continental South Asia
Ac4 Mongolia: border state of Central Asia
Ba Hong Kong, Malaysia, Thailand, Vietnam, Kyrgystan: clientelist new settler societies
Bc Brunei, the Philippines, Bhutan, Pakistan, Sri Lanka, Kazakhstan: state dominant clientilist societies
Ca Singapore, the Maldives: small isthmus/islands societies

It is important to note that this study uses materialism and post-materialism as very different concepts from that used by Ronald Inglehart (1977, 1989, 1997; Inglehart and Welzel 2005). The use of these concepts in this study is justified because they are based on prioritized life aspects in Asia. They are more encompassing of various life satisfactions, thus they are more widely and universally applicable. The types of society emerge from a comprehensive, systematic, and empirical analysis of daily life satisfaction from below. The outcome of this academic endeavor is an evidence-based typology of societies.

Some Future Prospects

Having surveyed, albeit somewhat selectively, an array of quality of life research conducted in Asia and on Asia, I am now in a position to make a few remarks about some future prospects in terms of substance, data collection, sampling methods.

Substantively, topics of quality of life research have been expanding steadily and will continue to do so. In this respect, the quality-of-life-focused AsiaBarometer survey has made a big impact. It covers the entire Asian societies except the Democratic People's Republic of Korea and Timor Leste. It allows open access to all the survey data and this fact not only enables researchers to make best use of AsiaBarometer data but also encourages researchers to execute new surveys full of original questions. As the definition of quality of life and well-being can expand in tandem with social change, this is inevitable. Asia's immense diversity and fast-changing dynamism make quality of life and well-being research in Asia to become a most alluring area of study.

New ways of data collection also encourages to expand the enlarged coverage of quality of life research. For instance, blood and neuron are two of the increasing attended human body components. Examining blood without blood-letting or -sucking is a daily routine now technically and safely carried out (Saito et al. 2012).

Examining neuron's change in brains is also a daily routine albeit with still expensive machinery (Wright and Schoff 2014). Quality of life and well-being are very delicate and sometimes difficult to measure. Progress in measurement technology enables now what was long regarded difficult to gauge, whether it is blood or neuron.

Methodologically, global sampling and national sampling methods should be re-constructed. Hitherto fore, the national sampling method has been used heavily since the 1950s. Yet progress in communication technology has blurred the distinction between population and sample. Random digital dialing (RDD) is a good example of such blurrification. Most seriously, when our interest lies in something only globally measured, the conventional procedure is to carry out national surveys and combine the results. When our interest is, say, interpersonal trust in social relations on the entire globe, global sampling is the correct way of choosing a sample of, say, 100,000 out of the entire global population of, say, 70 billions. Gilani (2014) has been testing national and global samplings to see whether global sampling is not only theoretically right but also right in terms of executing costs of sampling. I am moderately confident that use of Google Earth will be experimentally conducted in the near future for global sampling.

Thus, three lines of future prospects of quality of life and well-being research have been sketched out. Much remains to be done in all these areas.

References

Abdullah, Lazim (2014). "Malaysian Quality of Life Index", *Encyclopedia of Quality of Life and Well-Being Research*, Springer, pp. 3743–3748.

Alesina, Alberto, Arvind Devleeschauwer, William Easterly, Sergio Kurlat and Romain Wacziarg (2003). Fractionalization', *Journal of Economic Growth*, 8: 155–194.

AsiaBarometer Survey (2003 to 2008) https://www.asiabarometer.org/.

Chua, Hoi-Wai, Anthony Wong, Daniel T. L. Shek (2014). "Hong Kong, Quality of Life", *Encyclopedia of Quality of Life and Well-Being Research*, Springer, pp. 2920–2923.

Chiao, Y. Joan, Katherine Blizinsky (2010)."Culture –gene coevolution of individualism –collectivism and the serotonin transporter gene" Proceedings of the Royal Society B: Biological Sciences, 277(1681), pp. 529–537.

Coleman, James (1990). *Foundations of Social Theory*, Cambridge: Belknap Press.

Collet, Christian, Takashi Inoguchi (2012). "Is Globalization Undermining Civilizational Identities? A Test of Huntington's Core State Assumptions among the Publics of Greater Asia and the Pacific" *Japanese Journal of Political Science* vol.13, part 4, pp. 553–585.

Dorn, David, Justina A.V., Fischer, Gebhard Kirchgässner, and Alfonso Sousa-Poza (2007). 'Is It Culture or Democracy? The Impact of Democracy and Culture on Happiness', *Social Indicators Research*, 82(3) pp. 505–526.

Davey, Gareth, Ricardo Rato (2014). "Macau, Quality of Life" *Encyclopedia of Quality of Life and Well-Being Research*, Springer, pp. 3737–3740.

Epstein, David L., et al.(2006) 'Democratic Transitions', American Journal of Political Science, 50(3): 551–569.

Fukuyama, Francis (1997). *The End of History and the Last Man,* New York: Free Press.

Gilani, Ijaz (2014). "Polling Beyond the Nation-state: Regional and Global Polling Surveys," Keynote Speech at the Asian Network for Public Opinion Research, Niigata, Japan, November 24, 2014.
Huntington, Samuel (1993). 'The Clash of Civilizations?', *Foreign Affairs*, 72(3) pp. 22–49.
Hsiao, Hsin-Huang Michael, Po-san Wan (2014). "Public Attitudes Toward the State in Asia-Pacific Region" *Encyclopedia of Quality of Life and Well-Being Research*, Springer, pp. 5195–5203.
Huntington, Samuel (1996). *The Clash of Civilizations and the Remaking of World Order*, Simon & Schuster.
Inglehart, Ronald (1977). *Silent Revolution: Changing Values and Political Styles Among Western Publics*. Princeton, NJ: Princeton University Press.
Inglehart, Ronald (1989). *Culture Shift in Advanced Industrial Society*. Princeton, NJ: Princeton University Press.
Inglehart, Ronald (1997). *Modernization and Postmodernization: Cultural, Economic, and Poltical Change in 43 Societies*. Princeton, NJ: Princeton University Press.
Inglehart, Ronald and Hans-Dieter Klingemann (2000). 'Genes, Culture, Democracy, and Happiness', in Ed Diener and Eunkook Suh (eds.), *Culture and Subjective Well-Being*, Cambridge, MA: MIT Press, pp. 165–183.
Inglehart, Ronald & Welzel, C. (2005). *Modernization Cultural Change and Democracy: The Human Development Sequence*. New York, NY: Cambridge University Press.
Inoguchi, Takashi (2007). 'Clash of Values across Civilizations', in Russell Dalton and Hans-Dieter Klingemann (eds), *The Oxford Handbook of Political Behavior*, Oxford: Oxford University Press.
Inoguchi, Takashi, and Seiji Fujii (2013). *Quality of Life in Asia; A Comparison of Quality of Life in 29 Asian Societies*, Springer.
Inoguchi, Takashi Satoru Mikami, Seiji Fujii (2007). "Social Capital in East Asia: Comparative Political Culture in Confucian Societies" *Japanese Journal of Political Science*, vol. 8, part 3, Cambridge University Press, pp. 409–426.
Inoguchi, Takashi (2015)."Multiple Modes of Well-Being in Asia" in Wolfgang Glatzer, et al., eds., *Global Handbook of Quality of Life,* Springer and University of Mannheim, forthcoming.
Inoguchi, Takashi (2014a). "Asia, Quality of Life" *Encyclopedia of Quality of Life and Well-Being Research,* Springer, pp. 244–248.
Inoguchi, Takashi (2014b). "Japan, Quality of Life" *Encyclopedia of Quality of Life and Well-Being Research*, Springer, pp. 3425–3428.
Inoguchci, Takashi (forthcoming)."AsiaBarometer" in George Ritzer, ed., *Wiley-Blackwell Encyclopedia of Sociology*, 2nd edition, Wiley-Blackwell.
ISSP Research Group (2007). 'International Social Survey Programme (ISSP): Leisure Time and Sports, 2007' (Distributor: GESIS Cologne Germany ZA4850, Data Version 2.0.0 (2009-10-29)), available at http://www.issp.org, (accessed 11 August 2011).
Iwai, Noriko, Tokio Hotta.(2011). Family Values in East Asia: Acomparison among Japan South Korea, China, and Taiwan based on East Asian Social Survey 2006, Tokyo: Nakanishiya Publication.
Lin, Nan (2001), Social Capital: A Theory of Social Structure and Action, Cambridge: Cambridge University Press.
Kamo, Yoshinori, Makiko Hori (2014). "Marital and Family Satisfaction in 32 Countries" *Encyclopedia of Quality of Life and Well-Being Research*, Springer, pp. 3782–3790.
Kim, Seoyong (2014). "Cultural Capital and Quality of Life in Korea", *Encyclopedia of Quality of Life and Well-Being Research*, Springer, pp. 1374–1382.
Matsui, K. (2011). *Seinan Ajia no Sabaku Bunka (Dessert Culture in Southwest Asia)*. Kyoto: Jinbun Shoin.
Mikami, Satoru, Takashi Inoguchi (2008). "Legitimacy and effectiveness in Thailand 2003–2007: perceived quality of governance and its consequences on political beliefs" *International Relations of the Asia-Pacific,* vol.8 no.3, Oxford Journals, pp. 279–302.

Motobayashi, Yasuhisa (2006). *Bhutan to Kofuku Ron: Shuukyo Bunka to Girei (Bhutan and Happiness:Religious Culture and Rituals)*, Kyoto: Houzoukan.
Park, Chong-Min (2014). "South Korea, Quality of Life" *Encyclopedia of Quality of Life and Well-Being Research*, Springer, pp. 6233–6236.
Putnam, Robert (2000). *Bowling Alone: The Collapse and Revival of American Community*, New York: Simon & Schuster.
Saito, Yasuhiko, Xiaochun Qiao and Sutthichai Jitapunkul (2012). World of Association for Public Opinion Research, University of Hong Kong, 2012.6.14–16, "Health Expectancy in Asian Countries" in Jean-Marie Robine al, eds., *Determining Health Expectancies*, John Wiley & Sons, London, 2003.
Sasaoka, Shinya, Katsunori Seki (2011). "Democracy and Quality of Life in Asian Societies" *Japanese Journal of Political Science* vol. 12, part 3 Cambridge University Press, pp. 343–357.
Shin, Doh C., Nicholas Spina (2014). "Democracy, Faith in", *Encyclopedia of Quality of Life and Well-Being Research*, Springer, pp. 1534–1540.
Stolle, Dietlind (2007). 'Social Capital', in Russell Dalton and Hans-Dieter Klingemann (eds), *The Oxford Handbook of Political Behavior*, Oxford: Oxford University Press, pp. 655–674.
Tan, Soo Jiuan, Siok Kuan Tambyah (2014). "Singapore, Quality of Life", *Encyclopedia of Quality of Life and Well-Being Research*, Springer, pp. 5975–5982.
Tokuda, Yasuharu, Masamine Jimba, Haruo Yanai, Seiji Fujii, Takashi Inoguchi (2008). "International Trust and Quality-of-Life: A Cross-Sectional Study in Japan", *PLOS one*, 2008 December, vol.3 issue12.
Veenhoven, Ruut (2000). 'Freedom and Happiness', in Ed Diener and Eunkook Suh (eds.), *Culture and Subjective Well-Being*, Cambridge, MA: MIT Press, pp. 257–288.
Wangchuck, Ashi Dori Wangmo (2007). *Treasures of the Thunder Dragon: A Portrait of Bhutan*, New York: Penguin Global.
Wright, Nicholas and James L. Schoff (2014). "China and Japan's Real Problem: Enter the Fairness Dilemma," *The National Interest,* November 2.
Xing, Zhanjun (2014). "Personal Well-Being Index from Five Capital Cities in Mainland China", *Encyclopedia of Quality of Life and Well-Being Research*, Springer, pp. 4755–4759.
Yao, Grace (2014). "Taiwan" *Encyclopedia of Quality of Life and Well-Being Research*, Springer, pp. 6583–6586.

Chapter 15
South African Perceptions of the Good Life Twenty Years into Democracy

Valerie Møller

Introduction

South Africa celebrated 20 years of democracy in 2014. A key characteristic of a successful democracy may be whether citizens are given sufficient voice to express their views on how their lives are progressing and to hold their government accountable for creating the opportunities for society to prosper. Since the 1960s, quality of life researchers have made it their business to capture people's evaluations of their life situations that, in turn, inform governments how well they are performing. A substantial number of these researchers will have been inspired by Alex Michalos, who, as founder-editor of the oldest journal devoted to the measurement of quality of life, has led the way.

In 1996 and again in 2004, Alex Michalos visited South Africa to assist with the task of documenting the transition to democracy from a quality of life perspective. So-called 'roving conferences' were organised that enabled our distinguished visitor to meet researchers at universities and research organisations in three centres across the country: Durban, Cape Town and Pretoria in February 1996, and Cape Town, Pretoria and Grahamstown in the Eastern Cape in June 2004. The first conference aimed to awaken interest in quality of life and social indicators studies. The second marked the year in which South Africa celebrated its first 10 years of democracy as well as the 50th anniversary of my Institute of Social and Economic Research at Rhodes University.

At each one-day meeting, Alex Michalos, the unassuming philosopher, would break the ice by telling his favourite story, Aesop's fable of the man, the boy and the donkey. He would grin mischievously when he came to the moral of the story, that it is well-nigh impossible to please everyone all the time. But he never failed to

V. Møller (✉)
Institute of Social and Economic Research, Rhodes University, Grahamstown, South Africa
e-mail: v.moller@ru.ac.za

F. Maggino (ed.), *A Life Devoted to Quality of Life*, Social Indicators Research Series 60, DOI 10.1007/978-3-319-20568-7_15

please us with his story of 30 years of social indicators research. First we would hear about his idea of living in Paradise or in Hell from a well-being perspective (Michalos and Robinson 2012) and the distinction between positive and negative indicators. I still have a copy of the fine line-drawing Alex projected of a streetscape picturing a signpost giving the day's quality of life reading, a full 100 % QoL. Pharmacies in many parts of the world display the day's temperature in Celsius or Fahrenheit in flashing neon lights, but only Alex thought it just as important to know the degree of well-being in society. Alex's prescience that subjective well-being would in time take its rightful place in public accounts was vindicated when the Beyond GDP movement emerged in the new millennium (Stiglitz et al. 2009; Michalos 2011).

In the course of a conference morning Alex Michalos showcased the many approaches to measuring subjective well-being and different aspects of life as diverse as education and environmental protection. In the afternoon, members of the audience reported their first efforts to address quality of life issues in South Africa. Alex always listened attentively, offered encouragement and valuable advice, and recommended we continue our work. At the end of both conferences, he offered to publish our work, which resulted in 1997 in the first volume in Springer's Social Indicators Research Series with the title of 'Quality of Life in South Africa', followed 10 years later by an update on quality of life published in *Social Indicators Research* in 2007 (Møller 1997, 2007).

Alex Michalos returned to South Africa a third time in July 2006 to participate in the 7th International Society for Quality of Life Studies conference held at my university in Grahamstown. As a result of his enthusiasm and encouragement, South African researchers have warmed to the task of monitoring and evaluating changes in their society and by 2015, the number of South African scholars documenting South Africa's quality of life has grown prolifically. South African researchers have also made it their business to increase the data sources on offer. They now have access to longer-term repeat cross-sectional survey data, as well as panel-studies data, to monitor subjective well-being and objective indicators relating to the country's social and economic development (Møller and Roberts 2014a).

The 1997 volume on quality of life in South Africa, published after Alex Michalos' first visit, evoked the heady days following South Africa's first open non-racial elections in April 1994. At the time South Africa had gained the epithet of 'the land of miracles' with reference to the negotiated settlement that had avoided a civil war (Friedman and Atkinson 1994; Sparks 2003). The volume talked of South Africa's emergent social indicators movement, and covered topics of concern as well as hopes for the future. Concerns included poverty and inequality in society, the past experience of deprivation, crime, and trauma; hopes included the prospects for human development and optimism for the future. Two chapters reported on evaluations of well-being over time and whether the country was heading in the right direction. The second volume, which emerged from the 2004 roving conference, outlined major achievements and setbacks for the new democracy. It followed up on topics discussed in the first volume relating to poverty and inequality, crime, and updated trends in optimism. It also addressed new quality of life topics relating to health, notably the HIV/AIDS epidemic; migration, housing, and service delivery; and covered religiosity and truth and reconciliation in the 'rainbow nation'.

Chapter Outline

This chapter explores South African perceptions of progress after 20 years of democracy. The focus will be on the population group that was most disadvantaged before the coming of democracy, that is, black/African South Africans, who represent the majority in the population. I shall begin by outlining some events of 2014 and then present a set of social indicators that demonstrate some of the positive changes that have occurred in society since 1994. The positive review is contrasted by a more sober reflection on the state of the nation in 2014, and a set of social indicators on public opinions of government performance. The remainder of the chapter will selectively present personal views of individual and collective progress drawing on qualitative studies as well as quantitative survey results. The framework I've chosen to review the perceptions of life in the new South African over the past 20 years is the Multiple Discrepancies Theory (MDT) developed by Alex Michalos in the 1980s. A theory is said to be the most parsimonious tool to guide research. When Alex first presented his MDT in the 1980s, he confidently claimed that 'nobody has bound together as many hypotheses or articulated a theory of multiple discrepancies as systematically as I have here' (Michalos 2005, p. 306). I trust I shall be pardoned for using his set of MDT gaps as a guideline and organising principle when charting perceptions of quality of life in South Africa 'then' and 'now', rather than as scientific theorems to be tested rigorously.

Life Satisfaction Since the Birth of Democracy

The 'Miracle' of the 'First Dance of Freedom'[1]

There can be no doubt that expectations were high in the heady days following what was called the 'miracle' elections of 1994, when many South Africans voted for the first time in their lives. The following year the country won the Rugby World Cup with just a single player of colour to represent the 'rainbow nation' on the winning team. South Africa's new President Nelson Mandela had endorsed the team when he appeared on the field wearing their jersey and later led the nation in applauding their sports heroes in unison. Thereafter, the 'Madiba magic' – Madiba is Mandela's clan name, was coveted by sports teams to boost their luck, and the new government adopted sports as a vehicle for building social cohesion in the rainbow nation. Many

[1] The title of a chapter in Meredith's (2011, p. 162) historical account of the years following independence from colonial rule in Africa.

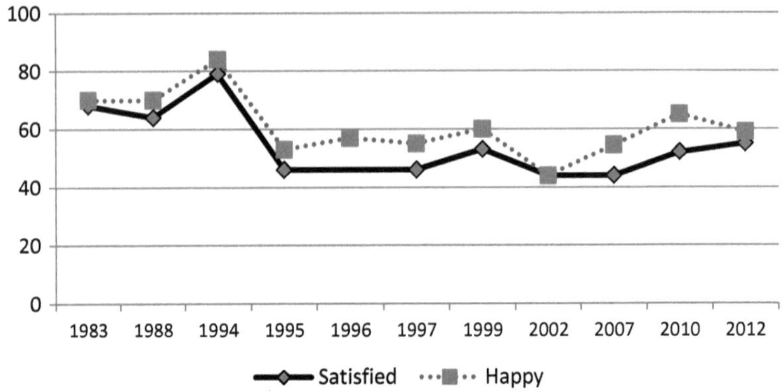

Fig. 15.1 Satisfied and happy South Africans, 1983–2012 (*Sources*: South African Quality of Life Trends Project (SAQoL, 1983–2010; HSRC South African Social Attitudes Survey (SASAS) 2012 (Percentages 'very satisfied/satisfied' and 'very happy/happy')) (Møller and Roberts 2014b)

South Africans still remember the pride and exhilaration they felt in the first few years of democracy when the country regained its international status in the world.

In the month following the first free elections of 1994, life satisfaction peaked. Figure 15.1 shows that four out of five South Africans, black and white, stated they were satisfied with life and happy, in response to a nationally representative survey for the South African Quality of Life (SAQoL) trends study.

However, the election euphoria faded rapidly after the 'first dance of freedom' (Meredith 2011) as the liberation movement that had become the ruling African National Congress embarked on the task of state-building. Since that time, life satisfaction dropped to between 45 and 55 %, on average, in six further waves of the study conducted between 1995 and 2012.

Fast Forward to 2014

In 2014, South Africa celebrated the 20th anniversary of the birth of democracy with great fanfare. It was also an election year. South Africans have gone to the polls every 5 years since 1994 to vote in national elections. In this fifth democratic election, the so-called 'born-frees', youth born after apartheid ended, were old enough to vote for the first time. As had been the case in all national elections since 1994, the 2014 election was declared free and fair. Exit polls found that voting procedures were firmly established and confirmed the competence of the country's electoral commission.

The election was again won by the ruling African National Congress (ANC), but with a reduced majority of 62 %, down from 65.9 % in 2009. The official opposition, the Democratic Alliance (DA) whose main support comes from white voters, increased its share of the vote from 16.7 to 22.2 %. The newly formed Economic

Freedom Front (EFF), launched by an expelled ANC youth leader, obtained 6.4 % of the vote.

In the first 20 years of democracy, South Africans have had four presidents, all members of the ruling ANC. The first 5-year term went to South Africa's revered struggle hero, Nelson Mandela, who had spent 27 years in prison before becoming the country's first iconic president. His term in office (1994–1999) focused on uniting the nation as the 'rainbow nation'. The Truth and Reconciliation Commission hearings, chaired by Archbishop Desmond Tutu, aimed to reconcile and heal the nation. South Africa's second president, Thabo Mbeki (1999–2008), spent most of his years as a political activist in exile, studying in the United Kingdom and undergoing military training in the Soviet Union. His term in office concentrated on building the economy, establishing macro-economic stability, and extending infrastructure and services to the previously under-served population. The country's vice-president, Kgalema Mothlanthe (2008–2009) took over from Mbeki's resignation before the end of his term. Jacob Zuma assumed the presidency in 2009 and retained the position when the ANC was re-elected in 2014. During his term of office the ANC adopted the National Development Plan that aims to eliminate poverty and reduce inequality by 2030.

The Good News Story in 2014

In the run-up to the national elections in May 2014, President Zuma's State of the Nation address and the ANC's election campaign focussed on the country's good news story. The country had seen many improvements since the advent of democracy. Service delivery featured prominently in the story: more households were living in formal housing and fewer were making do with informal housing in backyard shacks or shantytowns. Fewer murders were recorded, although the murder rate was still very high by international standards. The real gross domestic product per head had increased. A greater number of students were enrolled in universities. Standards of living had improved: the proportion of Africans living in poverty had decreased, largely due to social welfare being extended to just under 17 million people (Sethlatswe 2014).

South African writer and scholar, Jonny Steinberg (2014), singled out three outstanding achievements that South Africans justifiably could be proud of after 20 years of democracy: the roll-out of antiretroviral treatment to thousands of people living with the HI virus; free housing built for the poor throughout the country; and social protection for vulnerable people in the form of social grants – cash transfers in the form of old-age and disability pensions and child-support grants. He pointed out that nowhere in the world had a government issued free housing to over three million households and supported approximately one third of the population with a monthly income or stipend. Steinberg argued that the government was attuned to the needs of the people who had gained a voice in the new South Africa.

Many of the country's objective social indicators support this good-news story of South African achievements – Table 15.1 presents social indicators of change in select domains of life that denote progress in the lives of many South Africans between 'then' and 'now'.

The Other News in 2014

2014 was not only a year of celebration but also of sober reflection. While the ruling ANC party highlighted the achievements of its 20 years in government, political commentators, opposition parties, and the print and social media were more forthright in highlighting the country's problems and the government's shortcomings: although access to education had improved, the quality of public education was so poor that there was a shortage of skills; economic growth was insufficient to create enough jobs, particularly for school leavers; the unemployment rate stood at over 25 % or over 35 % if discouraged work seekers were included; health services were overstretched; infrastructure was crumbling due to lack of maintenance; an electricity crisis was looming; corruption was entrenched and ANC cadre deployment had seriously contributed to the loss of state capacity; affirmative action, aimed at fast-tracking transformation in society, had resulted in inexperienced people placed in positions beyond their competence; municipalities were in debt and lacked capacity to provide basic services.

One commentator referred to 2014 as South Africa's *annus horribilis*. Policy uncertainty, energy shortages and labour problems were crippling the economy and delaying foreign investment. The country narrowly avoided a recession, achieving only 1.4 % growth, while the rest of sub-Saharan African countries achieved growth rates of 5 % or more. National pride was dented when Nigeria claimed South Africa's place as the largest economy in sub-Saharan Africa. International agencies downgraded the country's credit ratings.

Prolonged wage-related strikes in the mining sector lasted for 5 months at the beginning of the year. Later in the year, South African Post Office workers went on strike for 3 months. Three state-owned enterprises, Eskom (the country's energy supplier), South African Airways, and the Post Office, fell into debt. For the first time since 2008, the country experienced electricity blackouts in November. Eskom announced that energy shortages would continue for at least 5 years until two new power stations then under construction were commissioned. Eskom's problems were seen as the result of incompetent leadership that had failed not only to plan for future energy needs but also to maintain existing power plants.

Political tensions increased within the ANC alliance in the run-up to the May elections. The ANC's trade union partner led a campaign to protest the government's introduction of electronic tolling on freeways in Gauteng Province, the country's industrial hub. It was the first time that middle-class South Africans were involved in collective protest action. So-called 'service delivery' protests continued in municipalities across the country (see Table 15.2). The protests were perceived as

Table 15.1 Select social indicators of social change and progress

	Date	*Then*	Date	*Now*
***Demographics*:**				
Population (millions)	1994	38.6	2013	53.9
Fertility rate	2001	2.92	2013	2.34
***Living standards, poverty and inequality*:**				
Share of black South Africans in highest Living Standards Measure, LSM10	2004	5 %	2012	25 %
People living on less than $2 a day	1996	16.2 %	2011	2.7 %
Gini coefficient:	Peak year:			
Total population	2003	0.67	2012	0.63
Black South African population	2003	0.61	2012	0.55
***Welfare*:**				
Total grant beneficiaries as share of total population	1996	6 %	2012/2013	31 %
***Health*:**				
Number adults receiving antiretroviral treatment	2005	101,416	2010	1,058,399
***Housing*:**				
Government subsidy housing units completed/under construction (cumulative)	1995/1996	135,229	2011/2012	3,383,998
Proportion of black households in formal housing	1996	52.5 %	2011	71.3 %
Households in RDP dwellings as proportion of formally housed households			2011	19.9 %
***Infrastructure services*:**				
Piped water in dwelling (% households)	1996	57.6 %	2011	83.8 %
Electricity for lighting (% households)	1996	79.8 %	2011	89.5 %
Proportion of poor households with access to free basic water (6000 l/household/month)	2001/2002	59 %	2010/2011	87 %
***Education*:**				
Black South African enrolment at universities (proportion of total headcount)	1995	50.2 %	2010	66.3 %
***Communication*:**				
Fixed line telephones per 100 people	2000	11.1	2012	7.9
Cellular phones per 100 people	2000	18.6	2012	134.8
***Safety and security*:**				
Murders per 100,000	1994/1995	67	2012/2013	31

Source: South Africa Survey 2012; South Africa Survey 2013 (SAIRR 2012, 2013)

Table 15.2 Public perceptions of government performance and protest action

	Date	*Then*	Date	*Now*
Government is performing well[a]	2000	72 %	2012	54 %
Country is going in the right direction[a]	2000	56 %	2012	46 %
Happy with delivery of basic services by government[a]	2004	77 %	2012	51 %
Major 'service delivery' protests[b]	2004	10	2012	173

Source:
[a]The Presidency, *Development Indicators 2012*, based on Markinor survey data
[b]Municipal IQ Hotspot Monitor, www.municipaliq.co.za, (SAIRR 2013, pp. 881–885)

a vehicle for citizens to voice discontent with local government. One community leader maintained that unless protests were accompanied by violence, they did not attract the attention of government.

Lastly, national leaders were involved in a number of scandals that undermined the credibility of some of the country's most respected oversight institutions. In some of the cases, recommendations by the public protector who had investigated wrongdoing were challenged, suggesting that the powerful were above the law. In August, the new EFF party demanded that the president should repay taxpayers' money spent on security upgrades at his private home, as recommended by the public protector. Riot police were called to quell the mayhem.

National opinion polls show there has been a decline in confidence in the government over the past decade (Table 15.2).

Depending on one's perspective of a glass half full or half empty, South Africa's twentieth year of democracy was either a year that celebrated achievements or one that courted failure. The next section examines how ordinary South Africans have viewed their life chances in the new South Africa over the past 20 years.

How's Life Since 1994

> ***Real Paradise***: If people's living conditions are good, and people accurately perceive and think about them, feel good, and act appropriately, we may describe that as Real Paradise.
>
> ***Fool's Paradise***: If people's living conditions are good, and people inaccurately perceive and think about them, feel bad, and act inappropriately, we may describe that as Fool's Paradise. (Michalos and Robinson 2012, p. 23)

Referring back to Alex Michalos' introduction to quality of life studies at our roving conferences, we might want to question whether people living in the new South Africa feel their lives have got better and they live in paradise or whether they have been 'fooled' by the promises of a 'better life' under democracy.

In this chapter, I shall try to present different viewpoints of the opportunities that democracy has offered to South African citizens. The evidence will be mainly from studies I've been involved in over this period, both of a quantitative and qualitative nature, including ones that have used less conventional measures of well-being.

Multiple Discrepancies as Drivers of Satisfaction

By way of frame of reference, Alex Michalos' (1985, 1991, 2005) theoretical framework, the Multiple Discrepancy Theory, provides a useful tool for creating some sense of order when presenting disparate views on 'how's life' in South Africa today. When listening to respondents' life stories and descriptions of why they rated their lives or aspects of their lives as satisfactory or not, we observed that they often made explicit the reference standards they were drawing on for their evaluations (Møller et al. 2014). The criteria used by our discussants when assessing their lives seemed to fit nicely into the framework proposed by the MDT.

Most readers will be familiar with the MDT, but to refresh memories, the theory as outlined by Alex Michalos in a 1985 paper posits seven 'perceived discrepancies' that respondents use when evaluating their current situation: how one's situation at present compares with those of <u>others</u>, to one's <u>best</u> situation in the <u>past</u>, to what one <u>expected</u> to have <u>by now</u>, to what one expects to have in <u>future</u>, and to what one <u>deserves</u> and <u>needs</u>. These six perceived discrepancies are conditioned by seven background characteristics or demographics which Michalos lists as 'age, sex, education, ethnicity, income, self-esteem, and social support'.[2] The seventh perceived discrepancy, between what one has and what one <u>wants</u>, serves as the mediator between all other perceived gaps and one's net satisfaction (see Michalos 1985, p. 376, Exhibit 14; Michalos 2005, p. 315, Exhibit 2).

A literature search conducted in the late 1980s already produced a list of some 90 publications that had employed some sort of gap or discrepancy hypothesis to explain happiness or satisfaction. The types of gaps and the domains under study varied widely and 79 % of tests were reported as successful (Michalos 1991, p. 310). The MDT has inspired many research efforts since that time. While Alex himself conducted an international student survey to test the performance of all seven posited discrepancies and their conditioners, many researchers have chosen to work with a selection of only one or two discrepancies that are assumed to be most relevant to a particular domain of life, such as the job situation and income. Here I shall examine, in turn, each of the reference comparisons that feature in the MDT gaps that are hypothesised to be drivers of net satisfaction, as they apply to the South African situation.

Source Materials

Material presented in this chapter is from select studies that span the period between 1994 and 2014 and the transition from apartheid to democracy. They include a 1970s survey (Hanf et al. 1981) – possibly the first to apply a happiness measure [3];

[2] Some 40 years later, the 2013 World Happiness Report uses 'social support', that is, someone to count on in times of trouble, in its list of conditioners or explanatory variables for happiness (Helliwell et al. 2013, p. 10).

[3] Michalos makes no distinction between happiness and life satisfaction; both measures evaluate overall well-being. In our South African studies, if forced to choose a single measure of well-being

a survey of the quality of life of township dwellers who had lost their jobs or were unemployed in the late 1980s (Møller 1993); the 2nd Carnegie poverty study conducted in 1993 (Ministry in the Office of the President 1995); a study of youth aspirations in the form of a letter-writing competition held in the second year of democracy in 1996 (Leggett et al. 1997); two nationally representative cross-sectional surveys – the 2010 wave of the South African Quality of Life (SAQoL) trends study (Møller 2013) and the 2012 South African Social Attitudes Survey (SASAS), which included a module on subjective well-being (Roberts et al. 2013); and two focus group studies that tested the understanding of the items that make up the Personal and National Wellbeing Indexes (International Wellbeing Group 2014) in the isiXhosa translation, fielded in 2012 and 2014 respectively.

The module on quality of life in the 2012 SASAS survey included two self-anchoring measures, Cantril's (1965) ladder-of-life and the less conventional Bernheim's Anamnestic Comparative Self-Assessment (ACSA) (Theuns et al. 2014). We asked respondents to first describe the end-anchors of the scale in their own words before rating themselves on the scale. We recorded and evaluated the descriptions of end-anchors: ACSA's best and worst periods of one's life and the Cantril ladder's best and worst imaginable life for self. The ACSA end-anchors have not always been recorded in the past, and to our knowledge, the full line of questioning used in Hadley Cantril's (1965) study of human concerns, that asks for and records respondents' descriptions of their concerns (hopes/aspirations and worries/fears) has not been replicated since the 1960s (Møller and Roberts 2014b).

The main focus in this chapter will be on the perceptions of black South Africans who were most oppressed under apartheid and therefore had the most to gain under democracy. Black/African South Africans represented a majority of 80.2 % in a population of 54 million in 2014, according to Statistics South Africa. Coloured South Africans accounted for 8.8 % of the total population, Indian/Asians for 2.5 % and white South Africans for 8.4 %.[4]

Reflecting on 20 Years of South African Quality of Life from a MDT Perspective

How do ordinary South Africans assess the progress they have made in their lives in the new South Africa over the past 20 years? This section inspects how South Africans weigh their lives relative to the reference comparisons outlined in the MDT theory.

---

for technical or funding reasons, we followed the McKennell and Andrews' (1980) distinction, using the more cognitive satisfaction measure when evaluating living conditions and the more affective happiness measure when examining more emotional issues such as national pride.

[4]Although the South African constitution guarantees equal rights regardless of race, gender or religious persuasion, apartheid-era racial categories continue to be used in everyday life, as well as in affirmative action quotas, the country's official statistics, and sample surveys that monitor attitudes, social change and transformation in society.

Relative Deprivation: SELF NOW Compared to What OTHERS Have

This MDT gap has roots in reference group theory (Merton and Kitt 1950) and goes by the popular name of social comparison theory (Michalos 1991, p. 50). The 'self now/other' discrepancy refers to people comparing where they stand in society or what they have achieved in life with the positions and achievements of significant or relevant others. Michalos and Robinson (2012) note that the ancient Greeks already made mention of the gains for personal happiness if one compared one's lot with the less fortunate. While downward comparisons may boost satisfaction with one's lot, upward comparison with those better off than oneself can act as incentive to catch up with the Joneses (or the South African Mkizes), but may also create frustration, dissatisfaction and feelings of inferiority.

In the South African scenario, apartheid policy sought to compartmentalise social comparisons to members of one's prescribed racial group. Geographic, job and social mobility was limited for black South Africans. The delay of the introduction of television may also have served to insulate black South Africans from aspiring to the lifestyles enjoyed in other parts of the free world. Nonetheless, domestic workers and gardeners would have had insight into how the more privileged lived.

Since 1994, many of our surveys found black respondents spontaneously expressing their sense of delight in the opening up of new opportunities, being treated as equals in society, and benefiting from affirmative action measures adopted by the ANC government. The new South Africa has become a consumer society and township dwellers represent an important market. Some of the black youth participating in our letter-writing study in 1996 reported that they relied on television advertisements to guide their consumer choices 'as seen on TV' (Leggett et al. 1997, pp. 97–113). Since 1994, upward social comparisons with more affluent members of society have become more common. For example, when describing their hopes for self, black respondents in the 2012 SASAS study made upward social comparisons:

> I [would] like to be one of the richest politicians. (Black male respondent, 29 years)
>
> I would like to have a big suburban house with a nice car so that I don't need to feel ashamed anymore. (Black male respondent, 48 years)

Other black respondents' upward comparisons were more modest:

> That the government can build an RDP [house] for me and offer me a toilet like other people. I will be happy. (Black female respondents, 55 years)

Perceptions of Progress: SELF NOW Compared to the BEST SELF One Has Had in the PAST

The MDT includes three temporal discrepancies. The first one refers to a retrospective comparison with the best previous situation one experienced in life (Michalos 1991, p. 51).

The 2012 SASAS survey used the less conventional Bernheim's ACSA (Theuns et al. 2014) as one of its measures of subjective well-being. Respondents were asked to describe the best and worst periods experienced in their lives, before rating where they stood at present relative to these periods, on an 11-point scale from −5 to +5. Both the numeric and the qualitative responses to ACSA are of interest for our review of perceptions of personal progress in the new South Africa.

Consider that the ACSA score might serve as a proxy measure of the 'self now/self past best' gap in the MDT. In this case, the gap is the distance between the ACSA score and the 'best time of life experienced in the past', the positive end-anchor of the scale.

Black respondents rated their lives worse than others on the ACSA scale, just above the mid-point. The black respondents' gap between their ACSA score and their 'best time of life' was 4.13 points. This 'self now/self best past' gap for black respondents of 4.13 points was wider than the gaps for the total sample (3.99) and for the subsamples of coloured (3.72 points), white (3.53) and Indian (3.24) South Africans.

Turning to the content of the best past experience as described by our respondents, we categorised best periods in life under 15 general headings and 70 more specific ones. Best times in life for black respondents revolved mainly around milestones and markers of achievements in life. In approximate order of frequency, achievements related to family life (births, marriage and harmony – approximately 447 mentions), employment (finding a job – 206), education (being in school, accessing a bursary, completing studies – 72), income (wages, social grants, and remittances – 63), and housing (mainly RDP subsidised housing – 53). Assets, grouped under the income heading, included mentions of consumer items such as one's first car, cellular phone, or television.

Of interest for the discussion here, some of the black respondents also remembered the heady days of the 'first dance of freedom' as the best time in their lives: the end of apartheid, voting for the first time, the Mandela presidency, the new ANC government. Sports achievements included the South African victory in the Rugby World Cup in 1995 and the hosting of the 2010 World Cup.

Perceptions of Personal Progress: SELF NOW Compared to What SELF EXPECTED TO HAVE BY NOW

The second temporal discrepancy included in the MDT refers to the sense of personal progress, that is, what one has now compared to what one expected to have now 3 years ago. Here the proxy measure for this discrepancy compares past and present ratings on the Cantril ladder of life. The SASAS 2012 survey asked respondents to rate their life situation 5 years ago and now, on the 11 rungs of Cantril's ladder of life (a 0–10 scale). Results indicated all South Africans experienced a sense of progress in their lives, in particular the black respondents (Møller and Roberts 2014b).

Table 15.3 Cantril's personal ladder-of-life scores: self 5 years back and now in 2012 (10 = highest score)

	Five years ago	Now in 2012	Difference
Black/African	4.42	5.06	+0.64
Coloured	5.45	5.82	+0.37
Indian/Asian	5.56	6.37	+0.81
White	5.94	6.44	+0.50

Source: SASAS 2012 (Møller and Roberts 2014b)

As shown in Table 15.3, black respondents on average placed themselves at 4.42 on the ladder 5 years back, and 5.06 at the present time. At both times, past and current, black respondents placed themselves lower on the ladder than their coloured, Indian and white compatriots. In fact, ladder ratings for 'self past' and 'self now' were in hierarchical order following the apartheid-era social pecking order, with black respondents worst off, white respondents best off, and Indian and coloured South African respondents in between. Important for this review, is that black respondents experienced greater progress than their white and coloured counterparts. The difference between 'self now' and 'self past' was +0.64 points on the ladder for black South Africans, compared to only +0.37 and +0.50 for coloured and white South Africans respectively.

To illustrate this sense of progress, we turn to examples from the focus group study on the Personal Wellbeing Index conducted in late 2012 with township dwellers in Grahamstown. Some of our discussants rated their life satisfaction close to the top score of 10, indicating they were 'completely satisfied'. They explained that their lives had turned out far better than expected (Møller et al. 2014).

> I am satisfied because I never thought I would have what I have now. (Female cashier, score 8)
>
> I've got everything I ever thought of having. I have two cars, this house, my wife and kids, a good job, [I'm] educated enough with my Honours degree, but I still wish for a Master's degree and still want to reach there. (Male nurse, score 9)

Optimism: SELF NOW Compared to What One Expects to Have in FUTURE

Michalos (1991, p. 52) reports that the influence of the discrepancy between the present situation and where people expected to be in 5 years' time was weak in many of his studies. He notes that using shorter time frames that can be predicted with greater certainty, say the next few weeks rather than 5 years hence, might be more powerful predictors. He thought the study context might dictate what time frame worked best.

It is perhaps telling that what may have been the first study to ever consult South Africans about their happiness, used a much longer time frame. The study that Hanf

Table 15.4 Cantril's personal ladder of life scores: self now in 2012 and in future (5 years from now)

	Now	Five years in future	Difference
Black/African	5.06	6.93	+1.87
Coloured	5.82	7.05	+1.23
Indian/Asian	6.37	7.57	+1.20
White	6.44	7.15	+0.71

Source: SASAS 2012 (Møller and Roberts 2014b)

et al. (1981) conducted in the mid-1970s on the country's prospects of peaceful change asked urban black South Africans to project how happy they thought they might be in 10 years' time.[5] The 10-year gap would have been an appropriate one at a time when the prospects of an end to apartheid seemed very distant.

Hanf and his colleagues found that both black and white South Africans expected the future to bring considerable changes in their destinies, but with very different outcomes. Whereas over half of white South Africans rated themselves as very happy or happy, only a little over a third thought they would still be happy in 10 years' time. Conversely, only one-fifth of the urban black South Africans in the study regarded themselves as happy, but over 60 % thought they would be happy in 10 years' time (Hanf et al. 1981, p. 420).

This constellation of different perceptions of 'self now' and 'expectations for the future' among black and white South Africans is still evident to a certain degree in 2012. In the SASAS survey of that year, black South Africans, who gave themselves the lowest rating on the Cantril ladder-of-life scale at present as shown in Table 15.3 above, thought they would stand significantly higher on the ladder in 5 years' time. Table 15.4 shows that once again the difference between the 'self now/future' ratings by black respondents is higher than that of other South Africans. The greatest difference between the 'self now/future' ratings is between black and white respondents.

Importantly, all South Africans see their situation improving in the future although at different rates.

South African Perceptions of Entitlements: SELF NOW Compared to What One DESERVES

The gap between what one has and what one deserves or merits has received attention in research based on equity theory. When I first read the Michalos report on his global study of student well-being to test his MDT theory, I was intrigued that the

[5] The item, which used a five-faces happiness scale from 'very happy' to 'angry and impatient' read: 'Which face shows the way most African people like yourself in [township] will most probably feel like in 10 years from now?' (Hanf et al. 1981, p. 467).

'self now/deserve' gap was a relatively strong predictor of net satisfaction among black South African students enrolled at the University of Zululand (Michalos 1991, p. 230). At the time, the results seemed to reflect the importance of equity in the student liberation movement and the strong feelings of injustice and relative deprivation among black South Africans in the 1980s. Fast forwarding to the new South Africa, the constitution adopted in 1996 enshrines equity for all people who live in the country.

Although the country's Gini coefficient, an indicator of inequality in society, is still very high (see Table 15.1), many South Africans feel they live in a more equal society than in the past. The 2010 wave of the SAQoL trends study, fielded soon after the successful hosting of the Fifa World Cup in South Africa, found that equality and equal opportunities was the third most important source of national pride for survey respondents, following after democracy and the country's sports achievements. Specific mention was made of equality in society, newfound equal opportunities in gaining access to education and jobs, and affirmative action policies that aimed to redress past inequalities. Noteworthy is that 13 % of black respondents were most likely to take pride in equality, followed by 9.9 % of coloured, 5.6 % of Indian, and 4.3 % of white respondents (Møller 2014).

Michalos (1991, p. 53) reported that many respondents in his own studies conducted in the 1980s appeared to have difficulties defining what they deserved. South Africans have no such problem. The quest for equity in South African society may have nurtured the strong sense of entitlement among ANC supporters, who look to the ruling ANC government to fulfil promises of the better life. When describing their hopes for self in response to the Cantril question in the SASAS 2012 survey, black respondents often named the ANC government as their benefactor:

> I wish the government can subsidise us with cows and seeds for our big gardens. (Black male respondent, 80 years)
>
> One day the government will build a house for me. (Black female respondent, 72 years)
>
> To be provided with a social grant for my grandchildren because I can't afford food for them. (Black female respondent, 58 years)

What do black South Africans expect from their country? The SASAS 2012 survey also replicated Hadley Cantril's questions on concerns for country, that represent the end-anchors of the ladder scale. The top-listed hopes and aspirations for country, mentioned by 5 % or more of black respondents, concerned employment, law and order (less crime), education, a decent standard of living, housing, an honest government free of corruption, good governance and wise leadership, an efficient government, national unity, economic growth, and good public health services.

Obviously, black South Africans make great demands of their government to provide education, jobs, housing, and a decent standard of living. The hope for an efficient government was often described in terms of the state as the provider of infrastructure and services. Concerning public health, it was hoped that antiretroviral treatment would continue to be available in public health facilities. Respondents worried that political infighting and corruption hampered good governance and detracted from implementing social development.

Given this strong sense of entitlement, it is not surprising that many ANC supporters feel they deserve more from their government. A SASAS 2012 respondent stated categorically:

> Government is not doing anything for us. (Black female respondent, 31 years)

When asked how satisfied he was with 'life in South Africa as a whole' in the focus group discussion on the National Wellbeing Index, a 72-year old black pensioner gave the following evaluation of his life over the past 20 years[6]:

> I was once satisfied in life after 1994 when we became free; we were all excited and happy. I was satisfied when RDP houses were built as I did not own a house before. These past years have brought dissatisfaction in my life. We grew up in poverty and suffered a lot during the apartheid era ... working very hard for little up to nothing in return. We also were involved in marching and toyi-toying[7] but we've seen no improvement and no reward to our struggle. The freedom we fought for has rewarded us with nothing. We are still poor, as pensioners there's a very little increase [in the state pension]. We are still hungry, only the educated get huge increases [in salaries] and they can take care of themselves; [they] even extend their houses. So, I am dissatisfied.
>
> Our leaders, I mean the [ward] councillors, are far apart from us. We hardly see them in our areas. They only get closer to us during voting period but after that they are nowhere to be found. Things decided upon in our ward meetings, none of them took place. Such things have made us unhappy and so I am dissatisfied. We wish that the Government would consider us for better life, especially old citizens.

The sense of entitlement is generally widespread in the black population, including the youth. In 2014, there was public outrage when the Minister of Human Settlements announced that the 'born-free' generation, those born after 1994, could no longer expect the government to build houses for them. Free housing was intended to right the wrongs of the past, the minister stated, and to give people dignity who had suffered under apartheid (City Press 2014).

Necessities in Life: SELF NOW Compared to One's NEEDS

The 'self now/self needs' discrepancy in the MDT refers to the mismatch between what a person needs by way of resources or capabilities, and what that person's social situation requires. This discrepancy, which has often been studied in relation to job situation and household income, points to the importance of the fit between a person and his or her environment. Maslow's (1970) hierarchy of needs, ranging from basic survival, at the one end, to higher order self-actualisation, at the other, comes to mind here (see also Hagerty 1999).

---

[6] Unpublished results from focus group discussions on the isiXhosa version of the National Wellbeing Index with township residents living in Grahamstown, Eastern Cape, South Africa, December 2014.

[7] Toyi-toyi is a dance that is used in political protests in South Africa.

Expectations that democracy would fulfil needs were raised already under apartheid. Jobs were a high priority need at the time and continue to be so under democracy, as documented in survey evidence over the past 25 years.

- In a survey of unemployed black township dwellers conducted in 1989, when the economic sanctions campaign against South Africa was biting, four in five respondents anticipated that they would have jobs when the economy recovered (85 %) and there would be 'jobs for all in a society without apartheid' (83 %) (Møller 1993, p. 227).
- In 1993, the 2nd Carnegie study of poverty conducted a household survey to inform the ANC government-in-waiting on the needs of the population (Ministry in the Office of the President 1995, p. 25). Survey respondents were invited to name up to three needs. The poorest 40 % of households identified jobs as the most important need before other basic necessities such as shelter, food and water. In order of importance, the identified needs were the following: jobs (named by 56 % of respondents), housing (34 %), food aid (31 %), piped water (41 %), electricity (29 %), schools (20 %), health clinics (16 %), and peace/end of the violence (12 %)
- In the 2010 wave of the SAQoL trends study, 63 % of all black respondents, and 70 % of the currently unhappy ones, said jobs, income or a better standard of living would increase their happiness (Møller 2013, p. 933).
- Similarly, black respondents in the 2012 SASAS survey were most likely to name jobs and employment as their chief concerns when asked to describe their hopes and fears for self and nation (Møller and Roberts 2014b).
- Over the past decade, all waves of the SASAS surveys conducted annually between 2003 and 2013 have consistently pointed to unemployment as the country's top-ranking 'most important problem', endorsed by approximately three quarters of the population on average (Davids et al. 2014).

Clearly, the ANC election promise of 'jobs for all' remains one of the highest priority needs for all South Africans.

Aspirations: SELF NOW Compared to What One WANTS

When introducing the MDT discrepancy between 'self now/wants', Michalos (1991, p. 49) notes that many theories of quality of life are telic in nature. Such theories posit that life satisfaction is the result of achieving one's aspirations, life goals or 'personal strivings' (Emmons 1986).

In 1996, a young black woman who participated in our letter-writing competition on expectations for 'my life in the new South Africa' penned her dreams for a middle-class lifestyle:

> I wish to be married by the rich man and I wish that we can give birth to two children (a boy and a girl) then I wish to have two cars, namely a BMW (new model) and a Venture.

I wish to build a big house with four (4) bedrooms, 3 (three) bathroom, two (2) toilets, two (2) garages, one (1) kitchen, dining room and sitting room. (Letter 111, Leggett et al. 1997, p. 107)

Some 16 years later, we asked respondents participating in the 2012 SASAS survey to describe their aspirations for self in response to the Cantril question on personal well-being. The top-listed aspirations that South Africans mentioned might be considered to stand in for the 'wants' in the MDT model.

To elicit these 'wants', we replicated exactly the original introduction that Hadley Cantril (1965, pp. 23–24) had used in his study of the Pattern of Human Concerns in the 1960s. Before asking his respondents to rate their standing on the ladder of life, he asked them to think of their hopes or aspirations for self. He stated that 'all of us want certain things in life…' (emphasis added), then asked respondents to describe their ideas of the 'best possible life' for self. This represents the positive end-anchor of his ladder-of-life.[8]

Hopes, or 'wants' for self, mentioned by more than 5 % of black respondents, in order of frequency were: employment, own house, own education, decent standard of living, life opportunities for one's children and grandchildren, family life, modern conveniences, and own business.

A few black respondents in the 2012 survey echoed the same middle-class aspirations that the young letter writer had dreamt of some 20 years earlier:

My dream is to have my own car and a big house. (Black female respondent, 43 years)

However, the majority of the top-listed aspirations mentioned by black respondents in SASAS 2012 may still be considered modest ones. People hope that getting an education will lead to a job, wage income will put food on the table for the family, and with regard to what Cantril called 'modern conveniences' – the government will provide an RDP house equipped with piped water and electricity.

To build me a toilet, that is all I ask and hope for. (Black female respondent, 57 years)

To get a job and a flushing toilet. (Black female respondent, 42 years)

I wish that I can get a job and have my own money so that I can be happy. (Black male respondent, 49 years)

That I can get an RDP house and also get a job. (Black female respondent, 50 years)

Not to worry about where the food comes from, I would be very happy, and having a house with electricity and water. (Black female respondent, 46 years)

In many cases the distinction between wants and needs is blurred – there is a strong overlap.

We *want* a good life. … We *need* food, water and electricity. (Black female respondent, 23 years, emphasis added)

[8] The full introduction to Cantril's ladder of life reads: 'All of us want certain things in life. When you think about what really matters in your own life, what are your wishes and hopes for the future? In other words, if you imagine your future in the BEST possible light, what would your life look like then, if you are to be happy? Take your time in answering; such things aren't easy to put into words.' Cantril specified that probes might also refer to 'dreams' and 'desires' (Cantril 1965, pp. 23–24).

Turning to the discussions on life satisfaction in the qualitative study on the Personal Wellbeing Index in 2012, the group of older black men were disenchanted with the government's broken promises of a better life for all. One of the men described his disappointment as follows (Møller et al. 2014):

> Before this new South Africa came into being, the government promised us employment and a lot of things that would make me feel free. … Instead, only poverty is ruling and more people are unemployed, including myself. The government promised people houses in which we find out that water penetrates into and we live in wet and miserable places. None of the things the government promised has been fulfilled … You'd feel that life in the apartheid era was better than the one we live in now, although it had its sorrows and hardships.
>
> The Bible has made us a lot of promises and God came through in those things. The president promised South Africa a lot of things but none has come through. You can't help but think of time wasted supporting this government for the change that never took place. It now seems worse than the apartheid era. (Unemployed discussant, 59 years)

Discussion and Conclusions

Satisfaction and Rising Expectations

Levels of life satisfaction in South Africa since the euphoric days following the birth of democracy in 1994 have remained stubbornly low, with no more than 55 % of the population stating they are satisfied on average. The flat trend line for life satisfaction seems to support the Easterlin paradox that achievements can never catch up with rising expectations and aspirations (Easterlin 1995). Perceptions of progress reviewed here, using Alex Michalos' Multiple Discrepancy Theory (MDT) as a guiding framework, suggest that the distinctions between the 'needs' and 'wants' of the majority of South Africans are blurred. The 'needs' of poor households identified in the 1993 poverty study reappear on the list of 'wants' identified in the 2012 SASAS survey, which replicated Hadley Cantril's line of questioning on hopes and aspirations for self.

South Africa's good-news story is that some 20 years on, many of these needs and wants have indeed been met for a large proportion of low-income households, as is evident from Table 15.1. Material success in life is a measure of dignity for South Africans who had been second class citizens in their own country in the past. Our respondents' recall of their 'best past' time of life in the SASAS 2012 survey often referred to achievements in material well-being. Standards of living have generally improved, as indicated by the Living Standards Measure (see Table 15.1), and a minority of the emergent black middle class may even have achieved their dreams of prosperity under democracy. However, if material aspirations or 'wants' represent one of the strongest drivers of life satisfaction, as hypothesised by the MDT, the flat trend line for life satisfaction suggests that many South Africans have not seen their life goals fulfilled. The disenchanted older black men who voiced their dissatisfaction with the new South Africa and its government are a case in point.

Our review highlights the importance of jobs and livelihoods as strong drivers of life satisfaction in the democratic era. Perceptions of the 'better life for all' is often equated with jobs for all, one of the ruling ANC's election promises. The unemployed men interviewed in the late 1980s expected to have work in a post-apartheid society. Twenty years later, respondents in the 2012 SASAS survey still hoped democracy would provide jobs. The following aspiration for self expressed by a 40-year old black respondent in the SASAS 2012 survey speaks for many:

> For South Africa to be a full-time democratic country. For everyone who lives in it to have a permanent job.

South African Exceptionalism

While the good news story of 2014 spells out South African achievements over 20 years, the alternative story speaks of challenges for the fledgling democracy. The rainbow nation has lost some of its authority as the poster child of democracy. Corruption already set in during the Mandela presidency. While President Mbeki ensured the country's macro-economic stability attracted foreign investment, the Zuma presidency has struggled to convince local and foreign investors that South Africa is open for business. The ruling party's strategy of cadre deployment, which puts political loyalty before competence, has contributed to loss of state capacity in state-owned enterprises. Executive interference has weakened the independence of key oversight institutions (Hartley 2014; Steyn 2015). Commenting on the first electricity blackouts in South Africa in early 2008, the editor of a business daily noted that South Africans never expected their country to go the way of the rest of Africa, that lived with regular electricity outages. The days of South Africa's exceptionalism in sub-Saharan Africa, might already be over, he suggested. In the same year, an authority on water resource management warned that a water crisis was looming for South Africa (Mpofu and Isa 2008).

Looking beyond South Africa's exceptionalism, one might be forgiven for making comparisons between the country's situation in its twentieth year of democracy and that of other sub-Saharan states after independence. Historian Martin Meredith (2011, p. 162) refers to the 'slippery slope' that many African states experienced some 20 years into independence in the 1970s and 1980s. He notes that initial achievements in social services such as education and health, were soon overshadowed by economic problems when global demands for their products declined. The infrastructure inherited from the colonial era crumbled after a decade of lack of maintenance. 'Most state corporations … were inefficiently managed, overstaffed, subjected to frequent political meddling and requiring huge government subsidies to keep them afloat' (Meredith 2011, p. 277–8). Meredith also points to Africa's problem of the Big Men who have dispensed patronage to ensure loyalty in order to remain in power. While the new middle-class elite with connections to power prospered, ordinary citizens remained poor.

Unlike their counterparts in many sub-Saharan states, South African presidents have not sought to extend their time in office. But the age of the country's political leaders, mainly struggle heroes, still contrasts with the much lower average age of the population. While the country's first president, Nelson Mandela was lauded as a wise and exemplary leader, current President Zuma, who has repeatedly pledged that the ANC will last till kingdom come, or Jesus returns, has been booed in public by disgruntled voters. The new opposition EFF's bold plans for instant gratification of needs and wants may have greater appeal to the youth than the ANC government's National Development Plan, which still remains to be implemented.

South African Entitlements

South Africa's population may be growing at a slower rate than in other countries south of the Sahara (see fertility rates in Table 15.1), but it still needs to provide for a large number of people whose needs were under-served in the past. Thirty per cent of the population are 15 years and younger. Frustration at the slow pace of change, coupled with the strong sense of entitlement, has fuelled discontent (see Table 15.2). New voters who feel they are deserving of the better life look mainly to the government to meet their needs and wants. While South Africa has led sub-Saharan Africa in providing social protection for the poor and vulnerable in society, there are also growing concerns that dependence on government hand-outs has stifled South African initiative and entrepreneurship. The editorial in a South African daily argues that 'the culture of entitlement that persuades all too many unemployed township dwellers that they can do nothing to improve their situation without state assistance has been encouraged by the governing party' (*Business Day* 2015).

Democratic Maturity

Nonetheless, the historical comparison may be over-stretched in many instances. The need for peace in South Africa, which featured as an item on the list of needs of poor households compiled in 1993, has been achieved. The country has experienced political stability since 1994. Poverty has been reduced and living standards improved, as shown in Table 15.1. Even if South Africa is still experiencing growing pains in the transition to democracy, it can build on strong foundations. Democratic institutions are firmly in place, while the constitution and courts safeguard human rights and the dignity of individuals. One of the most important pillars of democracy, freedom of speech and association is respected, and public opinion is valued.

When detailing South African 'wants', we referred to results from the SASAS 2012 survey that replicated Cantril's study of human concerns. Cantril advised social researchers to examine not only concerns mentioned by respondents but also ones that were *not* mentioned. Noteworthy is that 'freedom', one of the categories that Cantril used to classify human concerns in his 1960s study, was not utilised by respondents in the 2012 SASAS study. This omission suggests that freedom as a democratic right is now taken for granted by South Africans (Møller and Roberts 2014b). Similarly, the freedoms enjoyed since 1994 were mentioned as a source of pride in the 2010 SAQoL study (Møller 2014).

The openness with which respondents expressed their concerns about government in the 2012 SASAS survey, suggests that South Africans are confident in their rights to voice their views without intimidation. Looking back to the 1970s, Hanf and his colleagues (1981, p. 67) reported that black respondents were initially fearful to participate in their survey, and only gained confidence to talk about their aspirations after the student uprisings in Soweto in 1976. In the 1980s, some of our fieldworkers carrying out interviews for the unemployment study were arrested. During those turbulent years, we researchers soon learnt that an above-average non-response rate to a survey question indicated that it was considered a politically loaded item by our respondents, and answering it might endanger their lives.

South African Voice in an Inclusive Democracy

A further marker of inclusive democracy is that social researchers in the new South Africa regularly ask their respondents to evaluate national priorities and problems, in order to provide feedback to policy makers. Earlier, we referred to the public perception that unemployment was a top priority problem for the country in annual SASAS surveys conducted between 2003 and 2013 (Davids et al. 2014). In our analysis of MDT gaps, access to jobs featured as the 'needs', 'deserves' and 'wants' that respondents thought should be met. While the ANC government is still struggling with job creation and service delivery, it has been more successful in responding to other 'wants', such as public health, identified as a hope for the country in the replication of Hadley Cantril's questions in the 2012 SASAS study. Noteworthy is that the most dramatic drop in public perceptions of the country's problems relates to HIV/AIDS (Davids et al. 2014). Between 2003 and 2013, the percentage naming HIV/AIDS as a national problem dropped by 24 %, while the proportion satisfied with HIV/AIDS treatment increased by 29 %. Davids and his colleagues (2014) attribute the decline to government performance in response to the AIDS epidemic as of 2005. Steinberg (2014), cited in the introduction, claims that the roll-out of antiretroviral treatment in public health clinics is a good example of the power of voice that ordinary South Africans have gained as new democrats.

Although the focus of MDT is on the self, we also referred briefly to national hopes when discussing expectations of government to fulfil what voters feel they deserve, that is their entitlements in the new democracy. The greatest number of national concerns mentioned by South Africans in the 2012 SASAS survey referred to political and economic ones. While the majority of citizens will continue to be loyal to the erstwhile liberation movement, now the ruling ANC party, in elections, they are not afraid to make their government accountable for poor service delivery, lack of protection from crime and corruption. They hope for good governance to create better opportunities in life for themselves and their children and grandchildren.

Long-Term Optimism

Meanwhile, the majority of the South African population continue to be optimistic about future prosperity. Resilience in bad times and hope for the future may be the country's greatest resource in driving prosperity. Hanf and colleagues (1981) already noted the remarkable optimism of black South Africans in the 1970s. In both volumes on South African quality of life, inspired by Alex Michalos' visits to the country, Harris (1997, 2007) reports that the majority of South Africans, in particular black South Africans, are optimistic that the next year will be better than the present one. With reference to perceptions of progress for self on the Cantril scale from past to present to projected future in the 2012 SASAS survey, optimism continues to buoy black South African hopes of a better life under democracy.

Conclusion

Twenty years on, South Africa's multi-party democracy is still a work in progress. Its socio-economic and political foundations are sound and citizens are proud of their democratic rights and new found freedoms. Recent studies indicate positive perceptions of progress and appreciation of improvements in standards of living over the past two decades. But expectations of the 'better life for all' have risen and the country's achievements fall short of the aspirations of ordinary citizens. At the same time, there are definite signs that South Africa's democracy is gaining maturity. Voters are not tricked into thinking their government is performing optimally. While South Africans are not content to live in the philosopher's 'Fool's Paradise', they are resilient and still resolutely hopeful that one day they will live in a real 'Paradise'.

Acknowledgements Obviously, I am indebted to Alex Michalos for his interest in and support of South African quality of life studies. Three of the studies reported here were supported by the South African National Research Foundation: the subjective well-being module in the SASAS 2012 survey was supported by grant 77926 for research collaboration on quality of life between South Africa and Algeria; the two focus group discussions on the isiXhosa Personal Wellbeing Index and National Wellbeing Index were supported by NRF incentive funding grant 85343. I am grateful to my South African colleague, Benjamin Roberts, co-ordinator of SASAS at the Human Sciences Research Council, for the tabulations of the SASAS 2012 survey data. Views expressed are mine and should not be attributed to the NRF or any of my research partners and colleagues.

References

Business Day. (2015). Editorial – SA cannot deny its xenophobia issue. 27 January, p. 10.
Cantril, H. (1965). *The Pattern of Human Concerns*. New Brunswick, New Jersey: Rutgers University Press.
City Press. (2014) You've lost nothing to apartheid, Sisulu tells youth. 21 October. http://www.citypress.co.za/politics/youve-lost-nothing-apartheid-sisulu-tells-youth/ Accessed 26/01/2015
Davids, Y.D., Roberts, B. and Struwig, J. (2014). Fostering an inclusive development agenda in South Africa: Citizen voices and government policy responses. *Human Sciences Research Council policy briefs*, September.
Easterlin, R.A. (1995). Will raising the incomes of all increase the happiness of all? *Journal of Economic Behavior and Organization 27*, 1–34.
Emmons, R.A. (1986). Personal strivings: An approach to personality and subjective well-being. *Journal of Personality and Social Psychology 51*, 1058–1068).
Friedman, S. and Atkinson, D. (Eds.) (1994). *The Small Miracle: South Africa's Negotiated Settlement*. Johannesburg: Raven Press.
Hagerty, M.R. (1999). Testing Maslow's hierarchy of needs: national quality-of-life across time, *Social Indicators Research 46*, 249–271.
Hanf, Th., Weiland, H., and Vierdag, G. (1981). *South Africa: The prospects of peaceful change*. London: Rex Collings.
Harris, M. (1997). Monitoring optimism in South Africa. *Social Indicators* Research *41*, 279–304.
Harris, M. (2007). Monitoring optimism in South Africa. *Social Indicators Research 18*(2), 435–454.
Hartley R. (2014). The year we went backwards. *The Times*, Johannesburg, 19 December, p. 6.
Helliwell, J. Layard, R. and Sachs, J. (2013). *World Happiness Report 2013*. http://www.earth.columbia.edu/sitefiles/file/Sachs%20Writing/2012/World%20Happiness%20Report.pdf
International Wellbeing Group (2014). http://www.deakin.edu.au/research/acqol/iwbg/index.php
Leggett, T., Møller, V., and Richards, R. (Eds.) (1997). *"My Life in the New South Africa": A youth perspective*. Pretoria: HSRC Publishers. http://contentpro.seals.ac.za/iii/cpro/app?id=3922004803002071&itemId=1010393&lang=&service=blob&suite=def
Maslow, A.H. (1970). *Motivation and Personality*. New York: Harper and Row.
McKennell, A.C. and Andrews, F.M. (1980). Models of cognition and affect in perceptions of well-being. *Social Indicators Research 8*, 257–298.
Meredith, M. (2011). *The State of Africa: A history of the continent since independence*. London: Simon & Schuster/ Johannesburg: Jonathan Ball Publishers.
Merton, R.K. and Kitt, K.S. (1950). Contributions to the theory of reference group behavior. In: Merton, R.K. and Lazarsfeld, P.F. (Eds.). *Continuities in Social Research*. New York: John Wiley and Sons, pp. 40–105.
Michalos, A.C. (1985). Multiple Discrepancies Theory (MDT) (1985). *Social Indicators Research 16*(4), 347–413.
Michalos, A.C. (1991). *Global Report on Student Well-Being: Volume 1: Life satisfaction and happiness*. New York: Springer-Verlag.
Michalos, A.C. (2005). Multiple Discrepancies Theory (MDT). In Michalos, A.C. (Ed.), *Citation Classics from Social Indicators Research*, Dordrecht: Springer, pp. 305–371.
Michalos, A. C. (2011). What did Stiglitz, Sen and Fitoussi get right and what did they get wrong? *Social Indicators Research 102*(1), 117–129.
Michalos, A.C. and Robinson, S.R. (2012). The good life: eighth century to third century BCE. In: Land, K.C., Michalos, A.C. and Sirgy, M.J. (Eds.), *Handbook of Social Indicators and Quality of Life Research*. Dordrecht: Springer.
Ministry in the Office of the President, Reconstruction and Development Programme *(1995). Key Indicators of Poverty in South Africa*. Pretoria, South Africa.

Møller, V. (1993). *Quality of Life in Unemployment: A survey evaluation of black township dwellers*. Pretoria: HSRC Publishers.
Møller, V. (Ed.) (1997). *Quality of Life in South Africa*. Social Indicators Research Series Volume 1. Dordrecht: Kluwer Academic Publishers (now Springer). Reprinted from *Social Indicators Research 41*(1–3).
Møller, V. (Ed.) (2007). Quality of life in South Africa: Ten years into democracy, *Social Indicators Research 18*(2).
Møller, V. (2013). South African Quality of Life Trends Over Three Decades, 1980–2010. *Social Indicators Research 113*(3), 915–940.
Møller, V. (2014). Happiness, national pride and the 2010 World Cup. In: Sullivan, G.B. (Ed.), *Understanding Collective Pride and Group Identity: New directions in theory and practice*. London and New York: Routledge, pp. 110–123.
Møller, V. and Roberts, B. (2014a).South Africa, Quality of Life. In: Michalos A.C. (Ed.). *Encyclopedia of Quality of Life and Well-Being Research*. Dordrecht, Netherlands: Springer, 6218–6223.
Møller, V. and Roberts, B.J.(2014b). South African Hopes and Fears Twenty Years into Democracy: A Replication of Hadley Cantril's Pattern of Human Concerns. *Social Indicators Research* (accepted).
Møller, V., Roberts, B., and Zani, D. (2014). The Personal Wellbeing Index in the South African isiXhosa translation: A qualitative focus group study. *Social Indicators Research*, DOI 10.1007/s11205-014-0820-6.
Mpofu, B. and Isa, M. (2008) Expert warns of water crisis leading to instability in SA. *Business Day*, 25 November, p. 2.
Roberts, B., Struwig, J., Gordon, S., Ngungu, M. and Jordaan, A. (2013). *Quality of Life in South Africa and Algeria: SASAS 2012 tabulation report*. Pretoria: Democracy, Governance & Service Delivery research programme, Human Sciences Research Council.
Steinberg, J. (2014). Power of 'voice' steers state monopoly action. *Business Day*, November 28, p. 9.
Sethlatswe, B. (2014). Reflecting on twenty years. South African Institute of Race Relations *Fast Facts* No. 4, April / Issue 272, p. 1. www.irr.org.za
South African Institute of Race Relations (SAIRR) (2012). *South Africa Survey 2012*. Johannesburg.
South African Institute of Race Relations (SAIRR) (2013). *South Africa Survey 2013*. Johannesburg.
Sparks, A. (2003). *Beyond the Miracle: Inside the new South Africa*. Johannesburg: Jonathan Ball Publishers.
Steyn, R. (2015). Sobering reminder of how SA surrendered hard-won moral authority. *Business Day*, 6 January, p. 5.
Stiglitz, J. E., Sen, A., & Fitoussi, J.-P. (2009). *Report by the Commission on the Measurement of Economic Performance and Social Progress*. Paris. www.stiglitz-sen-fitoussi.fr
Theuns, P., Hofmans, J. and Bernheim, J.L. (2014). Anamnestic Comparative Self-Assessment (ACSA). In: Michalos, A.C. (Ed.), *Encyclopedia of Quality of Life and Well-Being Research*. Dordrecht: Springer Reference, pp. 166–169.

Chapter 16
Happiness and Sociability in a Nonrecursive Model: The US and Taiwan Compared

Ming-Chang Tsai

Researchers have regularly surveyed individuals' personal relationship and their effect on happiness. This reflects a long tradition within the social science to assert the significance of social ties or linkages in realizing 'well-being', defined in broad terms (Bruni 2007). In empirical research, important factors such as social capital, social skills and relationship network are cited as preconditions to better life quality (Graham 2009). However, this conventional practice neglects an equally important hypothesis that happiness can be a causal force to enhance various sorts of networking behaviors and consequently faciliate the building of interpersonal relations observed in the field. Veenhoven (2010) has recently demonstrated the limitation of a one-way notion of causality; for him, two-way causality is closer to the reality: "Capability is typically conducive to happiness, while happiness enhances capability" (Veenhoven 2010:350). In explaining how this casual interdependence is plausible, he maintains that happiness facilitates social activities and contact, as happy people have more chances to develop social skills than the unhappy, who may spend more time watching television. Also, happy people themselves constitute an amiable social context for others that find interactions more interesting or worthy, which encourages their willingness to meet happier people. There appears to be a virtuous cycle. Echoing an idea of two-way causality, Lyubomirsky, King and Diener's extensive review (2005) suggests that happiness is a strong factor of success, as it fosters adaptive and sociable behaviors, along with a positive affect and desirable cognition that help increase optimism, creativity and performance. Indeed, pioneers in the well-being study had long been concerned with a comprehensive assessment of the causes and consequences of subjective well-being (Michalos 2008; Lance et al. 1995).

Research that has explored the reverse causal directions, however, is scant in the literature. The consequences of subjective well-being have not been surveyed extensively, despite some critical exceptions (Veenhoven 2008). A few available

M.-C. Tsai (✉)
RCHSS, Academia Sinica, 128 Academia Road, Sec.2, Nangang, Taipei 11529, Taiwan
e-mail: mtsai304@gate.sinica.edu.tw

F. Maggino (ed.), *A Life Devoted to Quality of Life*, Social Indicators Research Series 60, DOI 10.1007/978-3-319-20568-7_16

findings were drawn mainly from experiments or quasi-natural settings. Samples often comprised select respondents with weak representiveness. Moreover, the estimation techniques used in these studies did not take the 'mutual influences' seriously enough. The literature as a whole lacks reliable evidence in assessing happiness' consequences (Oishi 2010; Veenhoven 2010). Hence there is an urgent need to investigate various consequences of happiness. More research should be conducted to test whether happiness can be a central dynamic factor in human life and action, besides regularly surveying happiness as an outcome of possession of income, material goods, or self-perceived discrepancies with others or between times (now and before) (Michalos 2008). Happiness studies can advance in policy influence when researchers show its favorable impacts on a plethora of life domains, in addition to representing it as a respectable, ultimate human goal (Hagerty et al. 2001).

This study aims to investigate the reciprocal causality between happiness and personal relationships. The techniques of structural equation modeling (SEM) (Hoyle 2012) are used to test nonrecursive models against recent data drawn from the US and Taiwan. Experts on life quality research expect that happiness can contribute to personal relationship building, while the latter also increases level of happiness. With reciprocal causality in mind, they seem to expect no substantial difference in the effect generated by either factor. Researchers from the cultural perspective might probe further and expect that in an individualist cultural context such as the US, personal happiness can weigh more in affecting the building of social ties, while in a collectivist cultural context like Taiwan, a person's embeddedness in social relationships determines subjective well-being more strongly than the reverse way around. The findings this study obtains indicate that happiness appears to be a decisive factor in affecting personal ties, while the reverse causality running from personal ties to happiness is less substantial in effect. This consequence of happiness is observed across the two cultural contexts. This study concludes that future research should construct adequate research designs to uncover the effect of happiness in various aspects of social life across countries and regions.

Theoretical Argument

Researchers on happiness have regularly surveyed a number of social relationship factors in explaining level of happiness. Only the more recent endeavors are reviewed herein for space's sake. Bjørnskov (2008) used a large set of social activities (bowling, camping, attending church, working on community projects, etc.) and factor analyzed them to obtain formal sociability and informal sociability. He found the two sociabilities to be strong predictors of life satisfaction in the US context (also Umberson et al. 1996). Church attendance, a proxy of interpersonal relationships, is also found to associate with Americans' happiness in studies that consider different experiences across sex, age and cohort groups (Yang 2008). Lim and Putnam's (2010) analysis of nation-wide panel data indicate that church attendance and congregational friendship help build networks in religious communities and enhance life satisfaction. In contrast, private or subjective aspects of religiosity have a scant influence on subjective well-being (see also Helliwell 2003).

Rodriguez-Pose and von Berlepsch (2014) turn their attention to people in 25 European countries. They further differentiated associational activities *a la* Putnam (2000) from participation in 'special interest groups' (Olson 1982). Their findings from a large pool of samples show that social interaction, norm (measured by social trust), and community sanctions (measured by a feeling of safety in the neighborhood, etc.) correlate with an individual's subjective well-being. While these social capital factors simultaneously contribute to individual happiness, it is informal social activities that constitute a primary determinant. Portela et al. (2013) mobilized a larger number of social capital proxies and obtained a similar result, concluding that compared to informal networks, formal networks show little effect on life satisfaction (but not happiness) among Europeans. They additionally note that political networks have no substantial influence on subjective well-being. Powdthavee (2008) replicates the favorable effect of meeting friends and relatives as well as talking to neighbors by analyzing a pooled data of the British households. In a study of a German panel, Winkelmann (2009) asserts that happier people tend to report they have an active social life, indicated by high frequency of visiting friends and relatives or engaging in voluntary work. In investigating Russians' 'emotional health', Rose (2000) shows trust to be a favorable factor, and memberships in formal or informal groups generates a similar benefit, despite that society's relatively low level of social capital.

Social capital is tied to better subjective well-being in Asia as well—perhaps a phenomenon unsurprising in this continent where strong ties feature in daily interactions, including business transactions (Hamilton 2006). Han et al. (2013) analyzed South Koreans and find a positive influence of organizational participation on individuals' scores on the Satisfaction with Life Scale (Pavot and Diener 1993). A pitfall of theirs is lack of evaluation of different indicators' relative weights in effect. Bian et al. (2015) investigated a large sample in the western region of China and replicate the favorable influence on happiness of social participation, social network (number of visitors at Chinese New Year, and the proportion of non-kin visitors). Chen (2012) combined two related items (i.e., the number of acquaintance contacts and the number of family member contacts during the last New Year holiday) as a proxy of social network to predict level of happiness. She obtained a consistent positive effect in Japan, South Korea, Taiwan and China (see also Chang 2009).[1]

[1] There are also notable research efforts that explore social capital and life satisfaction at an aggregate level. Bjornskov (2003, 2006) documented that social capital is a multifaceted phenomenon at the country level, such that social norms, social trust and associational activities can constitute distinct features of society, with trust being closely correlated with avowed satisfaction with life across more than 40 countries. However, recent studies using a larger size of country samples show that aggregated generalized trust has a decreased influence (Ram 2010). Recker (2013) provides interesting findings on the association between bridging (i.e., between group) social capital and assessment of quality life, both measured at the community level on the basis of small Iowa communities in the US. Since this study is concerned with micro-level association, I will only alert the readers to the relevant literatures.

The research findings across continents have arrived at several conclusions. Firstly, social network has been tapped into with a large variety of measures and proxies. There are several distinct components under this umbrella concept. Secondly, evidence obtained from cross-sectional or panel data across countries and regions suggests that not all social capital is equally important in enhancing subjective well-being. Thirdly, compared to formal organizational participation, informal social networks or *personal* relationships are more critical factors in well-being, either indicated by affective happiness or cognitive life satisfaction. Indeed, networking with formal organizations can be functional or instrumental. It often serves as a means to specific ends. It caters less to expressive needs, which are more likely to be met via intimacy and exchanges within informal relationships. Hence, sociability and subjective well-being are more closely linked.

These studies as a whole, however, lack due attention to a plausible reversed relationship in which happiness can operate to incur active social engagement or exchanges. This inattention is particularly unfortunate given that there have been major calls to explore causality from a two-way perspective (Lyubomirsky et al. 2005; Veenhoven 2010). Only a few studies have explored how happiness can be a precondition to various human activities and generate substantial outcomes. For instance, prosocial activities are more likely to happen after individuals have watched a happy movie (Wilson1981; Oswald 1996). Being satisfied from exchanges with others will lead to further reciprocation in a larger community (Oberholzer-Gee 2007). In low-quality marriage, unhappiness is responsible for lower self-esteem and health (Hawkins and Booth 2005). Cuffee et al. (2012) reports that patients who scored higher on a happiness scale tend to have better medication adherence in a sample of low-income African Americans with hypertension. This correlation is obtained when socio-economic backgrounds and difficulty in paying for medical care are controlled. These observations are somewhat scattered, and they were obtained with a research design too weak to assert happiness' status as an independent predictor.

Reciprocal Relations in Cross-Sectional Settings

Before I conduct estimation of a two-way causal model of happiness and sociability, a few clarifications are necessary. Firstly, it has been claimed that causal processes should be observed with panel data, which allow observation of "before and after" changes with time lags (Kline 2012). Survey projects collecting panel data on sociability are scarce. Most analyses relied on cross-section data that gathered information of social relationships and affect simultaneously. Yet, Wong and Law (1999) maintain that when the time interval between the causes and effects is sufficiently small, a cross-sectional nonrecursive model may be a viable representation of the reality. In my case, it should not take long for sociability to incur a pleasant mood, and happiness should stimulate a person to more frequently go out and meet intimate friends or neighbors without much hesitation—a long time lag is neither reasonable nor practical.

I construct a direct feedback model for gauging the relations between sociability and happiness, assuming that the two factors cause one another in a direct manner (*direct feedback*), without other factors mediating this feedback loop (*indirect feedback*). Estimation of reciprocal relations as such requires two essential considerations. Firstly, to identify a reciprocal model, one needs a special type of variable called 'instrumental variable' (IV). The IV's are needed to solve the difficulty arising from a situation that the regressor is correlated with the error term, known as the endogeneity problem (that is, sociability might covy with the residual of happiness). This "problematic" regressor necessarily occurs in a nonrecursive model (Paxton et al. 2011). For a solution, an instrumental variable is used for estimation and ideally it has to be (1) uncorrelated with the disturbances but (2) correlated with the variable for which it is an instrument (Paxton et al. 2011:17–18). A really good IV is hard to find. In this study, I rely on empirical testing when selecting certain IV's. More clarifications follow later.

The second necessity in the nonrecursive model is to specify the covariance between the disturbance terms of the endogenous variables. As a specification of covariation tends to generate outcomes that are different from a model without such specification, it is highly suggested that such a relationship always be specified in modeling (Wong and Law 1999). This specification also represents an important advantage of SEM over the conventional two-state least squares (TSLS) method in estimating mutual causal relations. The SEM method also allows latent variables with multiple indicators in specification, another advantage for choosing the SEM over the TSLS techniques for estimation (Hoyle 2012; Kenny and Milan 2011; see also Robbins 2012).

With these specification requirements in mind, I now start to introduce my research design and model specifications. The empirical analysis involves data from the US and Taiwan. A cross-country comparison is hence allowed to see whether the results produced from the nonrecursive model converge or are dissimilar in distinct cultural contexts. Additionally, I mobilized data from different waves of surveys in the US and Taiwan. This further enables a check of consistency on a time line.

Nonrecursive Model for the US

The data from the General Social Survey (GSS) are used for estimating reciprocal relations between sociability and subjective well-being. The GSS annually surveys Americans with regard to their attitudes, values positions and behaviors. Respondents comprise adults randomly selected across a large number of cities and towns and are representative of the general population (Smith et al. 2012). For measurement of sociability, the responses to three questions are used: How often does a respondent spend a social evening with (1) relatives; (2) someone who live in the neighborhood; and (3) friends who live outside the neighborhood (7-point scale from 'almost every day' to 'never') (see Appendix Table A.16.1 for summary statistics). This set of sociability measures is not equivalent to social networking, as it represents the typical bonding activities within close relationships. It does not reflect the bridging social capital ('weak ties') that extends well beyond the boundaries of kin and friends. Moreover, in comparison to certain popular measures of social capital that attempt to capture an individual's instrumental resources to be mobilized if needed (Lin 2001), the sociability indicators this paper uses clearly refer to the domain of interpersonal relationships.

To increase the reliability of measurement, I used two proxies for subjective well-being. The first is a feeling of enjoyment or pleasure, judging from one's own general conditions: 'Taken all together, how would you say things are these days – would you say that you are: (1) very happy, (2) pretty happy, or (3) not too happy?' Besides this often-used measure, I added another indicator of 'exciting life', by way of this question: 'In general, do you find life (1) exciting, (2) pretty routine, or (3) dull?' For both questions, the respondents were scored from 3 to 1 according to their level of positive psychology. People who feel life is exciting are a majority in the samples, whereas those reporting 'feeling very happy' comprised about one-third among the sampled Americans (see Appendix Table A.16.1).

Age and health serve as instrumental variables for the latent variable of sociability in the SEM, while financial condition performs the same function for the latent subjective well-being. Education is not an IV, as it has influence on both endogenous variables. The nonrecursive model is shown in Fig. 16.1 on the basis of pooled data from surveys conducted in 2002, 2004 and 2006 with a total sample size of 1640.[2] Note that financial condition is a latent variable comprising yearly household income (logarithm of a constant dollar measure) and an indicator of satisfaction with 'present financial situation' (3-point scale). An individual's interpersonal activities are not constrained by lower income in a significant manner. In the pooled data of 2008, 2010 and 2012 (see Fig. 16.2), for the latent sociability variable, I find education to correlate only slightly with sociability.[3] The two models presented seem to be appropriate for estimating nonrecursive relationships, as the statistics of the model fit show a good match between the constructed causal model and the data. For instance, the RMSEA (root mean squared error of approximation) and SRMR (standardized root mean squared residual) are both below the threshold of .08. Granted the large sample and degree of freedom herein, the fit is satisfactory (Hu and Bentler 1999).

It is particularly noteworthy to check the index of stability. In a recursive relationship, the effect of a variable for the 'dependent' variable (referring to its unstandardized coefficient) is cumulative: as it increases the effect on the latter, it simultaneously enlarges the effect of the latter on itself, and so on. These simultaneous changes

---

[2] Not all respondents in each survey were solicited to provide information on social activities and subjective well-being variables. In average, each survey provides about 500 subjects for pooling. As time lags were short and the differences between surveys were small, there is no need to apply specific techniques such as multilevel modeling for estimation.

[3] Other possibilities were experimented with but did not improve our estimation. For instance, a model with health serving as an instrument for sociability failed to converge, perhaps because it has a lower correlation with three original sociability variables (no higher than .10 for a social evening with relatives or neighbors for the pooled data (2002–2012); its correlation coefficient with a social evening with friends is slightly higher (.14).

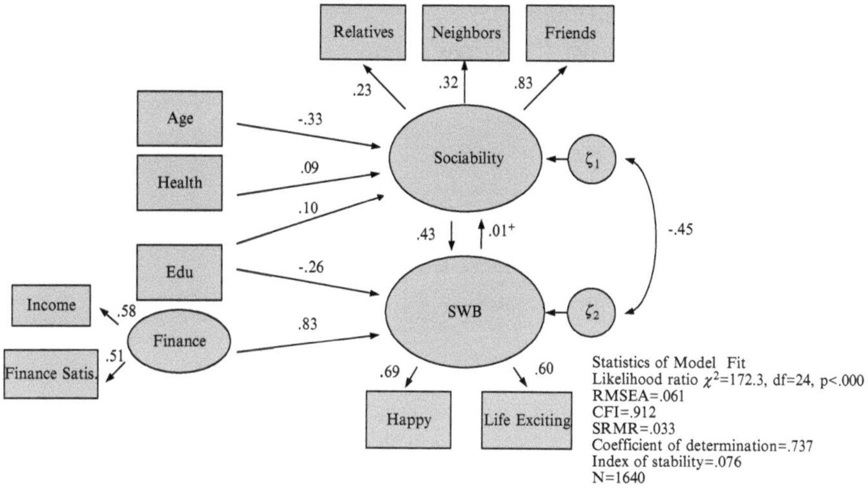

Fig. 16.1 Sociability and SWB in the U.S. (2002–2006) (Note: +indicate insignificance ($p > .05$))

might unfortunately lead to an explosive result. This brings the model into an 'unstable' situation. Alternatively, the simultaneous effects may become smaller in subsequent increments and converge on zero, a situation indicating stability of a model. This is an assumption of equilibrium in a stable model: the causation is assumed to occur in a finite amount of time, and after a certain period of time the estimated effects from reciprocal influences will complete its cycles over time and is damped out in effect. A standard procedure of stability checking is to compute the stability index, which is based on the matrix of coefficients for direct effects among all endogenous variables in the structural model (Kline 2006). The index of stability obtained from the proposed model is well below a threshold of 1.0, indicating a good equilibrium of the model (see Fig. 16.1).[4]

On the basis of these satisfactory statistics of model fit, I provide a number of important observations from Fig. 16.1 for the period of 2002–2006 (all coefficients are standardized). Firstly, age negatively associates with sociability, while better health and education produce positive effects. Secondly, in accordance with recent research findings (Stevenson and Wolfers 2013), an individual's financial condition strongly determines a feeling of happiness and exciting life. Thirdly, education appears to carry a negative *direct* effect for happiness. The model suggests that the indirect effect of education on happiness through sociability ($.098 \times .430 = .043$) only slightly moderates education's unfavorable impact. Hence, in general, the higher educated do not feel as happy as the lower educated in the US. Edgerton et al. (2012) propose that education's effect on subjective well-being is mediated by various mechanisms such as self-esteem and earnings. It is suggested that such

[4] The models also meet the requirement of identification by satisfying both order and rank conditions. Discussion of these technical issues is beyond the scope of this paper. See Kline (2004) and Paxton et al. (2011).

Table 16.1 R^2 for endogenous variables

	US (2002–2006)	US (2008–2012)	Taiwan (2005)	Taiwan (2010)
Sociability	.15	.28	.23	.27
Happiness	.50	.54	.26	.40

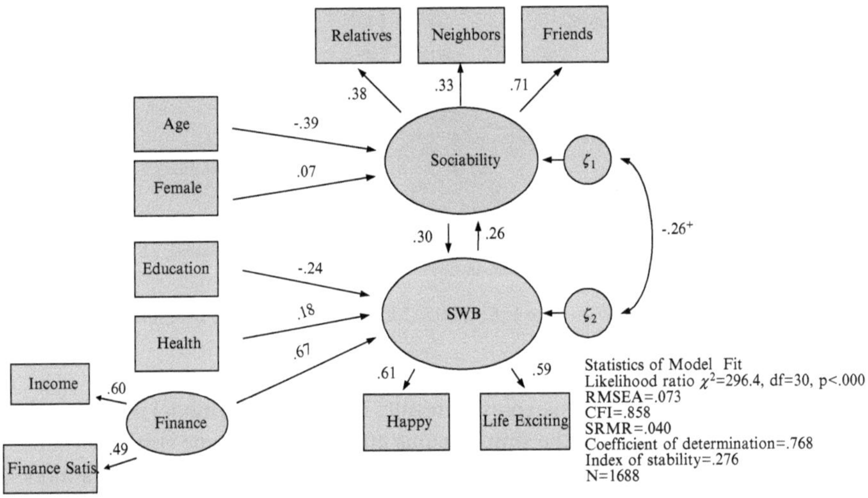

Fig. 16.2 Sociability and SWB in U.S. (2008–2012) (Note: +indicates insignificance (p>.05))

a specification be incorperated in order to more clearly understand education's intricate relationship with happiness. Fourthly, sociability does not exert an effect on happiness, while happiness increases the frequency of social evenings with kin and friends. I tested whether the two coefficients are equal, and the result rejects the null hypothesis ($\chi^2=7.1$, df = 1, $p<.01$). Lastly, the explained variance for the endogenous sociability variable is about 15 %, which is much lower than that for the endogenous subjective well-being variable (50 % of the variance explained) (see Table 16.1). Both R^2 are significant in a statistical sense, however.

Figure 16.2 shows the outcome from more recent surveys (pooling 2008, 2010 and 2012 data). The major difference is that health and education were found to be unrelated with sociability, so we replaced age and gender as instruments, as they perform better in the model. Females are more likely to have more social evenings than males do. Age is negatively correlated with the number of social evenings. Education continues to associate with happiness in a negative way, as was found from the previous result on Figure 16.1. The reciprocal influences between sociability and happiness are observed as both coefficients reach significance. The test of equality does not reject the null hypothesis ($\chi^2=3.7$, df = 1, $p>.05$).

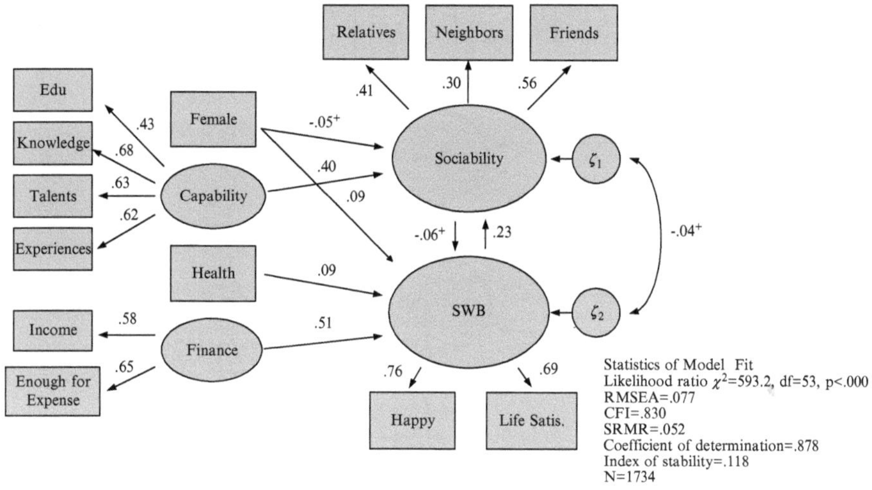

Fig. 16.3 Sociability and SWB in Taiwan (2005) (Note: +indicate insignificance (p>.05))

Nonrecursive Model for Taiwan

I additionally estimated a cross-sectional nonrecursive model for Taiwan to observe the pattern of mutual influences of sociability and happiness. I particularly note that the estimation is operated in a cultural context which has emphasized the significance of being embedded in real or fictive kin relations (Tsai 2006). Figure 16.3 show the result from the TSCS data for 2005. In response to the suggestion that an individual's capability should be considered a 'life-ability', which denotes how well a person is equipped to cope with problems of life and enhance his/her life quality (Veenhoven 2012), the model in Fig. 16.3 generates a latent variable that comprises education as well as three subjective evaluations of personal empowerment on the basis of the following survey items: (1) 'You like to use every opportunity to broaden your knowledge'; (2) 'You like to try your best to develop your talents'; and (3) 'You like to have all kinds of experiences in life' (level of agreement on 4-point scale).

For measurement of sociability, the TSCS survey provided three indicators: (1) 'In the past year, did you and your relatives get together often?' (6-point scale); (2) 'How many intimate neighbors visit you to chat?' (5-point scale); and (3) 'In the past year, did you and your friends get together often?' (6-point scale). The wording is somewhat different from those used in the GSS. Additionally, the 'friends' in the TSCS are not confined to those living *outside* of the neighborhood, unlike the GSS definition. Despite these differences, the three measures should capture an individual's personal relationships firmly. The latent variable of subjective wellbeing comprises two often-used elements of 'feeling happy' and 'being satis-

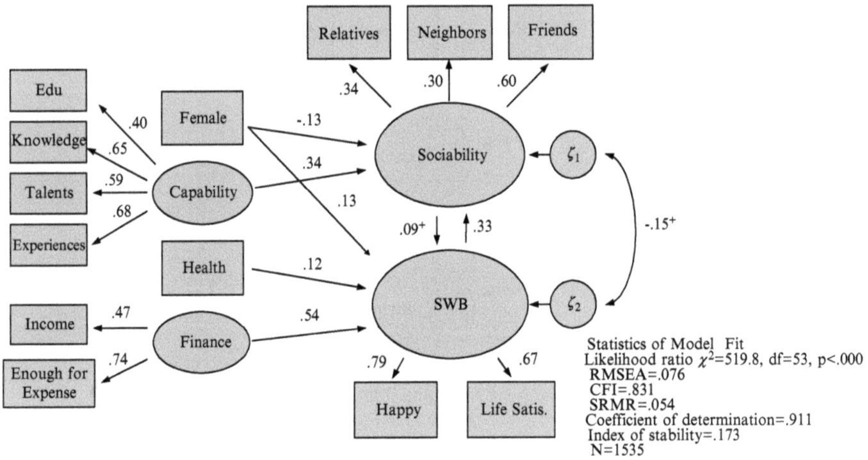

Fig. 16.4 Sociability and SWB in Taiwan (2010) (Note: +indicates insignificance (p>.05))

fied with quality of life' (see Appendix Table A.16.2) .[5] All statistics show a good model fit for Fig. 16.3. For an instance, the overall coefficient of determination is high at .878.

The result of the SEM estimation for the 2005 data indicates that sociability is highly affected by capability. However, females are not necessarily more active than males in building and maintaining social relationships. Better subjective well-being appears among females, healthier people,[6] and the higher-income group, a replication of earlier finding in the literature (Chang 2009; Dolan et al. 2008; Peifo 2007). With regard to the reciprocal relationship we are most concerned with, subjective wellbeing exerts a positive impact on sociability, while the reverse is not true. However, a test of difference for the two coefficients indicates that the discrepancy is not substantial in a statistical sense ($\chi^2 = 1.5$, df = 1, $p > .05$).

The estimation outcome from the 2010 TSCS data largely replicated those obtained from 2005 (see Fig. 16.4), except females' lower frequencies of meeting with kin, neighbors or friends. This gendered difference was not found in the 2005 estimation. The results from comparing males and females suggest more evidence is needed to conclude whether females are constrained in building wider networks or more ties even within intimate relationships. A feedback loop is not observed: while happiness stimulates sociability, sociability does not incur a similar favorable effect on happiness. However, the test of equality for the two coefficients does not

[5] The response categories for both happiness and life satisfaction differ slightly as the survey of 2005 used a four-point scale, while the 2010 survey used a five-point scale. The outcome appeared much the same, as only a small group of respondents (less than 3 %) placed themselves at the midpoint (see Appendix Table A.16.2).

[6] The health variable is a measure of the extent to which any discomforts or injuries affected the respondent's daily activities in the past 2 weeks. It is somewhat restrictive. I substituted another measure of 'perceived level of health' and obtained similar findings.

reach significance level ($\chi^2=.08$, df=1, p>.05). The model fit is satisfactory; and the index of stability shows the estimates are stable.

Discussion and Conclusion

It has long been argued that happiness depends far more on embedding in intimate relationships and wider social networks than on social positional characteristics (Portela et al. 2013; Recker 2013; Veenhoven 2014). Empirical studies have marshalled research findings to indicate the importance of social relations for happiness. This paper contends that a model of reciprocal effect can be more appropriate in specifying the intricate relationships between sociability and happiness. At a minimum, the potential effect which runs from happiness to sociability should be taken into consideration and incorporated into the research design in a more serious manner. Unfortunately, nearly all researchers in this field are not motivated to investigate the causal effect from a feedback loop perspective. This inattention necessarily prevents us from knowing the significance of happiness as an active factor, not merely in influencing specific dispositions and behaviors, but also in enhancing general human welfare. This paper hence contributes to the field of happiness studies by offering solid evidence for reciprocal causality on the basis of national probability samples recently drawn from the US and Taiwan populations.

I admit that this paper originates from a motivation to examine how likely happiness is to affect sociability given that a reverse loop is considered simultaneously in a context of SEM. The obtained outcome appears to show that a causal process running from happiness deserves more than special attention. In the US, sociability indeed leads to more happiness as is revealed for the two analyzed periods. In the 2008–1012 data, a loop appears clearly. In Taiwan context, for both 2005 and 2010 data, happiness is a significant predictor of sociability while the reverse feedback does not appear. In contrast, a causal path running from sociability to happiness is somewhat weak at best in the SEM modeling in this East Asian society. In sum, it is plausible that happiness leads to sociability, which happens in two cultures. Sociability may enhance happiness but it does so only under certain circumstances.

How do these main findings fit in the current debate, particularly in a comparative perspective that argues for an understanding of well-being in cultural contexts? Cross-cultural researchers suggest more attention, but not merely to the issue of conceptual equivalence of happiness-related concepts. Standard measures might not perform equally well across countries. It is argued that happiness features an intense feeling of excitement for Americans in an individualist culture; for East Asians it reflects a meaningful life, positive relationships, and social harmony, which are highly regarded in a tradition of collectivism. Thus, there is a distinction between amusement ('aroused positive emotions') and eudaimonia (a 'well-lived life') (Oishi 2010). Alternatively, it might be that some concepts of well-being are more acceptable in certain cultural contexts (Diener 2009). In responding to this argument, this study in reality adopts a specific measure of subjective well-being which features 'high-arousals' for American respondents, by tapping whether they feel life is exciting, in addition to a conventional one of 'general life satisfaction'. This 'cultural bias' embedded in the measures thus should satisfy culturalists.

The culturalists might additionally question the current research design as well as findings. They would expect that sociability should impact the subjective well-being among Taiwanese more than Americans since the former society typically represents strong value positions in collectivism. That is, social connectedness as indicated by interpersonal relationships is highly regarded in this society and therefore it is a source of happiness (Diener 2009; Lu et al. 2001; Lu and Gilmore 2004). I find this thinking somewhat intuitive. A high frequency of contacting with relatives, neighbors or friends might become a burden as a person is obliged to spend extra effort to maintain the relationships, thus offsetting benefits from ties and resources derived therefrom. In contrast, happy individuals apparently seek to meet close kin or friends quite frequently in the US (at least this was observed in recent data) and in Taiwan. Kitayama et al. (2000) suggest that intimate relationships are considered to be an individual's achievement and are indicative of a good internal self. Thus, happy people tend to expend considerable effort in increasing positive feelings when they are engaged with others in social activities. A consequence of happiness is hence to identify and meet the others who are selected into intimate relationships. Kitayama et al. (2000; Uchida et al. 2004) considers Americans to fit into this model, as their subjective feelings are constructed more through being directed to others (that is, inter-subjectively). However, there is no reason to reject the notion that Taiwanese or Asian populations also behave this way.

A natural sequel to this study is to conduct empirical testing of whether social capital has more substantial influence in living well, despite (or disregarding) its influence on feeling well. In contrast to sociability, which features affective ties with intimate kin and friends, social capital reflects resources in an organization of interpersonal linkages in which an individual is embedded, which can be mobilized to obtain certain goals through coordinated or cooperative actions (Coleman 1988; Putnam 2000). Social capital essentially entails an involvement in or even possession of a durable network of institutionalized relationships by way of acquaintances or recognition (Bourdieu 1985). Such linkage is more or less instrumental and for this reason, the specific consequences of it, such as useful information, job opportunities, and satisfactory salaries, have been much highlighted. But as Portes (1998) suggests, social capital is not a given but constructed through 'investment strategies' before an individual can use a reliable source and obtain benefits thereof. In simple words, 'to possess social capital, a person must be related to others' (Portes 1998:7). Yet, obviously, simply being with others does automatically bring about social capital. Many factors appear to operate in affecting access to social capital. Solidarity, trust, and exchange norms are cited as primary sources, among others (Portes 1998; Putnam 2000). A person's level of happiness can be considered as another primary factor. This necessarily brings up a need for further testing of a more complicated reciprocal causality between feeling well, social linkage, and living well. Ambitious researchers should find numerous extensions of topics out of the study presented here.

Appendix

Table A.16.1 Summary statistics for the US samples

	2002–2006	2008–2012
Female	52.68 %	53.61 %
Age	46.4 (17.1)	46.6 (16.7)
Health	3.0 (.80)	3.0 (.78)
Education		
Less than high school	12.44 %	12.09 %
High school	52.44 %	52.07 %
Junior college	8.48 %	7.88 %
Bachelor	17.20 %	17.36 %
Graduate school		10.60 %
Income (yearly household in constant dollars; base = 1986)	50383.1 (42508.0)	49364.6 (44561.8)
Financial satisfaction		
Not satisfied at all	26.65 %	29.98 %
More or less satisfied	44.51 %	44.61 %
Pretty well satisfied	30.35 %	25.41 %
Social evening		
With relatives		
Never	3.66 %	3.67 %
About once a year	6.34 %	6.99 %
Several times a year	18.54 %	17.65 %
About once a month	16.59 %	16.11 %
Several times a month	18.35 %	19.43 %
Once or twice a week	26.16 %	24.59 %
Almost every day	10.37 %	11.55 %
With neighbors		
Never	28.60 %	28.85 %
About once a year	10.24 %	10.25 %
Several times a year	13.90 %	13.27 %
About once a month	14.09 %	14.69 %
Several times a month	11.40 %	11.32 %
Once or twice a week	15.18 %	16.17 %
Almost every day	6.59 %	5.45 %
With friends		
Never	9.33 %	9.54 %
About once a year	7.26 %	7.23 %
Several times a year	16.22 %	17.48 %
About once a month	23.48 %	21.45 %
Several times a month	21.59 %	20.73 %
Once or twice a week	18.54 %	20.14 %
Almost every day	3.60 %	3.44 %

(continued)

Table A.16.1 (continued)

	2002–2006	2008–2012
Happiness		
Not too happy	9.51 %	12.26 %
Pretty happy	57.20 %	57.29 %
Very happy	33.29 %	30.45 %
Life is exciting		
Dull	4.63 %	5.39 %
Routine	43.48 %	45.02 %
Exciting	51.89 %	45.59 %

See Figs. 16.1 and 16.2 for sample sizes

Table A.16.2 Summary statistics for the Taiwan samples

	2005	2010
Female	50.00 %	48.55 %
Age	44.6 (16.9)	45.4 (16.8)
Income (monthly household)	7.97 (9.97)	8.67 (12.57)
Income enough for expenses		
Much less than enough	11.75 %	10.99 %
A little less than enough	18.79 %	17.54 %
Just enough	32.91 %	27.05 %
A little more than enough	32.35 %	39.04 %
Much more than enough	4.20 %	5.39 %
Education		
Less than high school	39.14 %	31.33 %
High school	29.00 %	29.03 %
Some college	9.80 %	10.13 %
University	17.94 %	24.21 %
Graduate school	4.12 %	5.31 %
Broaden knowledge		
Not at all	1.12 %	1.61 %
No	12.73 %	10.12 %
Yes	68.22 %	59.19 %
Very much	17.93 %	29.08 %
Develop talents		
Not at all	1.00 %	0.70 %
No	16.81 %	14.88 %
Yes	68.63 %	64.59 %
Very much	13.56 %	19.83 %
Experience new things		
Not at all	0.64 %	1.35 %
No	11.56 %	10.88 %
Yes	70.42 %	62.66 %
Very much	17.38 %	25.11 %

(continued)

Table A.16.2 (continued)

	2005	2010
Health (discomforts or injuries affected life in past 2 weeks)		
Very much	2.84 %	3.22 %
Quite a bit	3.17 %	3.43 %
Slightly	21.07 %	13.35 %
No	72.97 %	80.00
Sociability		
Got together with relatives		
Never	3.59 %	3.69 %
Seldom	33.89 %	30.34 %
Once every 2–3 months	31.10 %	29.34 %
Two to three times a month	15.52 %	22.48 %
Once every week	9.46 %	7.76 %
Two times or more every week	6.43 %	6.39 %
Neighbors came to visit		
None	11.46 %	21.90 %
Very few	34.39 %	32.40 %
Some	36.86 %	32.03 %
Quite a lot	9.51 %	5.91 %
A lot	7.78 %	7.76 %
Got together with friends		
Never	6.66 %	7.81 %
Seldom	28.61 %	23.91 %
Once every 2–3 months	20.41 %	17.69 %
Two to three times a month	18.41 %	25.77 %
Once every week	11.46 %	12.04 %
Two times or more every week	14.45 %	12.78 %
Happiness		
Life satisfaction		
Very unsatisfied	3.17 %	4.06 %
Fairly unsatisfied	22.05 %	13.93 %
Neither satisfied nor dissatisfied		2.53 %
Fairly satisfied	66.20 %	62.37 %
Very satisfied	8.58 %	17.10 %
Feel happy in daily life		
Not at all happy	2.05 %	4.70 %
Not very happy	9.69 %	20.69 %
Neither happy nor unhappy		2.22 %
Quite happy	66.64 %	54.83 %
Very happy	21.62 %	17.57 %

See Figs. 16.3 and 16.4 for sample sizes

References

Bian, Y., Zhang, L., Yang, J., Guo, X. & Lei, M. 2015. Subjective Wellbeing of Chinese People: A Multifaceted View. Social Indicators Research, 121, 75–92.

Bjørnskov, C. 2003. The happy few: cross-country evidence on social capital and life satisfaction. Kyklos 56, 3–16.

Bjørnskov, C. 2006. The multiple facets of social capital. European Journal of Political Economy 22, 22–40.

Bjørnskov, C. 2008. Social Capital and Happiness in the United States. Applied Research in Quality of Life, 3, 43–62.

Bourdieu, P. 1985. The forms of capital. In Handbook of Theory and Research for the sociology of education, edited by Richardson, J. G. New York: Greenwood, 241–258.

Bruni, L. 2007. The 'technology of happiness' and the tradition of economic science. In Handbook of the Economics of Happiness, edited by L. Bruni and P. L. Porta. Cheltenham: Edward Elgar, 24–52.

Chang, W.-C. 2009. Social capital and subjective happiness in Taiwan. International Journal of Social Economics, 36, 844–868.

Chen, W-c. 2012. How education enhances happiness: comparison of mediating factors in four East Asian countries. Social Indicators Research, 106, 117–131.

Coleman, J. S. 1988. Social capital in the creation of human capital. American Journal of Sociology, 94, s95–s120.

Cuffee, Y. L. et al. 2012. Does happiness predict medication adherence among African Americans with hypertension? Applied Research in Quality of Life, 7, 403–412.

Diener, E. 2009. Culture and Well-Being: The Collected Works of Ed Diener. The Netherlands: Springer.

Dolan, P., Peasgood, T. & White, M. 2008. Do we really know what makes us happy? A review of the economic literature on the factors associated with subjective well-being. Journal of Economic Psychology, 29, 94–122.

Edgerton, J. D., Roberts, L. W. and von Below, S. 2012. Education and quality of life. In In Handbook of Social Indicators and Quality of Life Research, edited by Land, K. C., Michalos, A. C. and Sirgy, M. J. Dordrecht: Springer, 265–296.

Graham, C. 2009. Happiness Around the World. Oxford: Oxford University Press.

Hagerty, M. R. Cummins, R. A., Ferriss, A. L., Land, K., Michalos, A.C. Peterson, M., Andrew, S., Sirgy, J. & Vogel, J. 2001. Quality of life indexes for national policy: review and agenda for research. Social Indicators Research, 55, 1–96.

Hamilton, G. G. 2006. Commerce and Capitalism in Chinese Societies. London: Routledge.

Han, S., Kim, H. and Lee, H.-S. 2013. A Multilevel Analysis of the Compositional and Contextual Association of Social Capital and Subjective Well-Being in Seoul, South Korea. Social Indicators Research, 111, 185–202.

Hawkins, D. N. & Booth, A. 2005. Unhappily ever after: effects of long-term, low-quality marriage on well-being. Social Forces, 84, 451–471.

Helliwell, J. F. 2003. How's life? combining individual and national variables to explain subjective well-being. Economic Modeling, 20, 331–360.

Hoyle, R. H. 2012. Model specification in structural equation modeling. In Handbook of Structural Equation Modeling, edited by R. H. Hoyle. New York: Guilford,126–144.

Hu, L., & Bentler, P. M. 1999. Cutoff criteria for fit indexes in covariance structure analysis: Conventional criteria versus new alternatives. *Structural Equation Modeling, 6*, 1–55.

Kenny, D. A. & Milan, S. 2011. Identification: a nontechnical discussion of a technical issue. In Handbook of Structural Equation Modeling, edited by R. H. Hoyle. New York: Guilford, 145–163.

Kitayama, S., Markus, H. R. & Kurokawa, M. 2000. Culture, Emotion, and Well-being: good feelings in Japan and the United States. Cognition and Emotion, 14, 93–124.

Kline, R. B. 2004. Principles and Practices of Structural Equation Modeling, 2nd edition. New York: Guilford.
Kline, R. B. 2006. Reverse arrow dynamics: formative measurement and feedback loop. In Structural Equation Modeling: A Second Course, edited by Hancock, G. R. & Mueller, R. O. Greenwich, CT: Information Age Publishing, 43–68.
Kline, R. B. 2012. Assumptions in structural equation modeling. In Handbook of Structural Equation Modeling, by R. H. Hoyle. New York: Guilford, 111–125.
Lance, C. E., Mallard, A. G. & Michalos, A. C. 1995. Tests of the causal directions of global-Life facet satisfaction relationships. Social Indicators Research, 34, 69–92.
Lim, C. & Putnam, R. D. 2010. Religion, social networks, and life satisfaction. American Sociological Review, 75, 914–933.
Lin, N. 2001. Social Capital: A Theory of Social Structure and Action. Cambridge: Cambridge University Press.
Lu, L. & Gilmour, R. 2004. Culture and Conceptions of Happiness: Individual Oriented and Social Oriented SWB. Journal of Happiness Studies, 5, 269–291.
Lu, L., Gilmour, R. & Kao, S.-F. 2001. Cultural Values and Happiness: An East-West Dialogue. The Journal of Social Psychology, 141, 477–493.
Lyubomirsky, S., King, L. & Diener, E. 2005. The benefits of frequent positive affect: does happiness lead to success? Psychological Bulletin, 131, 803–855.
Michalos, Alex. 2008. Education, happiness and wellbeing. Social Indicators Research, 87, 347–366.
Oberholzer-Gee, F. 2007. The helping hand-a brief anatomy. In Economics and Psychology: A Promising New Cross-Disciplinary Field, edited by B. S. Frey and A. Stutzer. Cambridge: MIT Press, pp.229–239.
Oishi, S. 2010. Culture and well-being: Conceptual and methodological issues. In E. Diener, D. Kahneman, & J. F. Helliwell, (Eds.), International differences in well-being. New York: Oxford University Press, pp. 34–69.
Olson, M. 1982. The Rise and Decline of Nation. New Haven: Yale University Press.
Oswald, P. 1996. The effect of cognitive and affective perspective taking on empathic concern and altruistic helping. Journal of Social Psychology 136:613–624.
Pavot, W. & Diener, E. 1993. Review of the Satisfaction With Life Scale. Psychological Assessment, 5, 164–172.
Paxton, P. M., Hipp, J. R. & Marquart-Pyatt, S. 2011. Nonrecursive Models: Endogeneity, Reciprocal Relationships, and Feedback Loops. Los Angeles: Sage.
Peiŕo, A. 2007. Happiness, satisfaction and socioeconomic conditions: some international evidence. In Handbook on Economics of Happiness, edited by Bruni, L. & Porta, P. L. Cheltenham: Edward Elgar, 429–446.,
Portela, M., Neira, I. and Social Capital and del Mar Salinas-Jiménez, M. 2013. Subjective Wellbeing in Europe: A New Approach on Social Capital. Social Indicators Research, 114, 493–511.
Portes, A. 1998. Social capital: its origins and applications in modern sociology. Annual Review of Sociology, 24, 1–24.
Powdthavee, N. 2008. Putting a price tag on friends, relatives, and neighbors: using surveys of life satisfaction to value social relationships. The Journal of Socio-Economics, 37, 1459–1480.
Putnam, R. 2000. Bowling Alone-the Collapse and Revival of American Community. New York: Simon & Schuster.
Ram, R. 2010. Social capital and happiness: additional cross-country evidence. Journal of Happiness Studies, 11, 409–418.
Recker, N. 2013. Bonds, bridges and quality of life in small towns. Applied Research in Quality of Life, 8, 63–75.
Robbins, B. G. 2012. Institutional quality and generalized trust: a nonrecursive causal model. Social Indicator Research, 107, 235–258.

Rodriguez-Pose, A. & von Berlepsch, V. 2014. Social capital and individual happiness in Europe, Journal of Happiness Studies, 15, 357–386.
Rose, R. 2000. How much does social capital add to individual health? a survey study of Russians. Social Science & Medicine, 51,1421–1435.
Smith, T. W., P. V. Marsden & Hout, M. 2012. General Social Survey, 2012 Merged Data, Including a Cultural Module [United States]. ICPSR35478-v1. Ann Arbor, MI: Inter-university Consortium for Political and Social Research [distributor], 2015-01-30. http://doi.org/10.3886/ICPSR35478.v1.
Stevenson, B. & Wolfers, J. 2013. Subjective Well-Being and Income: Is There Any Evidence of Satiation?American Economic Review, 103, 598–604.
Tsai, M.-C. 2006. Sociable resources and close Relationships: Intimate relatives and friends in Taiwan. Journal of Social and Personal Relationships, 23, 151–169.
Uchida, Y., Norasakkunkit, V. & Kitayama, S. 2004. Cultural construction of happiness: theory and empirical evidence. Journal of Happiness Studies, 5, 223–239.
Umberson, D, Chen, M. D., House, J. S., Hopkins, K. & Slaten, E. 1996. The effect of social relationships on psychological well-being: are men and women really so different? American Sociological Review, 61, 837–857.
Veenhoven, 2012. Happiness, also known as "life satisfaction" and "subjective well-being". In Handbook of Social Indicators and Quality of Life Research, edited by Land, K. C., Michalos, A. C. and Sirgy, M. J. Dordrecht: Springer, 63–77.
Veenhoven, R. 2008. Healthy happiness: effects of happiness on physical health and consequences for preventive health care. Journal of Happiness Studies, 9, 449–464.
Veenhoven, R. 2010. Capability and happiness: conceptual difference and reality links. Journal of Socio-Economics 39, 344–350.
Veenhoven, R. 2014. Sociology's blind eye for happiness. Comparative Sociology, 13, 537–555.
Wilson, D. W. 1981. Is helping a laughing matter? Psychology, 18, 6–9.
Winkelmann, R. 2009. Unemployment, social capital, and subjective well-being. Journal of Happiness Studies, 10, 321–430.
Wong, C.-S. & Law, K. S. 1999. Testing reciprocal relations by nonrecursive structural equation models using cross-sectional data. Organizational Research Methods, 2, 69–87.
Yang, Y. 2008. Social inequality in happiness in the United States, 1972 to 2004: an age-period-cohort analysis. American Sociological Review, 73, 204–226.

Part V
Training Quality of Life

Chapter 17
The Challenge of Teaching Quality-of-Life Theory and Research Methodology at the University: A View from South America

Graciela Tonon

Introduction

I consider Alex Michalos to be my professor. Not only have I learnt vastly from him in the scientific field but have, most importantly, received far more from him as a human being.

Thus, when Filomena Maggino invited me to collaborate in this book, I thought that the best way to honour him was by writing about my experience in the teaching of theory and research methods on quality of life to graduate and post-graduate university students, scholarship students, students working on post-graduate theses, and researchers from other South-American countries.

I wish to express my respect and admiration to a man whose work has strengthened the improvement of the quality of life of the human beings of his time.

Social Work and QOL

I began to teach quality of life, at a university level, more than a decade ago when I decided to incorporate it to the course *Theory and Method of Social Work I* which belongs to the Social Work Program at the Faculty of Social Sciences of Universidad Nacional de Lomas de Zamora, Argentina.

G. Tonon (✉)
UNICOM, Faculty of Social Sciences, Universidad Nacional de Lomas de Zamora, Provincia de Buenos Aires, Argentina

Manuel Arce 1189, C1408FKC Ciudad Autónoma de Buenos Aires, Argentina
e-mail: gracielatonon@hotmail.com

F. Maggino (ed.), *A Life Devoted to Quality of Life*, Social Indicators Research Series 60, DOI 10.1007/978-3-319-20568-7_17

This course is devoted to the study of the theory and methodology of Social Work within communities, and quality of life was included, in the year 2001, as one of the subject's theme units.

The syllabus of this course aims at the students' achievement of the theoretical-methodological knowledge required for social workers' professional practice in today's scenario of communities; it further aims at enhancing their knowledge and interpretation of the social reality, on the basis of an integration of theory and practice; as well as encouraging the development of a critical attitude together with a sense of commitment regarding the social reality in which they are likely to discover/construct possible strategies for professional development.

This has given way to an academic space for theory-practice integration which allows the treatment of subjects originated in the Social Work field as well as in other disciplinary fields (Political Science, Economy, Sociology, Psychology, among others). These latter, however, are particularized due to the fact that they are employed in the specific field of Social Work and are, therefore, characterized as thematic axes of daily professional practice, without disregarding the importance attributed to the context they operate in.

The aim of the subject is methodological, for it works on actual data, under the consideration that knowledge is socially distributed (Schutz 1974, p. 15). It stems from the conception that both theory and practice are an integrated whole, that they need and nurture one another, which implies that the relationship between them is characterized by solidarity rather than confrontation.

The course is introduced through theoretical-methodological input on Social Work, regarding it as a profession as well as a discipline; methodology of professional practice, its object, its aims, and the context of such practice; the incidence of externality on the definition of professional practice and Social Work as a profession oriented to public service. Regarding externality, we agree with Vélez Restrepo (2003, p. 19) in the sense that, in the process of its constitution, Social Work has been strongly marked by an external discursive relationship, constructed on the basis of mediation with the State, public enterprise, and state and private institutions/organizations.

In this pedagogical proposal, quality of life is introduced as a re-conceptualizing theoretical alternative to the study of the Social Work-social needs-social welfare relationship, as well as to the development of the professional role of social workers – including the construction of a conception of quality of life in a community, based on the fact that satisfaction with life in a community implies satisfaction with a number of situations; namely, security in streets and public places, social service, interaction among neighbours, infrastructure and equipment, public transport, capacity to work as well as enjoy leisure time in public spaces together with other members of the community, to exchange views and discuss mutual worries and problems (Tonon 2012, p. 22). Likewise, according to Bramston et al. (2002), quality of life in the community requires to major elements: community cohesion and people's sense of belonging to the community, both vital to the development of the social workers' professional practice.

We define *quality of life* as a multi-dimensional concept which involves a number of domains which people consider and experience in diverse forms according to the importance attributed to them in their individual lives, according to their expectations, their values, and their former experiences (Bramston 2002, p. 48). In this respect, Patrick et al. (2002, p. 7) have acknowledged that the effect of social relations, as well as of the relationship with the environment, have become subjected to mediatisation on account of the subjects' personal outlooks, i.e. by each of the subjects' interpretation of their context and situation.

Michalos (2007, p. 4) states that the quality of life of a subject or of a community may be conceived as a function within the present conditions of their lives, what the subject or community do with those conditions (considering that what is done is a function of the way in which those conditions are perceived), what they think and feel regarding those conditions, what they have done, and the consequences that will derive from them.

Casas (1996, p. 100), considers that the study of quality of life requires a consideration not only of perceptions, aspirations, needs and social representations that people experience in their environment, but also of the social dynamics in which all of these are immersed, as well as the services they are offered and the social policies they receive. Thus, quality of life becomes an outlook which includes both the traditionally called objective living conditions and the so-called subjective experiences, working on two levels: micro and macro, thus allowing the construction of a new outlook involving respect for human rights and integration of the more personal experiences to the political and community spheres.

The concept of community is examined from its different definitions and features, as well as the consideration of socio-territorial space, social participation, and the importance of university-community relationship. The concept is completed by the inclusion of major topics related to the characteristics of national and community contexts such as poverty, exclusion, inclusion, human capabilities, social and intra-categorial inequalities, cultural diversity, social participation, social citizenship, and access to social help programs. At this point it is worth considering the notion of well-being, not only from a personal perspective but also in social terms of collective groups, since the opportunities of a group are as important as those of each individual person (Royuela et al. 2003, p. 52).

Regarding Social Work, we coincide with Payne (1995, pp. 26–27) who points out that it is a socially constructed profession, born of the interaction of professional practice and more extensive social contacts, operated by three forces: those which create and control Social Work as an occupation, the ones that categorize people – who merely seek the help of a social worker – under the term "assisted", and those which constitute the more comprehensive social context in which Social Work is carried out. "Theory is not only an intellectual development, it also responds to the social forces which may, at a given moment, be generating Social Work, and many of which derive from practice" (Payne 1995, p. 295). Thus, there is more than one possibility of conceiving Social Work.

Over the years, and in various geographical locations, social workers have been using different theoretical propositions in relation to the different contexts of their professional practices, thus calling for reflection upon the choice of the theories applied in each case. A theory is far more than a set of findings for it offers explanations of certain phenomena and allows the development of a field of knowledge. Theorizing involves a lengthy process which not only implies the conception or intuition of ideas but also their formulation in a logical, systematic, and explicative scheme (Strauss and Corbin 2002).

In the 1990s, Payne (1995, p. 81) had already identified the different aims of the different theories regarding Social Work, namely: the theories that explain the nature and role of Social Work in society; the Social Work theories that describe its activities and aims; the tributary theories which interpret or describe the subjects' behaviour (such as the ones derived from the fields of Social Sciences, Psychology, Economy, Political Sciences, to name a few), and the theories on practice and methodology of Social Work. The author rounds off his idea by pointing out that the theories of Social Work are strategic by nature.

The axis of the social workers' professional practice are the subjects in need, the latter being the real protagonists of this professional practice; which makes the introduction of quality of life as a theoretical proposition highly commendable.

People have ways of perceiving the changes in their life circumstances which differ from the perceptions of the observers of the aforementioned circumstances, this situation also applying to professionals (Gullone and Cummins 2002). The perception is defined by Santuc (1999, pp. 333–334) as the recording of a foundation symbolic play, capable of enabling and guiding the possible exchanges among humans, thus creating a bond with the world and with others, establishing a deep feeling of being in this world bound by their other senses. It is then that the social workers' perceptions of the situations described by the subjects are likewise affected by the professionals' own subjectivity – their work being linked to their own lives, to their own history, and to their own personal forms of perception of that reality (Romero 1992, p. 45). In fact, reality is construction involving multiple outlooks and views both on the part of the observer and of the observed (Gonzalez Perdomo 2006, p. 30).

Since the late twentieth century, a process of migration and exchange of concepts and methodologies has been taking place in the field of the Social Sciences, which has both made an impact and enriched Social Work. Social workers apply specific theoretical knowledge in order to tackle reality resulting from a combination of concepts that often emerge from other disciplines, together with the philosophical concepts inherent of their profession, as well as with their numerous professional practices (very often non-systematized), which still contribute to the advances in the generation of new knowledge (Tonon 2001, p. 57). When making reference to the philosophical principles, historically upheld by Social Work, we are referring to the recognition of each person's individuality as a subject, respect for self-determination, being good listeners, refraining from passing judgement, encouraging the development of one's own potentialities and those of others with the object of finding solutions to problems and securing professional secrecy/confidentiality – in other words, respect for human rights.

Thus, including the theoretical proposition of quality of life allows a new outlook on the social needs which generate the daily demands that social workers deal with. Moreover, in our South-American context, when referring to social needs, we adopt the ideas of the Chilean writer Max Neef et al. (1986), the Father of the proposition known as "Development at a Human Scale", who considers that social needs are not a mere addition of individual needs. He further states that "needs, considered in a broad sense, not limited to mere subsistence, show the constant tension between deficiency and potentiality characteristic of human beings" (Max Neef et al. 1986, p. 34). He completes his idea by stating that the consideration of a relationship between needs and economic assets allows the construction of an objective discipline, whereas the inclusion of the forms which have, culturally, constructed the social groups in order to meet those needs (which he calls satisfactors) implies a subjective consideration (Max Neef et al. 1986 p. 36).

Following this idea of integrating objectivity with subjectivity, we present our Social Work students with the proposition of quality of life as a possibility to construct a new outlook on the social and political reality, as well as on the practice of their professional role.

As far as practice is concerned, our primary idea is that Social Work is considered as one of the so-called "helping professions" which are characterized by the lack of continuity and the temporal, social, and material uncertainty inherent of the cases they attend to, as well as by their lack of homogeneity, basically because the demands are made by the subjects in need of attention and, besides, because the demands grow at the same rate as the margin of satisfaction received (Tonon 2009, p. 413). Likewise, according to Ackoff (1993), it is important to mention that Social Work may be considered as a member of the group of professions which the above-mentioned author acknowledges to be defined by the subjects of attention, characterized by their dynamism, since the problems they tackle undergo a faster change than the instruments used for their treatment – thus demanding permanent up-dating on the part of the attending professional, as well as avoidance of constant repetition of the same kind of service.

Castel (2004) sustains that modern societies are constructed on insecure ground, for they are formed by subjects incapable of ensuring protection in their own environment. Fitoussi and Rosanvallon (1997) have characterized them from an individualistic point of view, i.e. the logics of the market, the subjects' internal retreat, increasing frailty of community ties, social atomization, and the value of autonomy. It is in this scenario that social workers act, which brings to mind the words of Lechner (2002) who characterized everyday life in the early twenty-first century as:

> ...accelerated to a lightning speed by thousands of anxieties and an endless succession of upheavals together with a permanent transformation of the working environment and the urban landscape, which render people breathless, unable to process change. (Lechner 2002, p. 55)

Social workers' professional practice, based on a theoretical proposition of quality of life, allows them to integrate objectivity with subjectivity, thus transcending the traditional antagonism between these dimensions. The consideration that whenever a subject seeks the attention of a social worker he/she is presenting in the same action both a concrete need (objective), together with a personal perception of this experience (subjective), represents the opening of a new path in professional practice. Quoting Martinez Pineda (2006), the subject is actor-author-producer of himself and of other projects in society.

In this respect, a decade-long experience in the teaching of quality of life to Social Work students demonstrates that the latter have valued, considered, and integrated this theoretical outlook with their post-graduate professional practices.

Childhood, Youth and QOL

The development of studies on quality of life has, furthermore, been included in a Seminar dedicated to the study of theoretical/practical integration regarding specific issues in the field of childhood and youth, which forms part of the Program Childhood and Family, at the Faculty of Social Sciences, Universidad Nacional de Lomas de Zamora, Argentina.

The object of this seminar is to encourage the students to deepen their knowledge on the diversity of daily situations, quality of life and welfare of boys, girls, and young people in Argentina and Latin-America, through the study of books and papers on the subject. Within this pedagogical space, information is offered on themes affecting boys/girls and young people, regarding situations of social risk, thus creating a space for reflection with the students in the identification of the peculiarities of the professional practice of graduated experts in childhood and family. Furthermore, students are likewise encouraged to study the alternative strategies of professional practice with an outlook on participation and the exercise of boys'/girls' and young people's citizenship, by initiating them in the study of research projects devoted to the study of daily life situations, quality of life, and the welfare of boys, girls, and young people.

The approached themes are related to the different life situations and social problems that boys, girls, and young people are afflicted with in our region, namely: inequality, exclusion, poverty, marginalization, diversity, family and social violence, childhood ill-treatment in the family circle, sexual and commercial exploitation, forced migration, and the traffic of boys, girls, and young people. Subsequently, through quality of life, students will sustain a new outlook thus allowing boys, girls, and young people to become leading actors of the piece as regards development; social, urban, communal, and political participation; and communal approach on daily situations.

Every semester, the aforementioned seminar receives colleagues from different countries in our region, devoted to the study of the quality of life of boys, girls, and young people. The students are introduced to the peculiarities of their own population groups in different cities and towns of Latin-America thus generating a centrifugal interchange of knowledge and possibilities for the construction of micro and macro-social strategies of professional practice.

Research Methodology and Quality of Life: Qualitative and Quantitative Methods

The Research Program of QOL was created in 2004 in the Faculty of Social Sciences, Universidad Nacional de Lomas de Zamora and, ever since that time, has developed research studies centered in quality of life, as well as the tutoring of research scholars and thesis Master's and Doctorate students of different universities in South-America.

Since 2004, to this day, 11 research projects have been developed,[1] 8 have been concluded, and 3 are in process of development (all of them centered in quality of life). These projects are research studies in which both quantitative and qualitative methods have been used; namely:

- Young people's satisfaction with their life in the country (2014–2015)
- Welfare of boys and girls in the Province of Buenos Aires. Argentine group working on the international project *International Survey Children Well-being* (ISCWeB), 2014–2016
- Quality of life and inequalities: an alternative proposition for its study and measurement (2013–2015).
- Quality of life and satisfaction with post-graduate studies (2012–2013).
- Quality of life and images of the future of young university students (2010–2011).
- Specificities in the development of the burn-out syndrome afflicting professionals in Argentina (2008–2009)
- Quality of labour life in social workers: the importance of context variables 2007
- Young people's quality of life: public participation and access to Public Health 2005–2006
- Values and quality of life of university students 2006
- A strategy for the improvement of quality of life: the university as a space for students' social integration 2005.
- Quality of life of young people living in Buenos Aires South Conurban 2004

The details of the research projects developed over the past decade have already been subject of comment in other books previous edited by Springer (Tonon 2011, 2012, 2015).

Thesis scholars for Doctorates and Master's Degrees from regional countries (Colombia, Peru, Argentina) have also received follow-up, in the fields of Psychology, Sociology, Health, and Education.

In this context, we would like to highlight the theses developed applying the qualitative method, considering that this type of studies are characterized by the fact that they are holistic and inductive, being their axes the discovery and comprehension. They are studies in which the subjects are the actual protagonists of the

[1] All of these papers have been directed by Dr. Graciela Tonon.

research processes which acknowledge the importance the actors attribute to context and significance.

Thus, the abovementioned theses have become pioneers in the methodological approach on the study of quality of life in Latin-America using qualitative methods:

- Satisfaction with life in the community: a study on youngsters from rural and urban communities in Ceibas (Province of Entre Ríos), and the Metropolitan Region of Buenos Aires.[2]
- Quality of life of middle-class boys and girls: case study in Santa Marta, tourist, cultural, and historic district, Colombia.[3]
- Health related quality of life of young people suffering from HIV/AIDS, at Señor del Milagro Hospital, Salta Capital.[4]

Post-Doctoral Studies in QOL

The Postdoctoral Studies in Quality of Life is a special research program dependent on UNI-COM[5] dedicated to the research on quality of life for doctors graduated in the field of Social Sciences in general, created in 2012 due to the lack of programs of this type in this region.

Postdoctoral studies demand research and transference activities for 300 h of work that may be fulfilled in a period of 6 months, with the possibility of developing part of the activities on an actual visit to the research center, and complying with the remaining activities by distance.

The participants are required to develop different activities:

(a) Participation in one of the research projects accredited by national institutions developed by UNI-COM in the quality of life field, in which their individual work will be registered.
(b) A working paper that will be edited by UNI-COM.
(c) A scientific article, to be presented in the *Journal Applied Research in Quality of life* or in other Journals which are state-of-the-art in the thematic field of quality of life.

---

[2] Author Lucía Zanabria Ruiz (Perú), Directed by Graciela Tonon, Doctorate in Psychology. Universidad de Palermo, Argentina. Approved, 2013.

[3] Author María Dilia Mieles Barrera (Colombia), Directed by Graciela Tonon. Doctorate in Social Sciences, Childhood, and Youth. Universidad de Manizales-CINDE Colombia. Approved, September, 2013.

[4] Author Milton Décima (Argentina), Directed by Graciela Tonon Master's Degree in Public Health. Faculty of Health Sciences. Universidad Nacional de Salta, Argentina. Finished March 2015.

[5] Institute of Social Research dedicated to the relation university-community in the Faculty of Social Sciences of Universidad Nacional de Lomas de Zamora, Argentina. Director Dr. Graciela Tonon.

(d) Participation as a guest professor for the abovementioned subjects which include the theme of quality of life.
(e) During their postdoctoral studies, the participants will be supervised directly by one of the members of UNI-COM group, specially designated for that purpose, considering the thematic area chosen.

Its Priority lines for 2013–2014 have been: young people's quality of life; qualitative studies in quality of life; urban quality of life, and quality of life and culture of populations from Asia and Africa. These priority lines are likely to be broadened and/or modified with a projection of several years.

In order to be selected for postdoctoral studies, the candidates must be accepted by the Postdoctoral Evaluation Committee, formed by three members who are doctors with expertise in the area and crediting postdoctoral studies, one of the requisites being membership of ISQOLS. Once their work is concluded, the participants will have 6 months' time to send their scientific productions. Once the aforementioned conditions have been fulfilled, the Postdoctoral Evaluation Committee must evaluate the papers.

So far, we have been visited by colleagues from Mexico, Colombia, Argentina, and Spain, devoted to the study of different population groups with relation to quality of life.

The post-doctoral themes are the following:

- The measurement and evaluation of the quality of life and inequalities (social, cultural, political and economic) of young people living in the rural area of the High Columbian Andean Mountain,[6] through replication of a questionnaire prepared to that end, administered by Tonon et al. (2013). Replication study of the abovementioned research entitled *Quality of life and inequality: an alternative proposition for its study and measurement* (2013–2015).
- Study of the quality of life of boys and girls between 8 and 10 years old in different towns of the Province of Buenos Aires,[7] Argentina, thus participating in the project *Welfare of boys and girls in the Province of Buenos Aires*, Argentine group working on the project *International Survey Children Well-being* (ISCWeB).
- Quality of life and quality of labor life of young people in Spain, the European Union, and Argentina,[8] probing into the social and economic determiners of inequality in quality of life and labor, which allows the elaboration of exhaustive indicators of quality of life and quality of labor life, based on the use of econometric models and the design of synthetic indicators.

[6] Dr. Antonio López López, COLCIENCIAS, Colombia.

[7] Dr. Claudia Mikkelsen, CONICET, Argentina.

[8] Dr. Noelia Somarriba Arechavala, Universidad de Valladolid, España.

Final Reflection

Teaching theory and research methods in quality of life implies the possibility of integrating the objective and subjective dimensions, considering that subjectivity is constructed on the basis of the daily interaction of the subjects as well as their interaction with their environment.

In this respect, the act of teaching is also a political act, which leads us to coincide with Lechner (2002, p. 120) in considering that the role of politics should not only be restricted to the solution of material problems, but also to develop an awareness of people's daily experiences. This proposition goes further in the line of thought developed by Martinez Pineda (2006) who expresses the need to conceive politics from a perspective that implies going beyond its pre-established fields of action, i.e., not being restricted to certain actors, organizations, or legitimized political forces (p. 136).

Thus, it is vital to teach students how to think, question, integrate knowledge, imagine new forms of analysis, to excel the traditional paradigm which teaches how to memorize information and concepts; the teaching of quality of life shows us the way towards integration. For, quoting Plascencia Castellanos (2006, p. 21) "the professor's profession is to profess a word he/she is committed with".

References

Ackoff, R. (1993) *Las fábulas antiburocráticas de Ackoff.* Buenos Aires. Granica.

Bramston, P. (2002) Subjective quality of life: the affective dimension. *Social Indicators Research* 16: 47–62.

Bramston, P, Pretty G. & Chipuer, H. (2002) Unravelling subjective quality of life: An investigation of individual and community de terminants. *SIR 59*–3 pp. 261–74.

Casas, F. (1996) *Bienestar social. Una introducción psico-sociológica.* PPU. Barcelona.

Castel, R. (2004) *La inseguridad social. Que es estar protegido.* Buenos Aires. Manantial.

Fitoussi, J-P and Rosanvallo, P. (1997) *La nueva era de las desigualdades.* Buenos Aires. Manantial

Gonzalez Perdomo, A. (2006) La interdiscplinariedad en la formación del pensamiento y el espíritu crítico que la guía. *Cuaderno de Sociología N° 40.* Universidad Santo Tomás. Bogotá. Colombia. pp. 17–33.

Gullone, E. and Cummins, R. (2002) *The universality of subjective well being indicators. A multi-disciplinary and multi-national perspective SIRS 16* Kluwer Academic Publishers. The Netherlands.

Lechner, N. (2002) *Las sombras del mañana. La dimensión subjetiva de la política.* Santiago. LOM ediciones.

Martinez Pineda, M. (2006) Disquisiciones sobre el sujeto político. Pistas para pensar su reconfiguración. En *Revista colombiana de Educación. N° 50.* Universidad Pedagógica Nacional. Primer semestre 2006. Bogotá Colombia. pp. 121–143.

Max Neef, M., Elizalde, A., Hopenhayn, M. (1986) *Desarrollo a escala humana.* Suecia. CEPAUR.

Michalos, A. (2007) *Education, Happiness and Wellbeing.* Paper written for the International Conference on 'Is happiness measurable and what do those measures mean for public policy?', at Rome, 2–3 April 2007, University of Rome 'Tor Vergata', organized by the Joint Research Centre of the European Commission, OECD, Centre for Economic and International Studies and the Bank of Italy.

Patrick, D, Edwards, T, Topolski, T, Walwick, J. (2002) *Youth quality of life: a new measure incorporating the voices of adolescents.* QOL Newsletter N° 28. Mapi Institute Lyon. Francia.
Payne, M. (1995) *Teorías contemporáneas del Trabajo Social. Una introducción crítica.* Barcelona. Paidos.
Plascencia Castellanos, G. (2006). Una propuesta deconstructiva de la universidad. En Plascencia Castellanos, G. (coord.) *Palabra libre condición de la universidad.* México D.F. Universidad Iberoamericana. pp. 19–45.
Romero, E (1992) La instrumentación del trabajador social. En *Revista de Trabajo Social N 61.* Pontificia Universidad Católica de Chile.
Royuela, V. Suriñach, J. y Reyes, M. (2003), Measuring quality of life in small areas over different periods of time. *SIR. 64–1.* Pp. 51–74.
Santuc, V. (1999) Desde donde mirar lo económico. En *Lo político en América Latina.* Scannone, J.C y Santuc, V. (compiladores) . Buenos Aires. Editorial Bonum. pp 303–342.
Schutz, A. (1974) *El problema de la realidad social.* Barcelona. Amorrortu.
Strauss, A. & Corbin, J. (2002) *Bases de la investigación cualitativa. Técnicas y procedimientos para desarrollar la teoría fundamentada.* Colombia. Universidad de Antioquía.
Tonon, G. (2001) Trabajo Social: profesión y disciplina. *Revista Saberes y Haceres, Año 3, Número 3.* Carrera de Servicio Social. Universidad Autónoma del Sur. Chile. pp. 46–58.
Tonon, G. (2009) Calidad de vida laboral de profesionales de la salud. *Vertex. Revista Argentina de Psiquiatría 88.* pp. 411–417. Bs. As. Editorial Polemos.
Tonon, G. (2011) Quality of life in Argentina. En Kenneth C. Land, Alex C. Michalos, and M. Joseph Sirgy (Eds.) *Handbook of Social Indicators and Quality of Life Research.* Dordrecht, Netherlands: Springer Publishers. Pp. 547–554.
Tonon, G. (2012) *Young people's quality of life and construction of citizenship.* Series SpringerBriefs in Well-being and quality of life research. Dordrecht, Heidelberg, London, New York: Springer.
Tonon, G., Rodriguez de la Vega, L, Maggino, F. & Anand, P. (2013) Questionnaire to study quality of life and inequalities. LOMASCyT Program . Universidad Nacional de Lomas de Zamora, Argentina.
Tonon, G. (Editor) (2015) Qualitative Studies in Quality of Life: Methodology and Practice. *Social Indicators Research Series* 55. Springer.
Vélez Restrepo, O. (2003) Reconfigurando el Trabajo Social. Perspectivas y tendencias contemporáneas. Bs. As. espacio Editorial.

MIX
Papier aus verantwortungsvollen Quellen
Paper from responsible sources
FSC® C105338

If you have any concerns about our products,
you can contact us on
ProductSafety@springernature.com

In case Publisher is established outside the EU,
the EU authorized representative is:
Springer Nature Customer Service Center GmbH
Europaplatz 3, 69115 Heidelberg, Germany

Printed by Libri Plureos GmbH
in Hamburg, Germany